Designing Gluten Free Bakery and Pasta Products

Marina F. de Escalada Pla • Carolina E. Genevois
Editors

Designing Gluten Free Bakery and Pasta Products

Springer

Editors
Marina F. de Escalada Pla
Universidad de Buenos Aires
Ciudad Autónoma de Buenos Aires
Buenos Aires, Argentina

Carolina E. Genevois
Universidad Nacional de Entre Ríos
Gualeguaychú
Entre Ríos, Argentina

ISBN 978-3-031-28343-7   ISBN 978-3-031-28344-4 (eBook)
https://doi.org/10.1007/978-3-031-28344-4

This Springer imprint is published by the registered company Springer Nature Switzerland AG
The registered company address is: Gewerbestrasse 11, 6330 Cham, Switzerland

To Dario, Montserrat, and Juan Francisco
– Marina

To German and Catalina
– Carolina

Preface

The intake of gluten from diet can induce several gastrointestinal disorders, such as celiac disease, allergy to wheat, and non-celiac gluten sensitivity. Nowadays the best treatment is the strict adherence to a diet without sources of prolamins and gliadins (wheat), secalin (rye), and hordein (barley). In addition, several studies have revealed that gluten-free (GF) diet may lead to nutrient deficiencies. Therefore, the formulation of GF foods, and in particularly those related to cereals, is a challenge to be solved considering different insights. A great effort has been performed by researchers and academics to improve technological and nutritional aspects of GF products based on cereal, evidenced by numerous articles published in international journals. This book comes to review the knowledge up to the moment regarding health disorders due to gluten intake and to summarise the main research advances in GF product development. Therefore, the reader can find in the different chapters a source of ideas for enhancing the healthy aspects of GF products and the GF food market expectations.

The aim of the book is to provide a tool for designing GF bakery products and pasta taking into account knowledge about gluten-related diseases as well as the research advances on traditional and non-traditional GF raw materials, bakery, and pasta processes. This can be particularly useful for food scientists and technologists who are looking for innovation in the market of GF ingredients and products. We hope to reach undergraduate and graduate students and researchers in Nutrition, Medical Sciences, Bromatology, Food Science and Technology, Food Engineering, Culinary Science, and Food Services, aiming to help them understanding how components and technological processes affect/improve the nutritional and/or sensory quality of GF products.

We understood that trying to reach this wide audience represented a real challenge and therefore we looked for help from colleagues and experts in this field. Finally, the book was organised into 10 chapters. In the first chapter, the medical and nutritional approach to the gluten-related disorders is summarised. From Chaps. 2 to 4, an exhaustive revision of raw material, which can be used in GF formulation, is detailed considering both traditional and non-traditional crops as well as new pretreatments and additives options. From Chaps. 5 to 8, different technological processes for baking and pasta production are presented considering traditional and emerging technologies as well as preservation alternatives through edible coatings. In Chap. 9, the sensory analysis of GF products is approached. The last chapter focusses on the regulation and labelling in the different regions and countries, since there has not been international consensus in this field until this moment.

Our grateful acknowledgement to every author and co-author for the effort and for the valuable contribution to this project. We highly appreciate the dedication for explaining in each chapter their own expertise and knowledge. We have enjoyed learning from the colleagues' chapters during the compilation and edition process of the manuscript. We hope, dear reader, you can go through the same experience when reading this book.

Buenos Aires, Argentina — Marina F. de Escalada Pla
Entre Ríos, Argentina — Carolina E. Genevois

Contents

Chapter 1
Everything That Must Be Known About the Relationship of Gluten to Human Health

Francesca Di Sario, Chiara Monachesi, Anil K. Verma, and Carlo Catassi

Abbreviations

Anti-tTG	anti-tissue transglutaminase antibodies
ATIs	Amylase-trypsin inhibitors
CD	celiac disease
DGP	anti-deamidated gliadin peptides antibodies
EATL	enteropathy-associated T cell lymphoma
EFSA	European Food Safety Authority (EFSA)
ELISA	enzyme-linked immune sorbent assay
EMA-IgA	IgA class anti-endomysial antibodies
ESPGHAN	European Society for Pediatric Gastroenterology, Hepatology, and Nutrition
FDA	Food and Drug Administration
FODMAPs	fermentable oligosaccharides, disaccharides, monosaccharides and polyols
GFD	gluten-free diet
GIP	gluten immunogenic peptides
GRD	gluten-related disorders
NCGS	non-celiac gluten sensitivity
RCD	Refractory celiac disease
T1DM	type 1 diabetes mellitus

F. Di Sario
Division of Pediatrics, DISCO Department, Polytechnic University of Marche, Ancona, Italy

C. Monachesi · A. K. Verma
Celiac Disease Research Laboratory, Polytechnic University of Marche, Ancona, Italy
e-mail: c.monachesi@univpm.it

C. Catassi (✉)
Division of Pediatrics, DISCO Department, Polytechnic University of Marche, Ancona, Italy

Mucosal Immunology and Biology Research Center, Division of Pediatric Gastroenterology and Nutrition, Massachusetts General Hospital, Boston, MA, USA
e-mail: c.catassi@univpm.it; ccatassi@mgh.harvard.edu

M. F. de Escalada Pla, C. E. Genevois (eds.), *Designing Gluten Free Bakery and Pasta Products*, https://doi.org/10.1007/978-3-031-28344-4_1

WA	wheat allergy
WDEIA	Wheat-dependent exercise induced anaphylaxis

1.1 Introduction

Gluten-related disorders (GRD) include celiac disease (CD) and other medical conditions like non-celiac gluten sensitivity (NCGS) and wheat allergy (WA) that are triggered by the ingestion of gluten-containing cereals, particularly wheat, and cured by the elimination of gluten-containing food from the diet. In this chapter we will briefly describe the clinical features of these disorders and point out how they can be differentiated and diagnosed in clinical practice. Finally, aspects related to the gluten-free diet (GFD), its nutritional quality, the gluten contamination issue and the impact of this treatment on daily life will be discussed.

1.2 Celiac Disease and Other Gluten-Related Disorders

1.2.1 Celiac Disease (CD)

CD is a chronic, autoimmune enteropathy triggered by the ingestion of gluten in genetically predisposed individuals. Gluten is the main protein component of wheat, rye and barley and is responsible for the baking properties of these cereals giving them cohesivity, viscosity and dough elasticity. Gluten includes two major protein fractions, i.e. gliadins and glutenins. Both gliadins and glutenins are rich in proline and glutamine that increase resistance to gastrointestinal proteolysis, since gastric, pancreatic, and brush border enzymes are deficient in proline endopeptidase activity. The final product of this incomplete digestion is a mix of peptides that may activate immune response (both innate and adaptive) leading to intestinal damage (Catassi et al. 2022).

Pathophysiology of CD

The etiology of CD is multifactorial and results from a complex interplay between genetic, environmental factors and immunological mechanisms. CD is strongly associated with the expression of specific human leucocyte antigen (HLA) class II molecules, i.e. HLA-DQ2 (HLA-DQA1*05:01-DQB1*02:01) and HLA-DQ8 (DQA1*03:01-DQB1*03:02). DQ molecules are expressed on the surface of antigen presenting cells (APC) and interact with selected gluten peptides generating an abnormal immune response (Megiorni et al. 2012). Although these predisposing HLA genotypes are present in most cases of CD (at least 95% of patients), their expression is necessary but not sufficient for the development of the condition. HLA alone does not fully explain genetic susceptibility and additional genetic factors may be involved. Gluten exposure is essential for the development of CD. In the intestinal lumen, gluten-derived peptides cross the epithelial barrier and reach the lamina propria where they are deamidated by tissue transglutaminase and presented by antigen presenting cells (APC) to CD4+ T-cells in the context of HLA-DQ2 or HLA-DQ8 molecules. The activation of CD4-lymphocytes produces high levels of pro-inflammatory cytokines leading to the typical mucosal damage of CD (infiltration of inflammatory cells, crypt hyperplasia and villous atrophy). Moreover, the T-cell mediated immune response activates B cells which secrete anti-gliadin, anti-endomysium and anti-tissue-transglutaminase antibodies (Kagnoff 2007).

Another important factor involved in CD pathogenesis is represented by increased gut permeability. In normal circumstances, intestinal epithelial barrier is poorly permeable to macromolecules. In CD the up-regulation of zonulin (a protein involved in the integrity of the Tight Junction system) causes an upregulation of the intestinal barrier function facilitating the translocation of gluten peptides into the subepithelial compartment (Fasano et al. 2000).

Epidemiology

CD is one of the most common life-long disorders affecting approximately 1% of general population worldwide with female and children predominance (Fasano et al. 2012; Singh et al. 2018). The incidence of CD has increased during the last decades due to the availability of sensitive diagnostic tools, awareness of the wide clinical polymorphism, and increased serological screening of individuals considered to be at high risk for the disorder. CD tends to be more common in people who have family history of CD, as well as in individuals with some genetic disorders (e.g. Down and Turner syndrome), IgA deficiency, type 1 diabetes mellitus (T1DM), thyroiditis and other autoimmune diseases, and inflammatory bowel diseases. From an epidemiological point of view, CD may be represented by an iceberg with the majority of cases, i.e. the submerged part of the iceberg, remaining undetected (Catassi et al. 1994).

Clinical Presentation

The clinical spectrum of CD is wide including symptomatic cases with intestinal and/or extraintestinal symptoms, subclinical forms which are occasionally diagnosed because of serological screening and potential cases (positivity of serum celiac autoantibodies and HLA-DQ2/DQ8 haplotypes, and a normal small intestinal mucosa at the small intestinal biopsy). Gastrointestinal symptoms include chronic diarrhea, steatorrhea, weight loss, bloating, flatulence, abdominal pain, abdominal distension and constipation. However, the majority of people with CD have signs and symptoms unrelated to the digestive system, including iron deficiency and microcytic anemia (because of iron malabsorption, chronic inflammation and resistance to oral iron therapy), bone disorders (osteopenia or osteoporosis as a result of impaired calcium absorption and vitamin D deficiency), hair loss, unexplained hypertransaminasemia, cutaneous manifestations such as dermatitis herpetiformis, mouth ulcers (aphtous stomatitis), tooth enamel defects, chronic fatigue, neurological disorders such as ataxia, peripheral neuropathy, epilepsy (mainly with occipital calcifications), endocrinologic dysfunctions, growth failure, gynecologic and fertility problems (Fasano et al. 2001). Loss of gluten tolerance can present at any age after the introduction of gluten, but symptoms differ in children and adults. Young children tend to have the more classical intestinal signs of CD, including growth problems, while older children and adults may present with symptoms that are non-specific or atypical.

Complications

CD complications are rare and affect approximately 1% of patients (Singh et al. 2018). Several studies demonstrated that a late diagnosis of CD (after the age of 50) and/or poor GFD compliance is associated with higher mortality compared to that of the general population (Rubio-Tapia et al. 2016). Complications of CD include refractory CD, ulcerative jejunoileitis, enteropathy-associated T cell lymphoma (EATL) and splenic hypofunction.

Refractory celiac disease (RCD) is characterized by the persistence of clinical symptoms and histological lesions after at least 12 months on a strict GFD. In most cases the absence of response is caused by intentional or unintentional gluten intake. RCD includes type 1 (IEL population has a normal CD3+CD8+ phenotype) and type 2 (presence of a monoclonal rearrangement of T cell receptor). The distinction between the two forms is imperative because of different therapeutic management and prognosis. Type II RCD is more aggressive and can lead to the development of intestinal lymphoma.

Ulcerative jejunoileitis is characterized by multiple ulcerations of the small bowel that can evolve in strictures and cause obstruction, bleeding and perforation with peritonitis. It is clinically characterized by abdominal pain, diarrhea, weight loss and low-grade fever. The recognition of this condition is important since mortality is very high.

The EATL is a rare and aggressive form of non-Hodgkin lymphoma. It is more common in men over 60 years and is often preceded by type 2 RCD. Unfortunately, these patients have a very poor outcome with a reported 5-year survival rate lower than 20%.

Hyposplenism (functional or anatomic) is often associated with CD affecting more than one-third of adult celiac patients. Due to splenic hypofunction CD patients are at risk of developing severe complications, such as thromboembolic events and encapsulated bacterial infections.

Diagnosis

The diagnosis of CD relies on a combination of clinical, serological and histopathological findings. In current clinical practice, IgA anti-tissue transglutaminase antibodies (Anti-tTG) (or IgG class in subjects with IgA deficiency) is the most useful marker for diagnosing CD with a 95% sensitivity and 97% specificity (Rostom et al. 2005). Anti-endomysial antibodies (EMA-IgA) are highly specific for CD (about 100% of specificity in active CD) but their determination is expensive and operator-dependent. Therefore, they are usually used as a confirmatory test. IgG anti-deamidated gliadin peptides antibodies (DGP), are useful in subjects with IgA deficiency and are the first marker that become positive in young children. HLA-DQ2 and HLA-DQ8 testing should not be used routinely but only in selected clinical situations, such as a screening test in high-risk individuals, due to their high negative predictive value.

In adult patients, an antibody positive test requires an endoscopy with small bowel biopsy for the definitive diagnosis of CD. The histological hallmark of CD is an increased intraepithelial lymphocyte count and a variable degree of villous atrophy. In children, according to the European Society for Pediatric Gastroenterology, Hepatology, and Nutrition (ESPGHAN) guidelines for diagnosis of CD, small intestinal biopsy may be omitted in children showing high titer of anti-TTG antibodies (higher than tenfold the upper normal limit) and EMA positivity (Husby et al. 2012).

Dietary Management

At present, the only accepted treatment for CD is the GFD (Kupper 2005; Ciacci et al. 2015). Strict adherence to the GFD normally leads to the resolution of symptoms (either intestinal and extraintestinal), normalization of serological tests and of intestinal villi architecture. Full normalization of both anti-tTG levels and histopathology may take over 2 years (severe small bowel lesions and high anti-tTG levels at diagnosis) (Monachesi et al. 2020). Additionally, a correct GFD is a key factor for decreasing risk of complications (particularly bone disorders, infertility and malignancy). Adhering to a GFD may have a negative impact on the quality of life, especially in adolescents, and may induce subtle vitamin and mineral deficiencies.

1.2.2 Non Celiac Gluten Sensitivity (NCGS) and Wheat Allergy (WA)

Non Celiac Gluten Sensitivity

NCGS is characterized by intestinal and extra-intestinal symptoms related to the ingestion of gluten (and potentially other wheat components) in subjects that are not affected by either CD or WA (Catassi et al. 2015). This entity has been described recently and many aspects of its epidemiology, pathophysiology, clinical spectrum and treatment are still unclear. Current evidence suggests that NCGS is more common in adults, particularly in females, but the overall prevalence in the general population is not clearly defined. As regards to disease mechanisms, experimental data suggest the role of an abnormal wheat-induced innate immune response. Clinical presentation of NCGS includes both intestinal (Irritable Bowel Syndrome like symptoms) and not intestinal symptoms. The most common intestinal symptoms are abdominal pain, bloating and alternating bowel habits (either diarrhea or constipation). Extraintestinal manifestations include headache, foggy mind (difficulties in concentrating), fatigue, joint and muscle pain, leg or arm numbness, dermatitis (similar to eczema), recurrent oral ulceration, anxiety and depression.

The latency between gluten ingestion and the appearance of symptoms is usually short, within hours or days. Unlike CD, patients with NCGS do not seem at risk for long-term complications.

Unfortunately, no sensitive and/or specific diagnostic biomarkers of NCGS have been identified so far. In contrast with CD, TTG, EMA and DGP antibodies are generally negative (except for an isolated positivity of first-generation antigliadin antibodies particularly of IgG class) and duodenal biopsies are either normal or show isolated duodenal lymphocitosis. Moreover, the CD-predisposing HLA-DQ2 and DQ8 genotypes are found in only 50% of patients with NCGS, and have no relevance for diagnosing this condition.

The diagnosis of NCGS is based on: (a) exclusion of CD and WA (b) defining patient's clinical response to the GFD (at least 6 weeks of GFD) and evaluation of the effect of reintroducing gluten by a double-blind, placebo-controlled challenge (Catassi et al. 2015). However, this approach is difficult to apply in daily clinical practice because of frequent self-diagnosis and treatment with GFD among patients. Moreover, since NCGS is not a chronic condition, gluten tolerance should be re-evaluated over time.

The only available treatment for NCGS is the GFD, although it is not already established if patients have to follow it on a life-long basis (Khan et al. 2020). Recently data suggest that other wheat components, particularly amylase-trypsin inhibitors (ATIs) and fermentable oligosaccharides, disaccharides, monosaccharides and polyols (FODMAPs) may be involved in triggering NCGS-like symptoms.

Wheat Allergy

WA is one of the most common food allergies. It is defined as a hypersensitivity reaction to wheat proteins triggered by an IgE-dependent mechanism. It shows greater prevalence in children while it is quite uncommon in adult population.

Symptoms typically occur within minutes to hours after the ingestion of wheat proteins and may be gastrointestinal (abdominal pain, bloating, nausea and vomiting, diarrhea), respiratory (bronchial obstruction, rhinitis), cutaneous (hives, atopic dermatitis). Rarely angioedema or anaphylaxis may occur (Inomata 2009). Wheat-dependent exercise induced anaphylaxis (WDEIA) is a particular type of WA which occurs when ingestion of wheat is followed within a short period of time by physical activity. Diagnosis of WA is classically based on skin tests (prick or patch technique and intradermal injections), measurement of total IgE and specific IgE antibodies (for example anti- wheat – barley and rye). However, since these tests are inadequately sensitive and specific, an open food challenge can be considered to confirm WA. WA can be transient, especially in children with predominantly gastrointestinal manifestations, or can persist as a lifelong disorder. Dietary allergen avoidance is the primary treatment for wheat allergy. Table 1.1 summarizes the main features and differential characteristics of gluten-related disorders.

Table 1.1 The main features of gluten-related disorders

	Celiac disease	Non Celiac Gluten Sensitivity	Wheat allergy
Time interval between gluten exposure and onset of symptoms	Weeks-years	Hours-days	Minutes-hours
Pathogenesis	Autoimmunity (Innate + Adaptive Immunity)	Immunity? (Iinnate Immunity?)	Allergic Immune Response
HLA	HLA DQ2/8 restricted (~97% positive cases)	Not-HLA DQ2/8 restricted (50% DQ2/8 positive cases)	Not-HLA DQ2/8 restricted (35-40% positive cases as in the general population)
Auto-antibodies	Almost always present	Always absent	Always absent
Enteropathy	Almost always present	Always absent (slight increase in IEL)	Always absent (eosinophils in the lamina propria)
Symptoms	Both intestinal and extra-intestinal (not distinguishable from GS and WA with GI symptoms)	Both intestinal and extra-intestinal (not distinguishable from CD and WA with GI symptoms)	Both intestinal and extra-intestinal (not distinguishable from CD and GS when presenting with GI symptoms)
Complications	Co-morbidities Long term complications	Absence of co-morbidities and long term complications (long follow up studies needed to confirm it)	Absence of co-morbidities. Short-term complications (including anaphylaxis)

1.3 Nutritional Considerations of the GFD

1.3.1 Gluten Exclusion in the Management of CD and Other GRD

Due to its nutritional properties, affordability, adaptability, and accessibility, over the last thousand years wheat has become a worldwide staple food. More than 25,000 different cultivars have been produced by wheat breeding, mostly consumed after processing into bread, pasta, noodles, bulgur and couscous. Wheat grain include three major components: starch, proteins, and cell wall polysaccharides, accounting for about 90% of the dry weight. Gluten is the main structural protein complex in wheat with equivalent toxic proteins in rye, barley, spelt, einkorn, khorasan wheat (usually marketed as Kamut), and triticale. The wide availability and functional properties of gluten proteins contribute to its wide use as an ingredient in food processing. Gluten is not a single protein but a mixture of proteins named prolamins, representing about 80% of the total protein content in grain. Gluten proteins are divided into two major fractions: (i) gliadins (monomeric, subdivided into ω-, γ-, and α/β-gliadin fractions), and (ii) glutenins (large polymers). The most immunogenic gluten fragment is the 33-mer peptide, which consists of 33 amino acids of the α-gliadin fraction (Lionetti et al. 2011; Sapone et al. 2012; Catassi et al. 2013). All the gluten-containing cereals are excluded in the GFD.

The only effective treatment for CD is a lifelong and strict GFD (Lionetti et al. 2011; Fasano et al. 2012). Unlike food allergies, CD does not always cause immediate and severe symptoms after gluten ingestion. This is why many patients following the GFD, mostly young and asymptomatic or with mild symptoms when diagnosed, tend to occasionally ingest amounts of gluten. The protracted ingestion of gluten traces (>10–50 mg/day) is sufficient to cause significant intestinal mucosa damage (Catassi et al. 2007), possible reappearance of CD specific autoantibodies in blood, increased risk of long-term complications such as osteoporosis and lymphoma (Lionetti et al. 2011). Based on the above daily threshold, a maximum tolerable amount of gluten of <20 parts per million (ppm) in gluten-free food has been calculated (Catassi et al. 2007), a threshold that has been endorsed by the major international regulatory agencies, e.g., the Codex Alimentarius, the US Food and Drug Administration (FDA), and the European Food Safety Authority (EFSA) (2008, 2013).

Nutritional problems may be found at both diagnosis and after starting the GFD. At diagnosis, deficiencies are the consequence of nutrient malabsorption caused by the intestinal mucosal damage with frequently low levels of iron, copper, folate, B12 vitamin and zinc. In the course of the GFD, the dietary problems are likely to be related to the reduced nutritional quality of the gluten-free products and inadequate alimentary choices.

1.3.2 Dietary Guidelines for a Balanced GFD

Following a strict GFD requires critical attention in the selection of gluten-free food, ingredients, and nutritional content. To avoid unintentional gluten exposures, it is extremely important for CD patients to look for the gluten-free label before buying processed gluten-free foods (2013). There are multiple organizations certifying gluten-free foods, complying with differing criteria for certification, from a level of gluten <5 ppm up to <20 ppm. Allowed fresh foods, that can be consumed confidently without extra screening, are fruits and vegetables, many kind of seeds, legumes and nuts in their unprocessed forms, eggs, lean, unprocessed meats, fish and poultry, amaranth, buckwheat, flax, rice, soy, corn, potatoes, millet, quinoa, teff, and alcoholic beverages produced from naturally gluten-free ingredients. Alcoholic beverages made from gluten-containing grains processed to remove gluten must carry a label stating that gluten content cannot be precisely determined and may contain some gluten traces. Foods labeled "gluten-free" may include naturally gluten-free food, processed food without gluten-containing ingredients, or food with a gluten-containing ingredient that has been processed to remove gluten.

Newly diagnosed CD patients are advised to receive dietary counseling on food labeling, and the most appropriate gluten-free foods (Penagini et al. 2013). The consumption of naturally gluten-free cereals and pseudo-cereals should be encouraged in CD patients. Amaranth, quinoa and buckwheat are an excellent option, since they are good sources of carbohydrates, protein, dietary fiber, vitamins (folate, riboflavin, vitamin C and vitamin E) and polyunsaturated fatty acids. Recent evidence showed that long-term introduction of selected uncontaminated and nonreactive varieties of oats can be safely included in the diet of patients with CD, with no deleterious effects at the clinical, serologic, or mucosal levels (Lionetti et al. 2018). Noteworthy, the inclusion of oats in the range of safe gluten-free options has many potential benefits for CD patients, being a good source of fiber (especially beta-glucans), iron, thiamine, B complex vitamins, providing a higher satiety value than other gluten-free cereals, and increasing the palatability and dietary variety.

A GFD is a nutritionally safe intervention that allows remission of the disease without any major risks. Apart from maintaining the above-mentioned safe limit of gluten intake (below 10–50 mg/day), a suitable GFD must also be nutritionally adequate to prevent micronutrients and fiber deficiencies, allow appropriate growth in children and pubertal development, and avoid long-term potential harms like hyperlipidemia, and hyperglycemia. Studies have shown sub-optimal intake of some nutrients over the long run, particularly fiber, calcium, iron, folate and other vitamins, with the GFD (Mariani et al. 1998; Lionetti et al. 2020).

GFD imbalance may occur because of the need of excluding several cereals or the different nutritional composition of gluten-free products as compared to their unrefined counterparts. In this regard, national/international food pyramids for food groups' consumption references and recommended energy and nutrient intake levels should be followed. Gluten-free raw materials result in gluten-free food which is less palatable than regular foods. The manufacturing of gluten-free products often requires the addition of additives such as hydrocolloids, and some macronutrients such as fats to mitigate the lack of gluten. Commercially available gluten-free products are quite expensive, and eating out can be socially challenging (Mariani et al. 1998; Valletta et al. 2010; Kabbani et al. 2012).

1.3.3 Adherence to the GFD

Frequent monitoring is crucial to promote adherence to GFD and early identification of nutritional deficiencies and/or metabolic imbalances. Several procedures are available to evaluate the compliance with the GFD, such as clinical symptoms monitoring, interview by an experienced dietitian, structured dietary questionnaires, serological tests (i.e. anti-tTG antibodies and DGP antibodies), intestinal permeability test, and small intestinal histology. Among the gluten-dependent biomarkers, serological tests are highly sensitive and specific for diagnosis, but not enough to detect occasional transgressions (Ludvigsson et al. 2018; Myléus et al. 2020). The use of serial biopsies is invasive and impractical for close monitoring. Normalization of serology and histopathology may take over 2 years, particularly in those with severe small bowel lesions and high anti-tTG antibodies levels at diagnosis (Sansotta et al. 2020; Monachesi et al. 2020). In recent years gluten immunogenic peptides (GIP) determination has gained scientific attention (Moreno et al. 2017). GIP are fragments of gluten proteins excreted in urine and in stools, detectable using specific monoclonal antibodies, particularly A1 or G12. However, there are some open questions about their clinical performance (i.e. latency between gluten exposure and appearance in stool/urine, and the relationship between the quantity of ingested vs eliminated gluten) (Monachesi et al. 2021a). So far, a reliable biomarker to test the adherence to the GFD in the long-term follow-up of CD patients is still lacking.

1.4 Gluten Contamination: Current Scenario and Advances

1.4.1 What Is Gluten Cross-Contamination?

Gluten cross-contamination occurs when a gluten-free grain/food item is directly or indirectly cross-contacted with a gluten-containing grain/food item. Cross-contamination can occur at various stages, for example when cereals are grown, harvested, processed, and/or bulk traded (Lee et al. 2014). Crop rotation is a beneficial farming practice, but this allows mixing of grains. Lentils grow in cooler climates similar to wheat and barley. Hence crop rotation between wheat and lentils increases the possibility of mixing the grains. Apart from this, transportation of grains in the same vehicle, use of shared harvesting equipment, and shared storage facilities cause cross-contamination (Lee et al. 2014).

1.4.2 Worldwide Status of Gluten Contamination of the GFD

In an early study, Gibert et al. (2013) showed a safe threshold level of gluten (i.e. <20 mg/kg gluten) in a wide range of commercially available European gluten-free food products (n = 205) (Gibert et al. 2013). However in recent years, studies from USA, Brazil, and Canada have shown a variable level of gluten contamination (i.e. 20.5%, 21.5%, and 9.5% respectively) in the locally available commercial gluten-free products (Koerner et al. 2013; Lee et al. 2014; Farage et al. 2017). In an interesting study, Farage et al. showed that 21.5% of commercially available Brazilian bakery products were cross-contaminated with gluten and not safe for CD patients (Farage et al. 2017). However, in another study the authors investigated gluten contamination in naturally gluten-free meals collected from food services in Brazil, and found a low occurrence of gluten contamination in naturally gluten-free preparations (Farage et al. 2019). A study conducted by Atasoy et al. reported a significant amount of gluten contamination (17.5%) in manufactured gluten-free products available on the Turkish market (Atasoy et al. 2020). On the other hand, recent

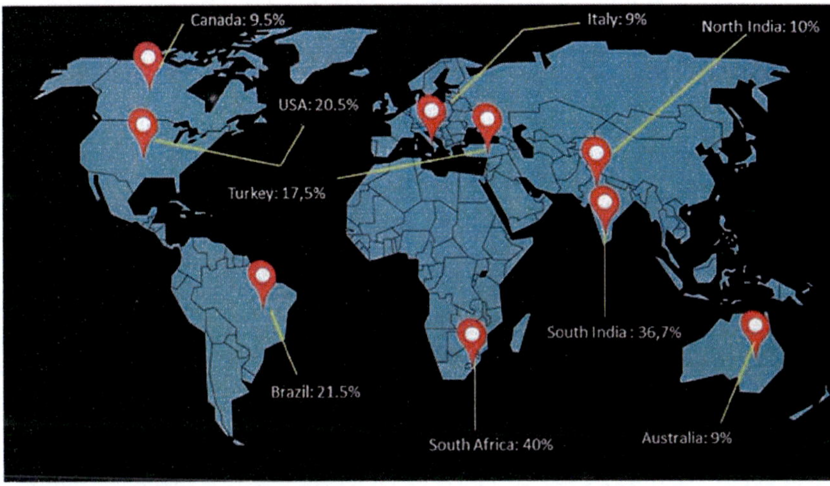

Fig. 1.1 Percentage of labelled gluten-free products containing gluten above the threshold limit (20 ppm) in different countries

studies from India found 10% contamination in labeled and 36.7% contamination in naturally gluten-free products (Raju et al. 2020; Mehtab et al. 2021). In a landmark large survey, our group showed a low level (9%) of gluten contamination in the gluten-free food products available in Italian supermarkets. This study also confirmed that naturally gluten-free products (lentil, oats) are at a significantly higher risk of gluten contamination as compared to certified gluten-free food products (Verma et al. 2017).

In a meta-analysis-based review article, Guennouni et al. reported that 15% of gluten-free food products contain gluten levels higher than the accepted safe threshold (>20 mg/kg). The study also confirmed that naturally gluten-free foods are significantly more often contaminated than labelled gluten-free products (Guennouni et al. 2021).

In summary, all these studies report the possibility of gluten contamination in products that are labelled as gluten-free (Fig. 1.1). These data show that there is an unmet need for a strict and universal gluten-free labeling regulations all over the world. A rule should also be imposed on the food manufacturers to declare the product ingredients on the package.

Is it possible to quantify the amount of contaminating gluten into the diet of the "average" celiac patient? Syage et al. estimated that treated CD patients on average consume up to 400 mg/day of gluten accidentally (Syage et al. 2018). However, this is likely to be an overestimation, at least talking about patients who do their best to comply with the requirements of the GFD. In another study from our group (Monachesi et al. 2021b) we quantified the accidental gluten contamination in the diet of Italian children. The results of this study found that gluten contamination in the daily diet is unusual and is usually below the safety threshold of 10 mg/day in the Italian pediatric population. This safe situation was achieved thanks to the high awareness of CD in this country (Monachesi et al. 2021b). However, unintentional gluten exposure is likely to be more common and needs further investigation in countries where CD awareness is not as high as in Italy.

1.4.3 Gluten Contamination in the Kitchen

See et al. in 2015 described four main ways of gluten cross-contamination, i.e. in the field, the factory or retail premises, restaurants, and home (See et al. 2015). During food preparation, gluten-free items may be contaminated in several ways. In a recent study conducted by Thompson et al. shared fryer, i.e. a fryer that uses gluten-free fries and oil but is used for cooking also gluten-containing food, has a high risk of gluten cross-contamination (Thompson et al. 2021). Cross-contamination at home can occur through shared kitchenware, the same cooking platform, and the use of gluten-containing food ingredients with gluten-free food ingredients. Miller et al. in 2016 reported that gluten-free foods should be kept at a minimum distance of 2 meters in a shared kitchen to avoid cross-contamination (Miller et al. 2016). A study conducted by Studerus et al. in 2018 confirmed that gluten cross-contamination in the kitchen environment may occur but using the same utensils for cooking gluten-containing food and gluten-free food generally does not cause cross-contamination in a domestic environment. However, the kitchen ladle used to cook gluten-containing pasta should be avoided for cooking gluten-free pasta.

Recently Weisbrod et al. (2020) have shown that the preparation of gluten-free food in close contact with gluten-containing food may not always cause gluten cross-contamination. In this study the authors investigated the gluten transfer and efficacy of washing methods during food preparation: (1) cooking pasta, (2) toasting bread, and (3) slicing cupcakes. They found that cooking gluten-free pasta with the water used to boil gluten-containing pasta is not safe but rinsing the pasta with fresh running water makes it safe to eat for CD patients. They also found that using the same toaster for gluten-containing and gluten-free bread does not cause cross-contamination and the use of the same knife to slice the gluten-containing and gluten-free cupcakes does not always cause cross-contamination (Weisbrod et al. 2020).

1.4.4 Methods to Detect Gluten Traces in Food Products

Several methods are available to measure traces of gluten in food items. However, no test is fully reliable so far. Nonetheless, the enzyme-linked immune sorbent assay (ELISA) test is considered a trusted method for this purpose (Verma et al. 2017).

Several antibodies (R5, A1/G12, α-20, MIoBS, DQ2.5-glia-α3, and Skerritt) have been developed to detect the gluten traces in food products (Verma et al. 2017;

Panda et al. 2019). All these antibodies use different gluten extraction methods and different gluten standards. That is why they show discrepancies in their gluten quantification results. Apart from these, matrix interference and antibody-binding affinities also cause variability in the ELISA results. There are no official reference materials approved, and there is no universal unit of measurement of gluten (Diaz-Amigo et al. 2013; Sharma et al. 2013; Hochegger et al. 2015; Osorio et al. 2019). However, these antibodies are highly specific for gluten traces. Gluten ELISA provides a satisfactory result in short time and it is an easy method to perform. Despite some limitations, the ELISA method is considered adequately reliable and the method-of-choice to detect gluten contamination in food products.

Among the developed gluten detection antibodies, R5 and G12/A1 (commonly known as G12 antibody) antibody ELISAs are the most frequently used gluten ELISA method. R5 antibody-based ELISA method is the most prevalent and is also a reference method for gluten estimation (Verma et al. 2017; Scherf et al. 2021). This method has been endorsed by the Codex Alimentarius as a Type 1 method to determine gluten in food (Scherf et al. 2021).

The R5 monoclonal antibody is raised against the omega Secalin from rye, and strongly recognizes the most toxic fragments of gliadin i.e. QQPFP, QQQFP, LQPFP, and QLPFP sequences (Osman et al. 2001). G12/A1 antibody-based sandwich ELISA is another frequently used ELISA method to detect gluten in foodstuff (Escarnot et al. 2018; Silvester et al. 2018). A1/G12 are highly sensitive monoclonal antibodies developed against the α2-gliadin 33-mer toxic peptide of the gliadin (Morón et al. 2008b). G12 antibody is claimed to have a broader specificity for the prolamins that are more toxic for CD patients (Morón et al. 2008a, b). It is restricted to the detection of the QPQLPY sequence of 33-mer toxic gliadin fragments, while A1 has a broader range of epitope recognition, and apart from the QLPYPQP sequence, it also recognizes two more sequences (QQPFPQP and QLPFPQP) (Morón et al. 2008b).

Some studies have assessed the performance of the R5 and G12/A1 antibodies-based ELISA methods and found that both antibodies work well and provide similar results (Bruins Slot et al. 2015; Hochegger et al. 2015; Yu et al. 2021).

1.4.5 Future Methods to Detect Gluten Traces in Food Products

Apart from these immunological methods (ELISA), in the last decades, several non-immunological methods have been developed to allow precise gluten quantification in food products (Osorio et al. 2019). Among these methods, DNA-specific genomics methods (i.e., PCR, QC-PCR, RT-PCR, real-time immune-PCR) are more sensitive than ELISA, but sometimes they show false-positive results and cannot be applied to hydrolysed food products (Osorio et al. 2019). Proteomics-based methods (i.e., column chromatography, gel permeation chromatography, MALDI-TOF

MS, LC-MS/MS, NIR spectroscopy) have also been established as a method to accurately quantify gluten (Mejías et al. 2014; Scherf et al. 2016). LC-MS/MS method is an extremely sensitive analytical technique that can effectively characterize, and quantify gluten fragments (Osorio et al. 2019). However, due to their respective drawbacks, such as complexity of the technique and difficulty in differentiating gluten and non-gluten proteins, these approaches are not regularly in use. In recent years, biosensors (gold nanoparticle-based immune sensors) were found to be a highly specific test for gluten quantification, but these tests require further validation (Khot et al. 2012; Vinci et al. 2019).

Despite these various tools, analysis of gluten contamination remains a significant issue. There is certainly a need to develop a reliable gluten tracking method with high accuracy and precision. This topic will be deepened in Chap. 10, because of its relevance in this book.

1.5 Conclusions

CD and other gluten-related disorders are common and affect humans worldwide with a wide array of clinical manifestations, both intestinal and extra-intestinal. Specific investigations and algorithms have been developed to correctly diagnose and treat these conditions, even though a biomarker of NCGS is still lacking. The GFD is the treatment of choice of gluten-related disorders. This is a safe nutritional intervention that is however difficult to maintain since gluten is a pervasive ingredient that may contaminate naturally or rendered gluten-free items.

References

Atasoy G et al (2020) Gluten contamination in manufactured gluten-free foods in Turkey. Food Addit Contam Part A 37:363–373

Bruins Slot ID et al (2015) Evaluating the performance of gluten ELISA test kits: the numbers do not tell the tale. Cereal Chem J 92:513–521

Catassi C et al (1994) Coeliac disease in the year 2000: exploring the iceberg. Lancet 343:200–203

Catassi C et al (2007) A prospective, double-blind, placebo-controlled trial to establish a safe gluten threshold for patients with celiac disease. Am J Clin Nutr 85:160–166

Catassi C et al (2013) Non-celiac gluten sensitivity: the new frontier of gluten related disorders. Nutrients 5:3839–3853

Catassi C et al (2015) Diagnosis of non-celiac gluten sensitivity (NCGS): the Salerno experts' criteria. Nutrients 7:4966–4977

Catassi C et al (2022) Coeliac Disease. Lancet 399:2413–2426

Ciacci C et al (2015) The gluten-free diet and its current application in coeliac disease and dermatitis herpetiformis. United European Gastroenterol J 3:121–135

Codex Alimentarius Commission (2008) In: Codex Alimentarius Commission. Foods for special dietary use for persons intolerant to gluten Codex STAN 118–1979. Codex Alimentarius Commission, Rome

Diaz-Amigo C et al (2013) Accuracy of ELISA detection methods for gluten and reference materials: a realistic assessment. J Agric Food Chem 61:5681–5688

Escarnot E et al (2018) Reactivity of gluten proteins from spelt and bread wheat accessions towards A1 and G12 antibodies in the framework of celiac disease. Food Chem 268:522–532

European Union (2011) Regulation (EU) No 1169/2011 of the European Parliament and of the Council of 25 October 2011 on the Provision of Food Information to Consumers, Amending Regulations (EC) No 1924/2006 and (EC) No 1925/2006 of the European Parliament and of the Council, and Repealing Commission Directive 87/250/EEC, Council Directive 90/496/EEC, Commission Directive 1999/10/EC, Directive 2000/13/EC of the European Parliament and of the Council, Commission Directives 2002/67/EC and 2008/5/EC and Commission Regulation (EC) No 608/2004. European Union, Brussels

Farage P et al (2017) Gluten contamination in gluten-free bakery products: a risk for coeliac disease patients. Public Health Nutr 20:413–416

Farage P et al (2019) Accidental gluten contamination in traditional lunch meals from food services in Brasilia, Brazil. Nutrients 11:1924

Fasano A et al (2000) Zonulin, a newly discovered modulator of intestinal permeability, and its expression in coeliac disease. Lancet 355:1518–1519

Fasano A et al (2001) Current approaches to diagnosis and treatment of celiac disease: an evolving spectrum. Gastroenterology 120:636–651

Fasano A et al (2012) Clinical practice. Celiac disease. N Engl J Med 367:2419–2426

Gibert A et al (2013) Might gluten traces in wheat substitutes pose a risk in patients with celiac disease? A population-based probabilistic approach to risk estimation. Am J Clin Nutr 97:109–116

Guennouni M et al (2021) Gluten contamination in labelled gluten-free, naturally gluten-free and meals in food services in low-, middle- and high-income countries: a systematic review and meta-analysis. Br J Nutr:1–15

Hochegger R et al (2015) Comparison of R5 and G12 antibody-based ELISA used for the determination of the gluten content in official food samples. Foods 4:654–664

Husby S et al (2012) European Society for Pediatric Gastroenterology, Hepatology, and Nutrition guidelines for the diagnosis of coeliac disease. J Pediatr Gastroenterol Nutr 54:136–160

Inomata N (2009) Wheat allergy. Curr Opin Allergy Clin Immunol 9:238–243

Kabbani TA et al (2012) Body mass index and the risk of obesity in coeliac disease treated with the gluten-free diet. Aliment Pharmacol Ther 35:723–729

Kagnoff MF (2007) Celiac disease: pathogenesis of a model immunogenetic disease. J Clin Invest 117:41–49

Khan A et al (2020) Nonceliac gluten and wheat sensitivity. Clin Gastroenterol Hepatol 18:1913–1922.e1

Khot LR et al (2012) Applications of nanomaterials in agricultural production and crop protection: a review. Crop Prot 35:64–70

Koerner TB et al (2013) Gluten contamination of naturally gluten-free flours and starches used by Canadians with celiac disease. Food Addit Contam Part A Chem Anal Control Expo Risk Assess 30:2017–2021

Kupper C (2005) Dietary guidelines and implementation for celiac disease. Gastroenterology 128:S121–S127

Lee HJ et al (2014) Gluten contamination in foods labeled as "gluten free" in the United States. J Food Prot 77:1830–1833

Lionetti E et al (2011) New clues in celiac disease epidemiology, pathogenesis, clinical manifestations, and treatment. Int Rev Immunol 30:219–231

Lionetti E et al (2018) Safety of oats in children with celiac disease: a double-blind, randomized, placebo-controlled trial. J Pediatr 194:116–122.e2

Lionetti E et al (2020) Nutritional status, dietary intake, and adherence to the Mediterranean diet of children with celiac disease on a gluten-free diet: a case-control prospective study. Nutrients 12:E143

Ludvigsson JF et al (2018) Outcome measures in coeliac disease trials: the Tampere recommendations. Gut 67:1410–1424

Mariani P et al (1998) The gluten-free diet: a nutritional risk factor for adolescents with celiac disease? J Pediatr Gastroenterol Nutr 27:519–523

Megiorni F et al (2012) HLA-DQA1 and HLA-DQB1 in celiac disease predisposition: practical implications of the HLA molecular typing. J Biomed Sci 19:88

Mehtab W et al (2021) Gluten content in labeled and unlabeled gluten-free food products used by patients with celiac disease. Eur J Clin Nutr 75(8):1245–1253

Mejías J et al (2014) Analysis of wheat prolamins, the causative agents of celiac sprue, using reversed phase high performance liquid chromatography (RP-HPLC) and matrix-assisted laser desorption ionization time of flight mass spectrometry (MALDI-TOF-MS). Nutrients 6:1578–1597

Miller K et al (2016) Catering gluten-free when simultaneously using wheat flour. J Food Prot 79:282–287

Monachesi C et al (2020) Slow decrease of antitissue transglutaminase antibody positivity in children with celiac disease after starting the gluten-free diet. J Pediatr Gastroenterol Nutr 71:49

Monachesi C et al (2021a) Determination of urinary gluten immunogenic peptides to assess adherence to the gluten-free diet: a randomized, double-blind, controlled study. Clin Transl Gastroenterol 12:e00411

Monachesi C et al (2021b) Quantification of accidental gluten contamination in the diet of children with treated celiac disease. Nutrients 13:190

Moreno M de L et al (2017) Detection of gluten immunogenic peptides in the urine of patients with coeliac disease reveals transgressions in the gluten-free diet and incomplete mucosal healing. Gut 66:250–257

Morón B et al (2008a) Toward the assessment of food toxicity for celiac patients: characterization of monoclonal antibodies to a main immunogenic gluten peptide. PLoS One 3:e2294

Morón B et al (2008b) Sensitive detection of cereal fractions that are toxic to celiac disease patients by using monoclonal antibodies to a main immunogenic wheat peptide. Am J Clin Nutr 87:405–414

Myléus A et al (2020) Rate, risk factors, and outcomes of nonadherence in pediatric patients with celiac disease: a systematic review. Clin Gastroenterol Hepatol 18:562–573

Osman AA et al (2001) A monoclonal antibody that recognizes a potential coeliac-toxic repetitive pentapeptide epitope in gliadins. Eur J Gastroenterol Hepatol 13:1189–1193

Osorio et al (2019) Gluten detection methods and their critical role in assuring safe diets for celiac patients. Nutrients 11:2920

Panda R et al (2019) Detection and quantitation of gluten in fermented-hydrolyzed foods by antibody-based methods: challenges, progress, and a potential path forward. Front Nutr 6:97

Penagini F et al (2013) Gluten-free diet in children: an approach to a nutritionally adequate and balanced diet. Nutrients 5:4553–4565

Raju N et al (2020) Gluten contamination in labelled and naturally gluten-free grain products in Southern India. Food Addit Contam Part A 37:531–538

Rostom A et al (2005) The diagnostic accuracy of serologic tests for celiac disease: a systematic review. Gastroenterology 128:S38–S46

Rubio-Tapia A et al (2016) Increased mortality among men aged 50 years old or above with elevated IgA anti-transglutaminase antibodies: NHANES III. BMC Gastroenterol 16:136

Sansotta N et al (2020) Trend of antitissue transglutaminase antibody normalization in children with celiac disease started on gluten-free diet: a comparative study between chemiluminescence and ELISA serum assays. J Pediatr Gastroenterol Nutr 70:37–41

Sapone A et al (2012) Spectrum of gluten-related disorders: consensus on new nomenclature and classification. BMC Med 10:13

Scherf KA et al (2016) Recent developments in analytical methods for tracing gluten. J Cereal Sci 67:112–122

Scherf KA et al (2021) Statement of the prolamin working group on the determination of gluten in fermented foods containing partially hydrolyzed gluten. Front Nutr 7:626712

See JA et al (2015) Practical insights into gluten-free diets. Nat Rev Gastroenterol Hepatol 12:580–591

Sharma GM et al (2013) Development of an incurred cornbread model for gluten detection by immunoassays. J Agric Food Chem 61:12146–12154

Silano M et al (2009) Toxic, immunostimulatory and antagonist gluten peptides in celiac disease. CMC 16:1489–1498

Silvester JA et al (2018) Cross-contamination with gluten by using kitchen utensils: fact or fiction? J Food Prot 81:1679–1684

Singh P et al (2018) Global prevalence of celiac disease: systematic review and meta-analysis. Clin Gastroenterol Hepatol 16:823–836

Syage JA et al (2018) Determination of gluten consumption in celiac disease patients on a gluten-free diet. Am J Clin Nutr 107:201–207

Thompson TL et al (2021) Gluten-free foods cooked in shared fryers with wheat: a pilot study assessing gluten cross contact. Front Nutr 8:652039

U.S. Food and Drug Administration (2013) Food labeling; gluten-free labeling of foods, final rule. Fed Regist 78:47154–47179. Available at https://www.federalregister.gov/articles/2013/08/05/2013-18813/food-labeling-gluten-free-labeling-of-foods

USA Dry Pea and Lentil Council. Chapter 3. USA dry pea, lentil & chickpea production. https://agresearch.montana.edu/wtarc/producerinfo/agronomy-nutrient-management/Pulses/USADryPeaCouncil%20FactSheet.pdf. Accessed 24 Mar 2022

Valletta E et al (2010) Celiac disease and obesity: need for nutritional follow-up after diagnosis. Eur J Clin Nutr 64:1371–1372

Verma A et al (2017) Gluten contamination in naturally or labeled gluten-free products marketed in Italy. Nutrients 9:115

Vinci G et al (2019) Noble metal nanoparticles applications: recent trends in food control. Bioengineering 6:10

Weisbrod VM et al (2020) Preparation of gluten-free foods alongside gluten-containing food may not always be as risky for celiac patients as diet guides suggest. Gastroenterology 158:273–275

Yu JM et al (2021) Analyzing gluten content in various food products using different types of ELISA test kits. Foods 10:108

Chapter 2
Raw Materials. Traditional and Non-conventional Cereals, Pseudo-cereals, Oilseeds and Legumes

Guido Rolandelli, Abel Farroni, and María del Pilar Buera

Abbreviations

DHA	docosahexanoic acid (22:6)
DSC	differential scanning calorimetry
EPA	eicosapentaenoic acid (20:5)
GAB	Guggenheim-Anderson-de Boer equation
GDW	D'arcy and Watt equation
MW	Molecular Weight
NMR	nuclear magnetic resonance
SEM	scanning electron microscopy
SFA	saturated fatty acid
Td	denaturation transition of proteins
Tg	glass-transition temperature
Tm	melting temperature
UFA	unsaturated fatty acid
XG	xyloglucans

G. Rolandelli · M. del Pilar Buera (✉)
Facultad de Ciencias Exactas y Naturales, Departamentos de Industrias y Química Orgánica, Universidad de Buenos Aires, Buenos Aires, Argentina

Instituto de Tecnología de Alimentos y Procesos Químicos (ITAPROQ), CONICET – Universidad de Buenos Aires, Buenos Aires, Argentina
e-mail: pilar@di.fcen.uba.ar

A. Farroni
Instituto Nacional de Tecnología Agropecuaria, Estación Experimental Agropecuaria Pergamino (INTA – EEA Pergamino), Pergamino, Argentina

M. F. de Escalada Pla, C. E. Genevois (eds.), *Designing Gluten Free Bakery and Pasta Products*, https://doi.org/10.1007/978-3-031-28344-4_2

2.1 Introduction

Seed proteins can be classified into three groups: storage proteins, biological active proteins (lectins, enzymes, and enzyme inhibitors), and structural proteins (ribosomal, chromosomal, and membrane proteins). The storage proteins, such as those prolamines and gliadines forming gluten, are the most abundant in many seeds and are, therefore, the key components of grain quality, with structural, technological and biological functionalities. These storage proteins generally comprise 5% or more of the total protein fraction. They do not have enzymatic activity and are stored in the seed surrounded by a vesicle or membranes to serve as a nitrogen source during germination (González-Pérez and Arellano 2009).

Gluten is a viscoelastic material generated after hydration and kneading of the complex mixture of gliadins and glutenins, which are proteins that are insoluble in water and in 0.5 M sodium chloride solution. The production of important foods (bread, pasta, noodles and many others) depends on gluten formation. In terms of technological abilities, gluten provides a special elastic continuous phase and the required texture to those foods, playing an important role in delaying starch retrogradation and product hardening during storage.

However, a lot of people are intolerant to the gluten proteins, present in certain cereal grains, mainly wheat, barley, oat and rye and their crossbred varieties and derivatives thereof (Rosell et al. 2014). Particularly, oat does not contain gluten proteins but is included in this group for cross contamination with the abovementioned cereals during storage or processing. The pathologies associated with gluten have increased in recent years worldwide. Prevalence of paediatric coeliac disease across Europe ranges from 0.1% to 3% (Roberts et al. 2021) with a worldwide prevalence estimate in 0.79% (Celdir et al. 2020). Most epitopes that trigger the coeliac disease have been described in gliadins, although some were found in the glutenin fraction (Rosell et al. 2014). The unique efficient treatment is a lifelong gluten-free diet. Nature offers a variety of cereals that are free of toxicity for gluten intolerant individuals, which include rice, corn, sorghum, millet, teff, and some specific wheat varieties. In addition, pseudocereals such as quinoa and amaranth are safe to be consumed by coeliacs.

In end-products gluten acts as a network that delays starch re-crystallization preserving their structure and texture. Due to these unique characteristics of gluten proteins, the development of gluten-free products is still a challenge for food technologists. Besides, population growth and consumers demand of novel and healthy foods, with plant proteins, small starch granules and functional ingredients, require the efficient use of available sources in each region. Cereals, legumes, and oil seeds (Rosell et al. 2014; Alvarez-Jubete et al. 2009), have become a choice of plant proteins source, and their usage value depends on their composition and on the organization of components (from molecular to macroscopic scale) in the storage organs.

2.2 Cereals That Are Traditionally Employed in Gluten-Free Products

Cereal grains (wheat, corn, rice, sorghum, and millet) are the fruit of monocotyledons temperate plants belonging to the Gramineae (Poaceae) family, which have a characteristic floral structure forming spikes (Taylor et al. 2014; Schoenlechner et al. 2008; Rouf Shah et al. 2016). They are easy to store because of their low water content and are an easy-to-handle food materials, having the ability to provide a great variety to the diet preparations. From a nutritional point of view, wheat, corn and rice provide with majority of the world food calories and about half of the proteins. They are also good source of micronutrients such as calcium, iron and of group B vitamins.

The most important gluten-free cereals are rice (*Oryza sativa* L.) and corn (*Zea mays* L.), which are essential part of the diet and for the preparation of traditional dishes in many countries in Latin America, Africa, and Asia (Ai and Jane 2016). Other cereals considered as "minor grains" are sorghum (*Sorghum bicolor* (L.)), millets (major species correspond to pearl (*Pennisetum glaucum*), foxtail, proso and finger millets), teff (*Eragrostis tef* and fonio) and canary seed (*Phalaris canariensis* L.), which are important for food security and health in at-risk communities in Africa, South America, and Asia.

Four main parts can be differentiated in cereal grains (Fig. 2.1): the endosperm, which represents approximately 80–85% of the grain weight, the embryo, responsible for 10–12% of the total mass, the outer cover, and the pedicel or flower stalk, that gather 5% and 1% of the total grain weight, respectively (Rouf Shah et al. 2016; Ai and Jane 2016). Each of these sections contain different types of nutrients. The bran is the multi-layered outer skin of the kernel, which is rich in fibre and supplies antioxidants, B vitamins, minerals like zinc, iron, magnesium, and phytochemicals (natural chemical compounds found in plants that have been linked to disease prevention). The embryo (germ) is the part of the seed that will give rise to the new plant. It is rich in lipids and proteins, lipophilic and hydrophilic vitamins (E and B, respectively), antioxidants, and contains single sugars. The largest portion of the kernel is the endosperm, in the interior of the grain, which contains the reserve

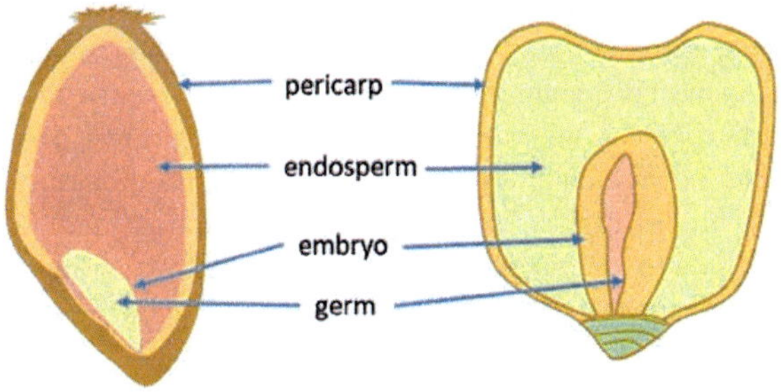

Fig. 2.1 General structure of the cereal kernels. (Adapted from Ai and Jane 2016)

carbohydrates (mainly starch), structural and storage proteins, and microcomponents like vitamins and minerals.

2.2.1 *Corn*

There are several varieties of corn, with diverse colors, shapes, sizes, hardness, and composition, which are used for a variety of purposes (Suriano et al. 2021). The "Flint" variety is highly valued at an industrial level for its hardness and pigment content, and is used to make flour and derived products, such as cereal bars, breakfast flakes, etc. (Farroni 2011; Cueto 2016). This variety emerged as a hybrid from germplasms of the original Silver-type varieties and Argentina is one of the main producers and exporters worldwide (Farroni 2011).

Wet milling is the main industrialization route for corn grain, from which corn starch and oil are mainly obtained, as well as derived products such as syrups and other caloric sweeteners. The by-products of this milling are used as fodder in animal nutrition. Dry milling, which represents a very small percentage of the industrial transformation of corn, produces corn flour, semolina, grits, and bran, which are used to produce foods such as breakfast cereals, snacks, baked products, among others.

2.2.2 *Rice*

Rice flour has 85–90% of starch, 7–8% of proteins, and very low contents of fat in a dry basis. As in most cereal grains, the bran contains significant amounts of B vitamins and minerals such as iron and calcium, and lysine is the limiting essential amino acid. In Asia, rice comprises the main source of proteins and energy of the diet (Juliano and Hicks 1996). Besides, rice bran contains high levels of bioactive compounds, such as phenolic acids with antioxidant activity, and its consumption has been related with lower cholesterol levels and antidiabetic and anticarcinogenic effects (Friedman 2013).

Rice flour is the most suitable commodity for gluten-free bakery applications due to its neutral taste, white colour, digestibility and hypoallergenic properties. Other attributes such as the low content of protein and the presence of easily digested carbohydrates can be additional benefits. The ratio of albumine-globuline-prolamine-glutelin is unique among the cereals, being 12S globulins its major storage proteins, with a high concentration of glutelins and low prolamins (Batterman-Azcona and Hamaker 1998). The main industrial applications of rice and rice flour include breads, cakes, baked products, infant formulas, breakfast cereals, snacks, and noodles.

2.3 Potential "Minor" Cereal Grains and Pseudocereals for Development of Gluten-Free Products

Several of the previously mentioned "minor gluten-free cereal grains" (sorghum, the millets, the Ethiopian cereal teff and canary seed) are distantly related to the *Triticeae* tribe cereals (wheat, barley, rye, oat). Also, some pseudocereals (i.e., amaranth, buckwheat, and quinoa) that are dicotyledonous plants (Wijngaard and Arendt 2006; Taylor et al. 2014), can also be used to produce gluten-free flours.

A very important feature of minor cereal grains and of the pseudocereals is their adaptation to grow in conditions with lower nutritional requirements as compared to main crops, and in arid or semi-arid environments, with low rainfall, high temperatures and to have short cultivation periods, which represent several advantages over other traditional cereal crops (Scanlin and Lewis 2017; Mahajan et al. 2021). For this reason, they are low-cost sources of energy for African and Asian populations, who consume them in typical dishes such as soups, stews, salads, breads, cookies, snacks, or pasta (Yousaf et al. 2021).

Some of these species, especially pseudocereals, have better protein and lipid contents and profiles than extensively used cereals (Table 2.1), with higher levels and a balanced proportion of lysine, methionine and threonine, and essential fatty acids like linoleic and linolenic acids that increase the nutritional pattern of foods (Thakur et al. 2021; Rosell et al. 2014; Alvarez-Jubete et al. 2009).

Additionally, these minor grains are characterised by being rich in many "health-promoting" phenolic phytochemicals, which exhibit antioxidant and free-radical scavenging activity (Przbylski et al. 1998; Dykes and Rooney 2006). Thus, the phenolic compounds in these grains may act in the prevention and reduction of oxidative stress, and have anti-cancer, anti-diabetic, anti-inflammatory, anti-hypertensive, and cardiovascular activities (Thakur et al. 2021). It has been proposed that breeding has selected those varieties rich in phytochemicals as they confer resistance to biotic stresses (Taylor et al. 2014).

Besides, nutritional improvements of sorghum and millets are being developed through conventional breeding and recombinant DNA technology to fight malnutrition in vulnerable populations. Varieties with increased lysine, provitamin A, iron or zinc contents, improved protein digestibility or mineral bioavailability through phytate reduction are being developed. These biofortified cereals need to have also good agronomic characteristics to be commercially useful and feasible for their adoption by farmers. The storage proteins and the amylose content are important in determining technological applications suitability. The storage proteins of these minor grains have the potential to produce a visco-elastic, wheat-like dough, similar to corn zein (Taylor et al. 2014).

Table 2.1 Proximate composition (g/100 g dry solids) of whole grains of cereals and pseudocereals

		Gluten forming	Starch, %	Amylose, % of starch	Proteins, %	Lipids, %	Dietary fibre, %	Ash, %
Cereals extensively used for human consumption	Wheat[a]	+	57–75	20–25	12–13	2–3	12–17	1–2
	Rice[a]	–	76–77	20–24	7–8	3–4	4–8	1–2
	Corn[a]	–	66–74	20–25	9–14	5–10	7–20	2–3
	Rye[g]	+	56–76	20–30	10–16	2–3	7–23	2–3
	Barley[f]	+	73–77	25–27	13–16	2	16–17	2–3
	Oat[e]	+	76	26–30	10–15	5–9	3–13	2–3
Minor cereal grains	Sorghum[a, c]	–	75–77	20–24	11–12	3–4	6–7	1–3
	Millet[c, d]	–	65–75	26–30	9–15	5–10	3–8	2–3
	Canary seed[b]	–	50–61	20–22	15–23	8–10	5–15	2–3
	Teff[a, i]	–	71–73	21–22	12–13	2–4	8–12	2–3
Pseudo-cereals	Buckwheat[a, c, h]	–	58–71	3–20	12–13	2–3	10–29	2–3
	Quinoa[a, c, h]	–	60–70	3–20	14–15	5–6	7–14	3–4
	Amaranth[a, c, h]	–	50–70	0.1–11	12–16	6–14	7–20	2–4

Range of concentrations were obtained from one or several references
[a]Rosell et al. (2014)
[b]Abdel-Aal (2021), Mason et al. (2018) and Patterson et al. (2018)
[c]Taylor and Emmambux (2008)
[d]Yousaf et al. (2021) and Dias-Martins et al. (2018)
[e]Biel et al. (2009)
[f]Asare et al. (2011)
[g]Nyström et al. (2008)
[h]Alvarez-Jubete et al. (2009)
[i]Zhu (2018) and Gebremariam et al. (2014)

2.3.1 *Pearl Millet (***Pennisetum glaucum***)*

Millet is a cereal that comprises a group of various types of crops, with different colors, shapes, sizes, and regions of origin. Figure 2.2 shows five of them. India is the largest producer with 10 million tons per year, followed by Nigeria and Sudan, with 7 and 4 million tons, respectively (Yousaf et al. 2021).

From the seven millet varieties, pearl millet (*Pennisetum glaucum*) is the most cultivated and contains higher levels of proteins and lipids than the rest (Dias-Martins et al. 2018; Yousaf et al. 2021). Its grains are oval, from which it derives its name, with a size of 3 or 4 mm. It stands out its lower carbohydrate content and higher levels of proteins and lipids compared to corn, with a larger germ (≈21% of the grain weight), responsible for its high lipid content (Table 2.1), which is difficult to separate (Mahajan et al. 2021).

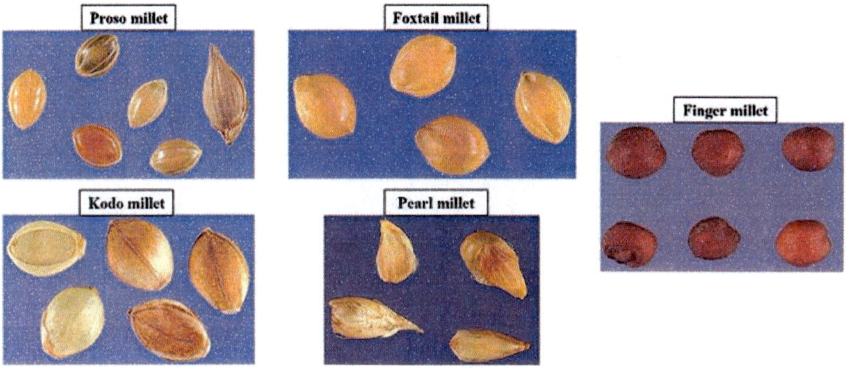

Fig. 2.2 Five types of millet crops. (Hurst S and Hernández J from USDA-NRCS 2022 Plants database https://plants.sc.egov.usda.gov/)

2.3.2 *Red Sorghum (*Sorghum bicolor *(L.) Moench)*

Sorghum is the fifth largest cultivated crop in the world, after corn, rice, wheat and barley. The main production regions are in Africa, America and Asia, with approximately 60 million tons per year (Rashwan et al. 2021).

Sorghum grain is around 4 mm long, mostly spherical in shape but flattened in the germ region (Taylor and Emmambux 2008). There are sorghums of different colors, from white to black, also with red and brown tones depending on the pigments (mainly polyphenols) present in the bran (Rashwan et al. 2021).

Sorghum is used as an ingredient in the preparation of snacks, cookies, soups, baked goods, malt for beer and it is also used as breakfast cereal or to produce cereal bars in its puffed grain version (Althwab et al. 2015). Although the use of sorghum as an ingredient for human consumption is growing annually, it continues to be very limited, and its main use is as feed for animals or for ethanol production (Awika and Rooney 2004).

One of the main limitations in the use of sorghum is the content of anti-nutritional factors in some varieties. Some of them include phytic acid, which reduces the bioavailability of minerals due to its ability to chelate multivalent metals. Trypsin inhibitors are antinutrients too and, of greater relevance, tannins, which reduce the digestibility of proteins. This negative effect of tannins lies in their ability to form complexes with proteins through hydrogen bonds and hydrophobic interactions: phenolic groups act as hydrogen donors to the carboxylic groups of proteins. These interactions can lead to protein precipitation if tannins are in excess (Rashwan et al. 2021). During processing of the grain, in stages of fermentation, soaking, cooking, among others, the levels of anti-nutritional factors are significantly reduced, making its consumption safe.

2.3.3 *Canary Seed (*Phalaris canariensis *L.)*

Canary seed is cultivated mainly in Canada and Argentina, with an annual production of 250,000 tons. Its cultivation is not widely developed, since it is mostly used as food for birds (Abdel-Aal et al. 2011). The main limitation in its use at an industrial level is the presence of small silica hairs called trichomes on the surface of the grain (Fig. 2.3a). Exposure or consumption of these silica hairs has been associated with the development of esophageal cancer and irritation of the skin and lungs (Abdel-Aal 2021). However, the problem is solved with the elimination of the trichomes, either mechanically or by genetic modification (Abdel-Aal et al. 1997), making their consumption safe in humans (Magnuson et al. 2014). Although the use of canary seed for food development is limited, it has been employed for the preparation of bakery products, breakfast cereals, cereal bars and pasta (Patterson et al. 2018).

Five varieties of canary seed have been developed without silica hairs, four with brown coloration (CDC Maria, CDC Togo, CDC Bastia and CDC Calvi) (Fig. 2.3b) and one with yellow pigmentation (CDC Cibo) (Patterson et al. 2018). Seeds have an elliptical shape and are 4 mm long and 2 mm wide (Mason et al. 2018; Abdel-Aal et al. 2011). The nutritional value of canary seed is higher than that of other cereals, due to its higher content of protein, fibre, and lipids (Table 2.1) (Abdel-Aal 2021; Mason et al. 2018; Patterson et al. 2018).

2.3.4 *Teff (*Eragrostis tef*)*

Teff is a cereal grown in Ethiopia and other countries that has low risk for coeliacs, has an excellent amino acid composition (including the eighth essential amino acids for humans), and very high fibre content (Table 2.1), making it suitable for gluten-free and health-promoting applications (Gebremariam et al. 2014; Zhu 2018). The functional properties of teff proteins have been studied and various teff-based food products have been developed (Zhu 2018). It is also a source of both bound and free

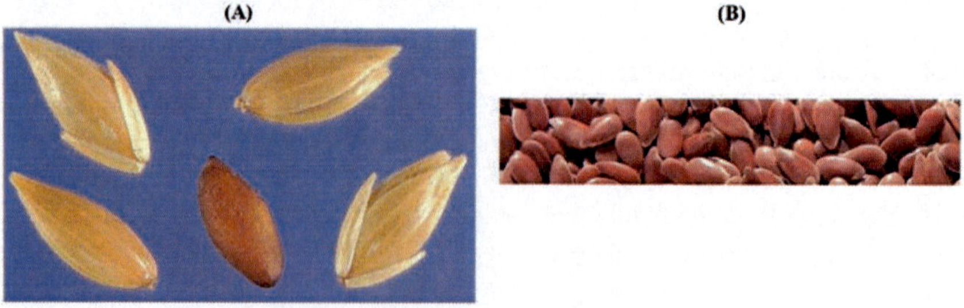

Fig. 2.3 Canary seed with trichomes (**a**) and genetically developed brown canary seeds without trichomes (**b**). (Hurst S from USDA-NRCS 2022 Plants database https://plants.sc.egov.usda.gov/)

polyphenols such as catechin, ferulic, rosmarinic, protocatechuic, and coumaric acids. Research opportunities exist to improve the status of teff as a sustainable crop and as a popular food item.

2.4 Special Features of the Composition of "Main" and "Minor" Cereal Grains and Pseudocereals

2.4.1 Grain Components

2.4.1.1 Starch

Starch is the major component (60–80%) of the endosperm of cereal grains (Table 2.1). It is made up of two types of high molecular weight polysaccharides: amylose and amylopectin. Amylose is mostly linear, formed by α-D-glucose molecules linked by α-1,4 bonds in a helical spatial arrangement with a hydrophobic interior (Zobel 1988; Mua and Jackson 1997). Amylopectin is formed by amylose arrangements with branches in α-1,6 bonds. Inside the granule, starch occurs in alternating semicrystalline and amorphous regions (Farroni 2011). The crystalline portion corresponds to associations of the linear amylose chains, while the amorphous region corresponds to the branches and is more susceptible to enzymatic or hydrolytic attack.

Type A crystalline form is predominant in native starch from cereals, which has a more compact arrangement of the amylopectin double helices than other crystalline forms (Mir et al. 2016; Singh et al. 2003). The proportion of amylose and amylopectin depends on the type of cereal, the variety, and the growing conditions (Zobel 1988; Mua and Jackson 1997). As shown in Table 2.2, in cereals and minor grains the typical amylose content of 20–26% is predominant, which is packed within a protein matrix. In waxy cereals varieties starch is composed mainly by amylopectin, having <5% amylose (Taylor and Emmambux 2008).

The modifications suffered by starch due to processing (grinding, cooking, associations with other components, etc.) is reflected in structural changes, which define the physical properties the final product (Sect. 2.8.2) (Chanvrier et al. 2005).

2.4.1.2 Proteins

Proteins of cereal grains are located mainly in protein bodies of the endosperm and in the bran. Prolamins are proline-rich storage glucoproteins which in wheat are called gliadins and glutenins and in maize are known as zeins. In contrast, the major storage protein in oat is avenalin, a globulin. Avenin is the oat prolamine similar to wheat gluten, which is only a minor component.

One common characteristic of cereal proteins is that they are deficient in the essential amino acid lysine, (Ai and Jane 2016), but they have a good proportion of

Table 2.2 Major fatty acids and protein fractions in cereals, minor grains and pseudocereals

	Major fatty acids in triacylglycerols (% of total)					Major protein fractions (% of crude protein)			
	16:0	18:1	18:2	18:3	18:2/18:3	Globulin	Albumins	Prolamine	Glutelin
Wheat[a]	17–24	18–21	55–60	3–5	11–20	Glob + alb 37–42		Gliadins 30–40 Glutenins 29–50	25
Rice[b]	23–24	42	33–36	1–2	16–20	12S fraction 6–13	4–6	2–7	79–83
Corn[c]	9–17	20–42	34–66	0.5–2	>20	3	3	Zeins 50–70	34
Sorghum[d]	10–20	30–40	30–50	1.5–1.7	>20	10–12	12–15	Kafirins 16–18	8–9
Pearl millet[e]	20–21	26–27	43–45	2.3–5.8	>20	43–49	11–17	21–25	13–19
Canary seed[f]	12	24	54	3	18	8	6	45	32
Teff[g]	13–18	23–31	44–50	6–7	6–7	3–5	23–31	3–6	45–60
Quinoa[h]	9–10	24–27	48–52	4–8	6.2	35–50 11S chenopodin	13–28 2S albumin	0.5–7	6–16
Amaranth[i]	20–23	18–38	35–55	0.4–0.9	2.7	20	40	2–3	25–30
Buckwheat[i, j]	10–18	20–37	34–39	2.2–2.7	2.6	8	44	10	15

[a]Morrison (1994)
[b]Amagliani et al. (2017) and Goffman et al. (2003)
[c]Batterman and Hamaker (1998) and Barrera-Arellano et al. (2019)
[d]Taylor et al. (2014) and Mehmood et al. (2008)
[e]Taylor and Emmambux (2008)
[f]Urbizo-Reyes et al. (2021)
[g]Satheesh and Fanta (2018) and Ahmed et al. (2021)
[h]Kozio (1992)
[i]Schoenlechner et al. (2008)
[j]Kim et al. (2004)

essential sulfur containing amino acids (methionine and cysteine) and high contents of tryptophan, phenylalanine and arginine, (Patterson et al. 2018; Abdel-Aal et al. 2011). Thus, these proteins meet the FAO nutritional requirements for adults, but not for infants or children (Dias-Martins et al. 2018).

Corn contains 8–9% proteins, of which approximately 60% corresponds to zeins (Table 2.2) and 75–85% of the total constitute α-zeins. These are in the center of the protein bodies and are of hydrophobic nature, with high amounts of glutamine and leucine (Batterman-Azcona and Hamaker 1998).

Rice and oats proteins have higher content of lysine than the other cereals. It is important to note that although the amino acid pattern of the proteins could be similar in different cereal varieties, significant differences have been reported in protein and starch digestibility among varieties (Acquistucci et al. 2009).

In sorghum and canary seed proteins are mainly prolamins (45%) and glutelins (32%) with around 14% of albumins and globulins (Table 2.2) (Abdel-Aal et al. 1997). Sorghum prolamines are called karphyrins (being α-type karphyrins more abundant than β and γ). They are cross-linked by disulfide bridges, making it difficult the access to proteases, which decrease their digestibility (Taylor et al. 2014).

Pearl millet has a relatively high content of proteins of the albumin and globulin type (25–26%), which are rich in essential amino acids, mainly leucine and isoleucine, and a lower proportion of proteins of the prolamine type (31–44%), which have lower nutritional quality (Taylor and Emmambux 2008). Nevertheless, its methionine and lysine content are low, as in the rest of the cereals.

The main characteristics of teff is its high protein content, with a better nutritional profile than the rest of the cereal grains.

2.4.1.3 Lipids

The total content of lipids in cereals is about 3–6%, and they are located mainly in the embryo and skin. The main fatty acids found in their triacylglycerols are linoleic acid (18:2), which is an essential fatty acid, oleic acid (18:1) and palmitic acid (16:0) (Strocchi 1982), with minor amounts of linolenic acid (18:3) (Table 2.2) (Abdel-Aal et al. 2020). In the most high-lipid grains, abundant amounts of vitamin E are also found (Taylor and Emmambux 2008; Mehmood et al. 2008). On the contrary, minor cereals such as sorghum and millet, contain higher lipids levels (up to 10%) (Table 2.1), but with higher unsaturated fatty acids than common cereals (Table 2.2). Particularly, higher levels of oleic and linoleic acid were reported (Torbica et al. 2021), generating increased 18:2/18:3 ratios in these minor crops when compared with rice or wheat (Table 2.2).

Lipids are susceptible to deterioration due to oxidation, mainly during milling and processing. Thus, in the production of cereal-based foods with low moisture content, the embryo is usually eliminated to avoid the production of rancidity due to oxidative process triggered by thermal process or developed during product storage (Cueto 2016; Farroni 2011). Modifications also occur during grains processing due to the formation of amylose-lipid complexes, in which the lipid material is included in the hydrophobic interior of the amylose helix (Jafari et al. 2017).

2.4.1.4 Fibre

Corn contains up to 6% fibre, composed mainly of cellulose (22%) and hemicellulose (70%), which are found in the husk of the grain. Cellulose is a linear polysaccharide, composed of β-D-glucopyranose molecules linked by β-1,4 bonds. Hemicellulose is made up of arabinoxylan and glucuronoxylan units, with different substituents in the chain, including arabinose, xylose, galactose, among others (Ai and Jane 2016). Bran or corn husk is included in food formulations to increase the dietary fibre content of products, which has health benefits, such as lowering the glycemic index, as well as control of triglyceride and cholesterol levels, prevention of cardiovascular diseases, type II diabetes, overweight and obesity (Sheng et al. 2018).

Of the total fibre in canary seed, which is mainly located in the shell, only a portion less than 1% corresponds to soluble fibre (Patterson et al. 2018).

2.4.1.5 Carotenoid Pigments

The yellowish coloration of some corns, particularly the Flint variety, is due to the xanthophylls located mainly in the shell (around 22 μg/g, of which 15.5 μg/g are lutein, 6 μg/g to zeaxanthin and 0.5 μg/g to β-cryptoxanthin). These carotenoids have antioxidant properties and protective effect to the eye from oxidative damage caused by the blue light (Rouf Shah et al. 2016; Sheng et al. 2018). α- and β-carotenes are found to a lesser extent in normal corn.

As for the group of minor grains, the presence of carotenoids is important in canary seed (11 μg/g). Among them, the husk of the grain contains considerable amounts of β-carotene (4900 μg/kg), lutein (2300 μg/kg) and zeaxanthin (500 μg/kg), without significant differences between brown and yellow varieties (Li and Beta 2012; Abdel-Aal 2021; Mason et al. 2018). The concentration of β-carotene (precursor of vitamin A, with protective effects on the skin and eyes), is higher than that found in corn (Li and Beta 2012).

Although their total content may decrease due to certain technological processes that involve mechanical and/or thermal energy (Cueto 2016), the consequent modifications can also improve the bioavailability of carotenoids (Ortak et al. 2017). Mechanical work and thermal treatments can favor the breakdown of the cellular structure that contains the pigments or also facilitate dissociation with the proteins interacting with them by hydrophobic forces, increasing its release, availability, or exposure (Ortak et al. 2017).

2.4.1.6 Polyphenolic Compounds

Polyphenols are secondary plant metabolites that have structures with one or more aromatic rings and one or more hydroxyl groups. They have important physiological activity as antioxidant and anti-inflammatory compounds and can reduce the risk of oxidative-related diseases (Rouf Shah et al. 2016). Additionally, they have implications in the preservation of food by protecting oxidizable structures.

The main polyphenols in corn are phenolic acids and flavonoids, which are preferably located in the husk of the grain. In the first group, derivatives of benzoic acid and cinnamic acid stand out, such as ferulic acid and *p*-coumaric acid, while in the second group anthocyanins prevail, such as cyanidin-3-glucoside or perlargonidin-3-glucoside. Although its content changes according to the variety, the highest values of total polyphenolic compounds are found in yellow maize, with 280–300 mg of gallic acid equivalent per 100 g of maize, on a dry basis (Sheng et al. 2018). It is important to remark the high anthocyanin content in blue-violet or red-pinkish corn, responsible for its distinctive pigmentation.

Polyphenolic compounds can be found free or bound to other components, such as fibre or proteins. For this reason, and in a similar way to carotenoids, technological processing can favor the release of these compounds and/or enhance their antioxidant properties (Kim et al. 2020; Călinoiu and Vodnar 2020).

Compared to corn, pearl millet has higher contents of polyphenolic compounds and higher antioxidant capacity (Dias-Martins et al. 2018). The shell of the canary seed also contains considerable amounts of polyphenolic compounds, mostly phenolic acids and flavonoids, which can be found free (protocatechic, *p*-coumaric and synapic acid) or bound (ferulic, caffeic and *p*-coumaric acid) to proteins, fibre or lipids. The combined form is predominant in canary seed (90% of the total) (Abdel-Aal et al. 2011) and without differences among the varieties. The flavonoids found in canary seed are derived from apigenin glucose, rhamnose and arabinose (Li et al. 2011).

The greatest differences between sorghum varieties are found precisely in the content and type of total polyphenolic bioactive compounds. Red sorghum presents the highest levels of pro-anthocyanins (condensed tannins) (Rashwan et al. 2021; Awika and Rooney 2004). The reported beneficial effects (antioxidant, anti-inflammatory, anti-diabetic, antihypertensive, etc.) of sorghum are attributed to these bioactive compounds (Taylor et al. 2014; Althwab et al. 2015).

2.5 Pseudocereals

2.5.1 Quinoa (Chenopodium quinoa Willd.) and Amaranth (Amaranthus sp.)

Quinoa and amaranth are pseudocereals belonging to the *Chenopodiaceae* family, which are dicotyledonous. They are cultivated mainly in the Andean region of South America, in countries such as Bolivia and Peru, which concentrate the largest world production, followed by Chile and Ecuador (Taylor and Emmambux 2008). Their main forms of consumption include the preparation of soups, or as expanded grains, as breakfast cereal or cereal bars. Quinoa flour is used for the preparation of bakery products such as cookies, pasta, baked goods or, through fermentation processes, quinoa-based alcoholic beverages are obtained (Navruz-Varli and Sanlier 2016; Nowak et al. 2016).

Amaranth and quinoa seeds have a size varying between 1 and 3 mm. The embryo has a circular shape and combines with the seed coat to form the bran

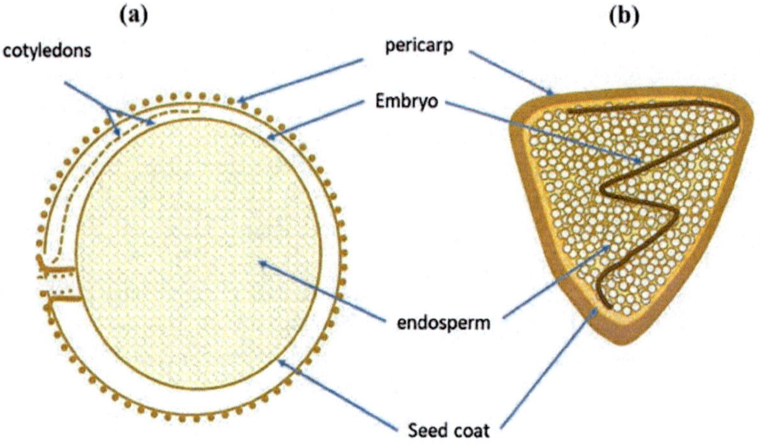

Fig. 2.4 Scheme of the quinoa and amaranth (**a**) and buckwheat (**b**) grains. (Adapted from Alonso-Miravalles and O'Mahony 2018)

fraction (Fig. 2.4a), which is relatively rich in lipids, fibre, proteins and ashes and surrounds the starch-rich perisperm (Taylor and Emmambux 2008; Scanlin and Lewis 2017).

2.5.2 *Buckwheat* (**Fagopyrum esculentum** *M.)*

Buckwheat is an herbaceous dicotyledonous plant of the *Polygonaceae* family. Thus, it is not closely related to wheat and it is not a cereal. Russia and China are the main producers of buckwheat, although cultivation has gradually spread to other parts of the world with similar climatological characteristics. In contrast to quinoa and amaranth, buckwheat grain has a triangular grain shape (Fig. 2.4b), and starch crystals are stored in the endosperm, as in common cereal grains. The embryo is rich in fat and protein and extends through the starchy endosperm (Kim et al. 2004).

It can be consumed as a grain, but it is commonly used to make flour that is part of many dishes. In France it is used to make crepes. Japanese gastronomy also uses this grain in a classic preparation such as soba noodles. It is also used for the preparation of semolina or cakes. In the West it was considered food for cattle and a typical food for peasants, but in Asia this plant has always been valued, both for its nutritional capacity and for its healthy properties (Winjgaard and Arendt 2006; Przbylski et al. 1998).

2.5.3 Nutritional Aspects of Pseudocereals

Certain nutritional and functional properties of amaranth, quinoa and buckwheat are better than those of cereals, due to their high protein, fibre and lipid content (Table 2.1) and good essential amino acid profile.

2.5.3.1 Starch

Starch is the main carbohydrate in quinoa and amaranth and, as opposed to cereals, it is located mainly in the perisperm in the form of small granules of 1–3 μm in diameter (Taylor and Emmambux 2008). Their lower amylose content (3–20%) compared to other traditional crops (Table 2.1) gives these starches greater stability to the freeze-thaw process, resistance to retrogradation and lower gelatinisation temperatures, which favors their use as a thickening agent and developers of creamy textures in low-fat products (Scanlin and Lewis 2017; Navruz-Varli and Sanlier 2016).

2.5.3.2 Proteins

While gluten-free cereals rice and corn are low in protein, fibre, and folate, quinoa, amaranth and buckwheat are high in protein and show a favourable fatty acid composition (Hager et al. 2012). Proteins' content is higher in the embryo. Regarding their composition, 37% belongs to the globulin type and 35% is represented by albumins, with the most important being 11S globulin (Table 2.2). The relative predominance of globulins and albumins to prolamines and glutelins in pseudocereals is of technological importance. Albumins and globulins are highly soluble in water and in dilute salt solutions, which can be an advantage for food formulation purposes, particularly for the production of plant-based beverages (Alonso-Miravalles and O'Mahoney 2018). Besides, the amino acid profile of pseudocereal proteins have significantly better nutritional quality than that of rice or corn, being high in lysine and low in glutamic acid and proline (Kozioł 1992; Bressani and Ligorría 1994; Li and Zhang 2001; Schoenlechner et al. 2008). For example, the protein quality of quinoa is similar to casein, it is rich in lysine and other essential amino acids such as cysteine, methionine, threonine, histidine and arginine (Taylor and Emmambux 2008; Vilcacundo and Hernández-Ledesma 2017).

The particular amino acid profile of buckwheat may also have cholesterol-lowering effects (Li and Zhang 2001), which could be attributed to the low digestibility of buckwheat protein. This can partly be explained by the abundance of thermally resistant trypsin inhibitors and tannins in these seeds (Wijngaard and Arendt 2006). Since protease inhibitors in buckwheat have shown allergenic reactivity with symptoms such as asthma, urticaria, wheezing and anaphylactic shock (Wijngaard and Arendt 2006), its potential allergenic reactivity needs to be considered when designing foods containing buckwheat (Li and Zhang 2001).

2.5.3.3 Lipids

Amaranth and quinoa lipids are concentrated in the seed embryo and are in the range of 5–6%, which represents more than twice the content found in wheat. They are composed mainly of oleic acid (20–30%), with α-linolenic and palmitic acid in minor quantities (10%) (Table 2.2) (Navruz-Varli and Sanlier 2016; Vilcacundo and Hernández-Ledesma 2017).

The fatty acid profiles of amaranth, quinoa and buckwheat are characterised by a high degree of unsaturation, which is desirable from a nutritional point of view. The unsaturated/saturated ratios are 2.7, 6.2, and 2.6, respectively, due to their high linoleic and oleic acid content. The consumption of diets high in monounsaturated fatty acids (mainly oleic acid) has been linked to a decreased incidence of cardiovascular disease (Field et al. 2003). It is also worth noting the relative high proportion of α-linolenic acid (C18:3, n-3) found in quinoa (9–12%), and its low linoleic: α-linolenic ratio. Linoleic acid (C18:2, n-6) is in proportion of 50–55%. Linoleic and α-linolenic acid and their long-chain derivatives have different metabolism, and often opposite physiological functions (Simopoulos 2001). A diet with a high n-6/n-3 ratio promotes many diseases (cardiovascular, cancer, osteoporosis) and inflammatory and autoimmune diseases, whereas an increased n-3 fatty acid intake reduces the biological markers associated with the above-mentioned diseases (Simopoulos 2001). The current n-6/n-3 ratio in western countries diet has been estimated to be in the range 14:1–20:1 (Field et al. 2003), which is far from the recommended levels of 5:1–10:1. Among these pseudocereals, quinoa's n-6/n-3 ratio, at 6.2, falls within the recommended values (Table 2.2).

2.5.3.4 Fibre

Dietary fibre is another component of physiological relevance found in abundant amounts in the pseudocereal seeds. 78% of the total fibre content of quinoa corresponds to the insoluble fraction, composed mainly of homogalacturonans, xyloglucans (XG) and cellulose, while the soluble fibre (22%) is made up of homogalacturonans and arabinans (Scanlin and Lewis 2017).

The intake of fibre (which is beneficial to the maintenance of health) in the gluten-free diet is considered inadequate and experts recommend a higher intake of whole grain cereals as opposed to refined grains (Kupper 2005; Thompson et al. 2005). Therefore, the incorporation of these seeds in the diets of coeliac patients would alleviate the deficit in fibre intake and would also increase the overall consumption of whole grains.

2.5.3.5 Polyphenols

Quinoa and amaranth have considerable amounts of polyphenolic compounds, such as phenolic acids and flavonoids, which have antioxidant properties and the ability to reduce the risk of non transmissible diseases such as diabetes, cancer, cardiovascular diseases, among others (Repo-Carrasco-Valencia et al. 2010). These benefits are highly valued by consumers. However, the processing to which the grain is subjected, such as washing, cooking, roasting, etc., can affect the levels of these compounds, limiting the extent of their beneficial properties (Nickel et al. 2016).

2.5.3.6 Mineral Content of the Seeds

In general, pseudocereals seeds contain higher levels of calcium, magnesium and iron compared with wheat. Zinc and iron are important in quinoa and the calcium content of buckwheat is approximately twice than that found in quinoa and wheat. In amaranth seeds, the levels of phosphorus, calcium, potassium and magnesium are generally higher than those of cereals (Bressani and Ligorría 1994). Since these minerals have been shown to be deficient in gluten-free products and in the gluten-free diet (Kupper 2005; Thompson et al. 2005), the use of pseudocereals or their fractions as ingredients in gluten-free products could help improve the mineral profile of this type of diet.

2.6 The Potential of Legumes for the Development of Gluten-Free Products

2.6.1 Main Legumes Used for Human Consumption

Legumes are plants of the Fabaceae (or Leguminosae) family, the third largest and economically important plant family, which fruits or seeds are also called legumes. When used as a dry grain, the seeds are known as pulses. Leguminosae family includes the plants that produce beans, soybeans, peas, chickpeas, peanuts, lentils, and lupins. Also, guar and many species of *Prosopis* (mesquite, vinal, carob, tamarind, alfalfa, fenugreek and clover) are Fabaceae.

They are grown agriculturally, primarily for human consumption, for livestock forage and silage, and as soil green fertilizer. A remarkable characteristic of leguminous plants is the presence of nodules that contain symbiotic nitrogen fixing *Rhizobium* bacteria. For this reason, they play a key role in crop rotation. Legumes are a healthy and affordable source of protein and provide excellent nutritional support to humans and animals.

The average protein content in legume crops (20–40%) is two to three times than that of wheat and rice. Of the total carbohydrates, up to 85% is composed of starch, while dietary fibre constitutes anywhere from 10% to 20% of the weight of dried legumes (Table 2.3). Seed starch levels widely vary across legumes, being about 50% of its dry weight in pea (*Pisum sativum* L.), and very low in soybean ($\leq$0.91%) (Wilson et al. 1978) and in the seeds of the forage plant *Medicago truncatula* ($\leq$1–2%) (Song et al. 2017).

Legume starch molecules are packed into dense granules which maintain more parts of the cell walls intact, creating a physical barrier that leaves few ends for the enzyme amylase to access. In some legumes, the relatively high amylose content may contribute to this effect. These effects reduce starch digestibility, which is known as resistant starch (RS) that it is not immediately digested into glucose in the small intestine and functions much like dietary fibre (Tayade et al. 2019). Legumes are a very good source of RS (20–30% on dry basis). RS is transferred to the large intestine where it is fermented by the microbiota, producing healthy metabolites for the intestinal function (Dhital et al. 2016). In comparison, cereals have a higher amount of starch (Tables 2.1 and 2.3), and very limited resistant starch, releasing more glucose in the blood (Tayade et al. 2019). However, it is to be noted that the ratio of RS is different in the raw grains than in flours and it also changes according to the cooking conditions (boiled, cooled, reheated and on the retrogradation degree). In boiled lentils, chickpeas and beans seeds the RS was between 10% and 16% of the total starch, while in their flours between 34% and 55% of the starch was resistant (García-Alonso et al. 1998).

Another important compositional characteristic of legumes to produce gluten-free products is the presence of hydrocolloids that generates a matrix that delays starch re-crystallization. As discussed before, one of the main challenges in the development of gluten-free cereal-based products is related to the need of improving their structural properties (Gallagher et al. 2004; Moore et al. 2004; Schober et al. 2005), and several research works have explored the use of gums to act as gluten-replacers. One of the main type of polysaccharides obtained from the endosperm of some seeds from plants of the Leguminosae family are galactomannans, which function as energy reserves. Chemically, galactomannan molecules are neutral, constituted of a linear chain of β-1,4 linked β-D-mannopyranose units (M) with α-1,6 branches of α-D-galactopyranose units (G) (Labeau 2012). The galactose content, ratio and its distribution in the galactomannan skeleton, the M:G ratio and the molecular weight (MW) depend on the source and influence the physicochemical and rheological properties of each gum. It must be considered that some legumes belonging to the subfamily *Faboideae*, such as soybean, store relatively small amounts of galactomannan in a thin endosperm (Buckeridge et al. 2000). Examples of galactomannans are listed in Table 2.3. The four most commercially important galactomannans in the food and non-food industries are guar gum, tara gum, locust bean gum and fenugreek, being guar by far the most produced galactomannan, with M/G ratio of 1.8–2/1, and very high MWs. Guar is a renewable abundant raw material and guar derivatives constitute an attractive sustainable alternative to polyacrylamides and other synthetic polymers used in oil field, cosmetics, agrochemicals, food, paper coating, textile, and explosives (Srivastava and Kapoor 2005; Labeau 2012).

Table 2.3 Composition of major legumes (%, dry basis)

Common name	Systematic name	Crude protein	Lipid	Carbohydrates	Dietary fibre	Minerals	Main polysaccharide
Peas[a]	*Pisum sativum*	23–26	1.4	53.7	19–26	2.5–3.0	ND
Garden bean[a]	*Phaseolus vulgaris*	24.1	1.8	54.1	19.2	4.4	Arabinose-rich pectins, β-glucans, galacturonans, arabinans
Chickpea[a, b]	*Cicer arietinum*	22.7	5.0	54.6	10.7	3.0	ND
Faba bean[b]	*Vicia faba*	31–38	1–2	43–49	14–16	3–4	ND – (branched polysaccharide)
Mung bean[c]	*Phaseoulus aureus*	26.7	1.3	51.7	21.7	3.8	Arabinogalactan, hemicellulose B; mung bean polysaccharide
Lentils[d]	*Lens culinaris*	28.6	1.6	57.6	11.9	3.6	Pectic polysaccharides containing arabinose, glucose, and galacturonic acid
Lupin[f]	*Lupinus albus*	31–35	4–6	39	16	4–5	Galactans
Locust bean - carob[e]	*Ceratonia siliqua*	7–24	1.5–7.5	31	40	1.5–5	Galactomanan M/G = 3.5–4:1
Guar[g]	*Cyamopsis tetragonoloba*	24–27	3	53–55	12–14	4–5	Galactomanan M/G = 2:1
Fenugreek[h]	*Trigonella foenumgraecum*	25–30	7–9	45–55	20–25	3–4	Galactomanan M/G = 1:1
Mesquite[i]	*Prosopis pallida*	9.5	1	57.6	29.6	2.3	Galactomanan M/G = 1:1
Vinal[j]	*Prosopis ruscifolia*	35–40	5–6	54–57	40–53	3–4	Galactomanan M/G = 1.6
Alfalfa[k]	*Medicago sativa*	30–38	7–13	32	26	4–5	Galactomanan M/G = 1.2:1
Tara[l]	*Caesalpinia spinosa*	54	14	19	7	6	Galactomanan M/G = 3:1
Cassia[m]	*Cassia tora*	14	16	58	8	5	Galactomanan M/G = 2.5–5:1
Tamarind[n]	*Tamarindus indica*	13–27	4–16	50–57	7–9	2–4	Xyloglucan, glycosaminoglycan galactoxyloglucan

(continued)

Table 2.3 (continued)

Common name	Systematic name	Crude protein	Lipid	Carbohydrates	Dietary fibre	Minerals	Main polysaccharide
Red clover[o]	*Trifolium pretense*	18–26	2–3	42	21–23	7–9	ND
"*Chañar*" seed[p]	*Geoffroea decorticans*	21.6	47.2	20.1	–	2.9	ND
"*Chañar*" whole fruit flour[q]	*Geoffroea decorticans*	6.5	6.3	36	15	2.9	ND

ND not determined
[a]Belitz et al. (2009)
[b]Khan et al. (2015)
[c]Hou et al. (2019)
[d]Nomura et al. (2021)
[e]Dakia et al. (2008)
[f]Erbaş et al. (2005a)
[g]Sharma et al. (2016)
[h]Mathur and Mathur (2005)
[i]Gonzales-Barron et al. (2020)
[j]Freyre et al. (2010)
[k]Ullah et al. (2016) and Giuberti et al. (2018)
[l]Del Re-Jiménez and Amado (1989)
[m]Adamu et al. (2013)
[n]Bagul et al. (2015)
[o]Petrović et al. (2014)
[p]Lamarque et al. (2000)
[q]Costamagna et al. (2013)

2.6.2 Non-conventional Legumes with Interesting Properties

Fenugreek is the dried seed of the leguminous plant *Trigonella foenumgraeceum* (*Fabiaceae*). The pods split easily and are threshed to free seeds, which are winnowed, cleaned, and further dried. Their characteristic components are trigonellin and δ-cadinene. One of the main industrial uses of fenugreek is the mucilage or gum obtained from its seeds that presents stabilizing, emulsifying and thickening properties (Salarbashi et al. 2019).

Brea tree (*Cercidium praecox*) (Ruiz and Pav. Burkart and Carter) is a South American species with a wide distribution, from Mexico to the North and West of Argentina that grows through arid corridors of the Andes. The glaucum subspecies is endemic to Argentina, from very arid areas from Jujuy to Río Negro. It is very ornamental in flowering, with a vascular exudate (rubber, brea gum) traditionally used by the peasant communities of the most arid zones since its chemical properties are like those of Arabic gum. Brea gum is allowed by current legislation in Argentina and it has many applications as thickener and protecting agent.

Gleditsia amorphoides Griseb., Taub. "espina corona" and *Gleditsia triacanthos* L. grow spontaneously in forests and jungles in the North of Argentina and adjacent regions of Bolivia, Paraguay, Brazil, and Uruguay. Espina corona is one of the closest forest specie of *Ceratonia silicua* L., also from the *Fabaceae* family, whose seeds are used to obtain locust bean gum (LBG), which is a common food ingredient. Espina corona gum is highly used in dairy products like milk protein gels and yoghurts for its rheological properties, and as a stabilizing and thickening agent (Galante et al. 2019; Pavón et al. 2014).

Vinal (*Prosopis ruscifolia* Griseb.) is an extensively growing tree from the North-East of Argentina. It can grow under extreme ambient conditions and develop spontaneously in deforested lands (Bernardi et al. 2010). Many species from *Prosopis* family contain galactomannan gums in their seeds with structures and functionalities that are close to those of common and widely used galactomannans such as guar gum (Busch et al. 2015). They are also a source of polyphenols (Sciammaro et al. 2016).

Tamarindus indica L. is a native tree of tropical Africa, particularly Sudan, where it grows wild. It is also widely distributed throughout the tropics, from Africa to Asia, Australia and the rest of Oceania. As for Latin America, it grows in Mexico, Central America and the Colombian Caribbean, which are the largest producers and consumers of the fruit. Its seeds are an abundant and cheap available by-product of tamarind pulp industry. They are rich in protein, containing high amount of many essential amino acids (isoleucine, leucine, lycine, methionine, phenylalanine, and valine). Seeds are also good source of essential fatty acids and minerals, particularly calcium, phosphorous and potassium, which levels are relatively high compared to other legumes. Tamarind seed kernels contain 46–48% of XG, a jelly forming polysaccharide called jellose that can be obtained in abundance and is comparatively cheaper than other gelling agents (Bagul et al. 2015). Tamarind XG is commonly known as 'tamarind gum' and it is commercially available as an ingredient for rheological control of aqueous phase for thickening, stabilizing, and gelling in food. The most common applications are as a stabilizer in ice cream, mayonnaise, and cheese. When XG is added to starch, the mixtures yield high paste viscosity and pseudo-plasticity degree. The partial substitution of tapioca starch by XG improved starch gelatination and delayed retrogradation during storage of pastes at 5 °C (Bagul et al. 2015). It improves the crispness and thickness of biscuits. Tamarind seed contains also other polysaccharides, glycosaminoglycan and a galactoxyloglucan that are used to stabilize suspensions and dispersions. These seeds have huge potential to be explored in terms of food, pharmaceutics, and industrial benefits.

2.7 Oilseeds

2.7.1 Major Oilseeds

Oilseed crop consumption has increased drastically in the last decades due to an increased demand for food and non-food industrial applications (Rahman and de Jiménez 2016). Unlike cereals and legumes, oilseed crops are of the most diverse types. Despite this, at present, a few crop species such as soybean (*Glycine max*), oilseed rape (*Brassica napus*) and sunflower (*Helianthus annuus*) dominate the international edible oilseed market. With oil palm (*Elaeis guineensis*) and olives (*Olea europaea*), which are obtained from the fruit pulp, they compose the five major oil crops that account for ~80% of world oil production (Arrutia et al. 2020).

While in cereals and pseudocereals the main reserve component is starch, in oilseeds the main reserve is of lipidic nature. Vegetable oil is obtained by pressing the seeds and then extracting the oil. The oil content ranges from as low as 10–15% of the weight of coconuts to >50% of the weight of *Sesamum indicum* seeds and *E. guineensis* kernels. On the other side, protein content is very high in soybeans (~40%) but is much lower (15–25%) in most other oilseeds and is still lower in some other oil-bearing crops (Arrutia et al. 2020). The cake or meal obtained separated from the oil in the extraction is a rich source of proteins: sunflower and peanut meals contain 40–50% and 50–60% proteins, respectively. Other oilseed meals contain 35–45% proteins (Table 2.4). In oilseeds proteins, leucine and valine are the two essential amino acids that are present at the highest concentrations, while methionine, cysteine, and tryptophan at the lowest ones (Kotecka-Majchrzak et al. 2020). These values are strongly affected by the oilseed variety and production conditions.

The importance of the use of oilseeds in the production of gluten-free foods relies not only in the nutritional improvement but also in the structural aspects of the food products (Zampronio Zorzi et al. 2020). For example, soy flour is one of the most complete in terms of their amino acid profile, and it also strengthens the matrix thanks to its cohesive properties (Genevois and de Escalada Pla 2021). Chia seeds and flaxseeds are used in the bakery industry such as the development of gluten-free

Table 2.4 Protein content and fatty acid composition of various oilseeds

Oil seed	Systematic name	Protein (% d.b.)	Lipid content (% d.b.)	Fatty acid (g/100 g lipids)						
				16:0	18:0	18:1	18:2	18:3	20:1	22:1
Canola/ rapeseed[a, d]	*Brassica* sp.	40–45	18–25	4–6	1–2	57–65	17–22	3–7	0.6–0.7	0
Flaxseed high linolenic[a]	*Linum usitatissimum* L.	18–20	34–44	5	3	16	15	60	0	1
Flaxseed low linolenic[a]				10	5	16	65	2	0	0
Camelina[a, b]	*Camelina sativa*	23–27	31–38	8	3	17	23	31	0	3
Safflower[a]	*Carthamus tinctorius* L.	13–17	41	7	2	14	77	0	0	0
Sunflower[a]	*Helianthus annuus*	21	43	6	4	17	72	0	0	0
Soybean[c]	*Glycine max*	37	20–25	14	2	19–23	56	4	0	0
Sesame[h]	*Sesamum indicum*	18	50	8–12	5–6	36–42	42–48	0	0	0
Peanut[i]	*Arachis hypogaea* L.	16–36	36–54	8–15	1–7	31–60	20–45	0	1–3	0
Grapeseed[j]	*Vitis vinifera*	10–16	8–20	7	3.5	14	75	0.2	0.4	0
Watermelon[e]	*Citrullus lanatus* L.	31–40	24–25	14	1–6	18–19	59–64	0.1	0.2	0
Wild almond[g]	*Prunus scoparia* L.	25	50	7	3	67	22	0.1	0	0
Chia[f, h]	*Salvia hyspanica* L	35–41	10–11	6–7	3–4	7–8	18–20	66–67	0	0
Coconut[h]	*Cocos nucifera* L.	11	48	8	3	6	1.6	0	0	0
Olive[k]	*Olea europaea*	17	19–25	15	2	69	12	0.8	0	0
Chañar[l]	*Geoffroea decorticans*	20–27	45–50	7–9	6–7	31–43	35–53	–	–	–

[a]Jaeger and Siegel (2008)
[b]Kirkhus et al. (2013)
[c]Belitz et al. (2009)
[d]Matthaus et al. (2016)
[e]Angelova-Romova et al. (2019)
[f]Akinfenwa et al. (2020)
[g]Givianrad et al. (2013)
[h]Kotecka-Majchrzak et al. (2020)
[i]Singh et al. (2021)
[j]Garavaglia et al. (2016) and Yang et al. (2021)
[k]Al-Bachir and Sahlou (2017)
[l]Salinas et al. (2020)

products for their high water-holding capacity and the presence of a mucilage that generates a gel-like texture when mixed with water that has rheological properties similar to guar gum (de Lamo and Gómez 2018). Besides, chia seed protein hydrolysates have demonstrated to present health-promoting bioactivity, such as antioxidant and anti-microbial properties. Similarly, rapeseed and sesame proteins have been included in the development of functional and gluten-free products for their nutritional value and their bioactivity, such as antioxidant and antithrombotic properties, and protection of cardiovascular and immune systems (Kotecka-Majchrzak et al. 2020; Difonzo et al. 2021). Lignans are antioxidants present in important quantities in flaxseed and sesame and have shown antitumour properties. They are stable at baking conditions; thus, these oilseeds can be incorporated in baked gluten-free products to increase their functionality (de Lamo and Gómez 2018). Sunflower protein concentrate, which is the meal obtained after oil extraction, was used in a gluten-free bread formulation at different concentrations and compared with pea flour (Zampronio Zorzi et al. 2020). The resulting products were sensorially accepted and those containing sunflower meal had higher protein contents than those made with pea flour. Besides, they presented lower hardness values and higher moisture contents than breads containing pea flour during storage up to 21 days, which indicates improved stability in time. Coconut meal is valuable for its high dietary fibre contents and amounts of magnesium, potassium and calcium, while olive meal is rich in antioxidants such as phenolic acids (Difonzo et al. 2021). The addition of okara, which is the main by-product from soybean wet milling, to bakery products such as noodles and bread presented hypoglycemic effects which was attributed to its high fibre contents (Difonzo et al. 2021). The addition of up to 14–16% of chia, flaxseed or sunflower flour was reported to improve the nutritional properties of bread for their increment of tocopherols, minerals, fibre and omega-3 fatty acids contents while keeping good sensory acceptability (de Lamo and Gómez 2018). These benefits increased when oilseeds were incorporated as flours, but this negatively affected the oxidative stability due to the higher exposure of the labile antioxidants and unsaturated fatty acids. Regarding this, delay of starch retrogradation was reported with the addition of oilseeds for their high lipid contents, but, in those cases, lipid oxidation prevailed over the textural characteristics for the definition of the shelf-life of bread or biscuits (de Lamo and Gómez 2018).

2.7.2 Non-conventional Oilseeds

With a continuous increase in population, the demand for high-quality seed oils is also increasing. To meet this demand, there is a need not only to surge the production of the major oilseed crops but also to diversify the sources by popularizing and rising the production of minor crops. In this section several non-conventional oilseeds are introduced, and their main characteristics are presented for their potential inclusion in gluten-free formulations.

2.7.2.1 Wild Almond (*Prunus scoparia* L.)

Wild almond species is distributed as an oilseed in Western and Central Asia and constitutes an important crop in Iran. *P. scoparia* seeds are considered an important source of protein but wild almonds are also used in various industrial products, such as soaps, paints, and biodiesel (Sorkheh et al. 2016). Despite its great advantages in comparison with other wild almond germplasm, including low bitterness, evergreen habitus, and high yields of seed and oil, *P. scoparia* suffers from a lack of improvement program through modern breeding efforts (Sorkheh et al. 2016).

Oil quantity and quality in wild almond is comparable to that of other oilseeds such as sunflower, safflower and linseed. Their oils are rich in both oleic and linoleic acid and contain about 10% of saturated fatty acids (Givianrad et al. 2013). The high oleic acid content makes wild almond oil suitable for cooking purposes while the high linoleic acid content makes it nutritionally valuable, being a potential source of edible seed oils (Sorkheh et al. 2016). Wild almond oil also has considerable amounts of β-sitosterol, which lowers cholesterol levels and has antioxidant and anticarcinogenic properties and tocopherols, mainly α-tocopherol, which are important for oil stability and their nutritional value (Givianrad et al. 2013).

2.7.2.2 Camelina (*Camelina sativa* L. Crantz)

Camelina is an underexploited, but promising oilseed crop that may be well-suited for organic cropping. Camelina is a low-input and short-seasoned oilseed crop, with low nutrient requirement, no seed dormancy, and fewer problems with insect damage than rape and turnip rape. The seed quality makes it relevant for both edible oil and animal feed, but so far, the market is limited as well as the agronomic knowledge (Zanetti et al. 2021).

Camelina seeds contain up to 30% of proteins, with high contents of essential amino acids like leucine, valine, lysine, phenylalanine and isoleucine and 45% of oil. The oil is particularly high in the omega-3 fatty acid α-linolenic acid (18:3) (Table 2.4), which constitutes 35–45% of the fatty acids. α-linolenic acid is converted to some extent to the long-chain omega-3 fatty acids eicosapentaenoic acid (EPA, 20:5) and docosahexanoic acid (DHA, 22:6) in the body, and it has been shown that intake of camelina oil compared to rapeseed oil gives significantly higher serum concentrations of 18:3, EPA, and DHA, as well as a decrease in serum cholesterol in hypercholesterolemic subjects (Kirkhus et al. 2013). Camelina seeds have an omega-3/omega-6 ratio of 1.3–2.6 which is valuable for human health and its regular consumption could help in increase the levels of omega-3. The health benefits of EPA and DHA are well documented, including protective effects on cardiovascular disease and autoimmune and mental disorders, but there is also a growing body of scientific data supporting the idea that 18:3 may exert beneficial effects by other mechanisms rather than simply acting as a precursor for EPA and

DHA. Camelina oil also contains phytosterols known to have a cholesterol-lowering effect and natural antioxidants such as tocopherols (vitamin E), carotenoids and phenolic compounds (Zanetti et al. 2021). The oil is also considered to be more stable toward oxidation than other highly unsaturated oils, probably due to the high levels of γ-tocopherol (90% of the total). Also, phenolic compounds such as chlorogenic acid may contribute to the protection against oxidation (Kirkhus et al. 2013).

Natural antioxidants and phospholipids are best preserved in cold-pressed oil, but crude camelina oil has a distinct smell and taste that may be difficult to find acceptance among consumers. Studies should be performed to remove undesirable flavor and at the same time ensure both a long shelf life and high nutritional quality. The limited industrial applications of camelina oil are in salad dressings, as cooking oil, and margarines. Nevertheless, the long-term consumption of bread containing camelina seeds probed to have benefits on intestinal health, for its contents of lignin, fibre, and mucilage, confirming its potential to be included at large scale for the development of novel products (Zanetti et al. 2021).

2.7.2.3 Watermelon (*Citrullus lanatus*)

Watermelon is one of the major under-utilized fruits grown in the warmer part of the world at an industrial scale. The juice or pulp from watermelon is used for human consumption while rind and seeds are major solid wastes. The rind is utilized for products such as pickles and pre-serves as well as for extraction of pectin, whereas seeds are a potential source of protein and lipids. Watermelon seeds are used for oil production at the subsistence level in Nigeria, in several other African countries, and in the Middle East. In Nigeria, such seeds are used for oil extraction by small local farmers but not on an industrial scale for oil or protein production (Moaddabdoost Baboli and Safe Korodi 2010).

The dry seeds of watermelon have been reported to contain on average about 32 g of protein and 51.4 g of fat per 100 g sample, with high levels (60%) of linoleic acid (Table 2.4). Some reports about the fatty acid composition of oils from some varieties of watermelons acknowledge its good quality (Table 2.4), presents a unique flavour and compare well with those of soybean and sunflower oils. Thus, it might be an acceptable substitute for highly unsaturated oils for cooking or frying purposes and to take advantage of its health benefits for the contents of phytosterols and antioxidants, like carotenoids, phenolic compounds and tocopherols (Biswas et al. 2017). This also explains the reported induction time of 5.8–6.7 h at 110 °C for a highly unsaturated oil (Moaddabdoost Baboli and Safe Korodi 2010; de Conto et al. 2011; Biswas et al. 2017). The utilization of watermelon seed for oil production could provide extra income and at the same time help to minimize waste disposal problems.

2.7.2.4 Grape Seed (*Vitis vinifera* L. ssp.)

The berries of *Vitis vinifera* L. ssp. are appreciated worldwide for the production of wine and for the nutritional properties of the raw and dried fruit. The by-products have risen interest for the pharmaceutical properties of their derivatives, such as peel and seed extracts. For instance, grape seed extract (aqueous or alcoholic) has a high antioxidant potential; its beneficial effects include the modulation of antioxidant enzyme expression, protection against oxidative damage in cells, antiatherosclerotic and anti-inflammatory effects, and protection against some cancer types, in both humans and animal models (Yang et al. 2021; Garavaglia et al. 2016).

Grape seed is a by-product of winemaking process that contains 8–20% of oil (dry basis) (Table 2.4). Oil content is traditionally extracted using either organic solvents or mechanical techniques. Cold pressing is a method of oil extraction that involves no heat or chemical treatment and hence may retain more health beneficial components. Although the yield is usually lower compared to solvent extraction, in cold-pressing there is no concern about solvent residues in the oil, resulting in a safer and more consumer-desired product (Yang et al. 2021; Garavaglia et al. 2016; Rombaut et al. 2015).

Grape seed oil composition is related to grape vine variety, environmental factors and maturation degree of the seeds. Due to grape seed oil pleasant flavor, the interest in its use in culinary preparations and a functional food product has increased, especially because of its high levels of phenolic compounds, tocotrienols, unsaturated fatty acids (UFAs), and phytosterols. Grape seed oil contains linoleic (58–78%) and oleic (14–20%) as the main fatty acids, while saturated ones remain at 10% (Table 2.4). Besides, high amounts of phenolic compounds (catechin, epicatechin, trans-reverastrol and procyanidin B1) are also present (Yang et al. 2021; Perumalla and Hettiarachchy 2011; Rombaut et al. 2015). Thus, the addition of grape seed to gluten-free formulations improved the total phenolic contents and antioxidant activity (Kapcsándi et al. 2021) and the nutritional value of the final bakery products, while at the same time modified some physicochemical properties like color, texture and sensory acceptance (Levent et al. 2020).

2.7.2.5 Chañar (*Geoffroea decorticans* Gill.ex Hook. et Arn. Burkart)

Chañar is a native legume tree which grows in arid or semiarid regions of South America, reaching heights up to 10 m. Its fruits (of about 1.5–3 cm) are drupaceous, rounded and reddish-brown in color. Ripe fruits are consumed raw or in preparations like a very sweet flavored syrup known as *arrope*. Due to its ability to colonize the lands used for grazing, chañar is considered a plague and is deforested. However, the fruit could be used to prepare flour-based gluten-free foods, with considerable fibre content, satisfying population health needs, and taking advantage of a nutritional resource with economic potential (Costamagna et al. 2013; Lamarque et al. 2000). It could be a source of polysaccharides, for application in food and pharmaceutical industries. Although it is currently not cultivated or harvested and is little exploited in its natural habitat, chañar may cover the current interests in sustainably with the adequate use of non-timber resources from forests. Chañar polysaccharide, which structure has not been fully determined, is a branched polymer with potential applications in food and pharmaceutical industries (Salinas et al. 2020) for edible film preparation, as thickener or encapsulation agent.

Moreover, chañar almonds, which are discarded during the production of arrope, contain about 50% lipids and are a potential source of edible oil, mainly composed by mono- and polyunsaturated fatty acids (oleic and linoleic acids). The ratio between unsaturated and saturated fatty acids (UFA/SFA) of chañar almond oil was in the range of 4.5–4.7, presenting an adequate balance for human consumption (Table 2.4) (Lamarque et al. 2000).

2.8 Some Important Physical Properties to Be Considered for the Development of Gluten-Free Foods

2.8.1 *Water Sorption Isotherms*

Water adsorption isotherms are typically constructed by the isopiestic method, which consists of exposing small portions of the samples in hermetically sealed containers with saturated solutions of specific salts that impart a precise relative humidity or water activity (a_w) to the environment. After the equilibrium, the water content of each sample exposed at the varying relative humidities is evaluated for the construction of the isotherms (Greenspan 1977).

There are different types of isotherms depending on the characteristics of the systems. In cereals, oilseeds and legumes, type II predominates, with a sigmoidal shape, in which it is possible to determine three zones associated with different relationships between water and solids (Van den Berg and Bruin 1981). In the first zone ($a_w \approx 0$–0.25) water molecules are closely associated with the solids, mainly with the most hydrophilic compounds. This water is not available to act as a solvent or plasticizer. The percentage of water associated with the upper limit of a_w of this zone is known as hydration limit, or "monolayer" water and indicates the water content that completely covers the polar groups of the exposed surface of the food (Furmaniak et al. 2009). This parameter is important since deterioration reactions at this moisture are minimal, except for lipid oxidation (Labuza and Dugan 1971). The second zone ($a_w \approx 0.25$–0.75) contains the water that has a less intense degree of interaction with the solids than in the first zone, due to the shielding effect of the molecules most involved with the solid. The name "multilayer" is usually attributed to the water molecules that compose this zone, since they are located above the first layer of water molecules closely associated with solids. Finally, in the last zone ($a_w \approx 0.75$–1) water molecules with a lower degree of association with solids and with greater mobility is present. These are water molecules that act as a solvent, can freeze and allow microbial growth.

There are widely used mathematical models to characterise adsorption isotherms over the entire range of water activity, which are the Guggenheim-Anderson-de Boer (GAB) equation (Van den Berg and Bruin 1981) and the D'arcy and Watt (GDW) equation (D'arcy and Watt 1970). Both equations provide information on the water hydration limit and on certain parameters related to the heat of sorption (in GAB equation) and on the sorption kinetics of primary and secondary sorption sites (GDW). In addition, GDW offer data on the microstructure of the material. From these mathematical models, it is possible to relate the obtained parameters with water relationships in terms of physicochemical quality and microbiological stability (Table 2.5).

2.8.2 Thermal Properties and Supplemented Phase/State Diagrams

Since the '80 Slade and Levine (1991) leaded the rescarch and Food Polymer Science approach that helped to understand many phenomena occurring in food systems due to phase and state transitions, emphasizing the role of glass transitions and water plasticization in foods as central themes. Since then, supplemented temperature/composition phase diagrams were used to interpret and control the changes of physical properties and serve as a reference to define process and storage conditions (Buera et al. 2011; Roos 2020). These diagrams can be obtained by determining the temperatures at which phase and state transition take place, at a given solids/water ratio. They include the non-equilibrium glass-transition temperature (T_g) curve and equilibrium ice-melting and solubility curves.

In the case of the materials discussed in this chapter, the most relevant transitions to define technological applications are starch melting or gelatinisation temperature (T_m), denaturation transition of proteins (T_d) and other thermally defined phenomena (such as entangled polymer flow, reaction zone and softening), and glass transition temperatures (T_g). When the temperatures corresponding to these transitions are plotted as a function of solids concentration (or water mass fraction), the obtained diagram provides a very complete picture of the expected changes upon heating.

Gluten-free dehydrated product materials (either extruded, freeze or spray-dryed), can be in amorphous or partially crystalline state. The temperature range at which the amorphous phase undergoes the state change from glass to supercooled liquid, with consequent material softening, is called the glass transition temperature (T_g), and depends on several factors, mainly on the composition and on water content (Roos 2010, 2020; Fan and Roos 2017). The T_g of a material decreases with the increase in its water content, being able to reach T_g values below room temperature if the water content is enough (Fan and Roos 2017; Cova et al. 2012).

Starch gelatinization is the most important transformation that occurs during the manufacture of cereal-based foods. In general, it is the process in which the starch granules go from an ordered structure to a disordered one, given by heating in the

Table 2.5 Sorption parameters for gluten-free seeds fitted by GAB and GDW models

		GAB			GDW				
		M_0	C	k	M_e	K	k	w	References
Cereals and pseudocereals	Corn	9.6	16	0.64	13	6	0.8	0.5	Rolandelli et al. (2022)
	Wheat bran	6.9	62.6	0.83	10.6	0.61	0.8	0.38	Li et al. (2021) and Furmaniak et al. (2011)
	Rice	8.6	21	0.1	15	4.3	0.9	0.2	Toğrul and Arslan (2006) and Zhang et al. (2016)
	Semolina	11.8	4.2	0.65	16.7	3.1	0.9	0.22	Erbaş et al. (2005b) and Furmaniak et al. (2011)
	Millet	9.5	0.66	0.8					Raji and Ojediran (2011)
	Quinoa	8	19	0.7	9	10	0.7	0.8	Rolandelli et al. (2022)
Oilseeds	Rapeseed	3	9	60	ND	ND	ND	ND	Lazouk et al. (2014)
	Flaxseed	6	6.5	5.6	ND	ND	ND	ND	Lazouk et al. (2014)
	Sunflower	5	6	21	ND	ND	ND	ND	Lazouk et al. (2014)
	Melon seeds	2.3	12.5	0.73	ND	ND	ND	ND	Silva et al. (2015)
	Grape seeds	3.1	17.0	0.69	ND	ND	ND	ND	Silva et al. (2015)
Legumes	Pea	8.6	8.3	0.84	5.7	55.1	0.01	1.05	Vertucci and Leopold (1986)
	Soybean	ND	ND	ND	4.4	118	0.04	0.95	Socorro et al. (2010)
	Chickpea	6.0	7.0	0.9					Boucheham et al. (2019)
	Faba bean	6.0	6.3	0.84	9.6	6×10^{-4}	0.99	0.34	Boucheham et al. (2019) and Furmaniak et al. (2011)
	Lupine	5.0	6.3×10^{-5}	0.47	ND	ND	ND	ND	Vázquez et al. (2003)

ND not determined

presence of enough water, which guarantees its consumption and digestibility (Wang et al. 2021; Singh et al. 2003). Because of gelatinization, structural modifications occur, such as a decrease in crystallinity, and conformational and association changes between macrocomponents, which will define the mechanical, textural,

Table 2.6 Some literature references about thermal transitions of cereals and legumes components as a function of water content that provide data to generate phase/state diagrams

	Material	Compound	References
Cereals and pseudocereals	Rice	Starch	Ring et al. (1987) and Wang et al. (2021)
	Corn	Starch Protein	Mestres et al. (1988), Wang et al. (2021), Madeka and Kokini (1996) and Zhang et al. (2015)
	Sorghum	Starch	Ubwa et al. (2012)
	Millet	Starch	Ubwa et al. (2012)
	Quinoa embryos	Protein	Matiacevich et al. (2006)
Legumes	Soybean	Starch Protein	Zhang et al. (2015), Monnet et al. (2019) and Bengoechea et al. (2007)
	Pea	Starch Protein	Singh et al. (2008), Zhang et al. (2015) and Pelgrom et al. (2013)
	Faba bean	Starch	Ring et al. (1987)
	Phaseoulus vulgaris	Protein	Sun et al. (1998)

microstructural and sensory properties of the products (Jebalia et al. 2019; Chaunier et al. 2007; Chanvrier et al. 2005). When gelatinized starch cools, the thermal energy of the system decreases, and the amylose and amylopectin molecules tend to re-associate through hydrogen bonding. This generates cross-linking of molecules and the reappearance of crystalline regions that can ultimately lead to gel formation or precipitation (Wang et al. 2021). This process impairs the quality of starchy products and is called retrogradation, affecting food organoleptic properties (Gulati et al. 2020). Retrogradation is faster in gluten-free materials, since gluten acts as a physical buffer and retrograded starch is indigestible, constituting part of resistant starch.

The supplemented state diagrams for cereal proteins (Madeka and Kokini 1996; Kokini et al. 1994) and soy proteins (Morales and Kokini 1998) have been reported. Monnet et al. (2019) proposed a generic representation of starch and proteins phase/state transitions to help a rational formulation of legume-enriched cereal products. Table 2.6 shows some helpful information on the transitions of starch and proteins and their glasses as a function of water content for some of the discussed materials, in order to depict the state diagrams for single components or more complex systems as whole flours. In this late case several thermal events are possible to occur when heated as a function of temperature and water content.

Phase and state transitions and chemical reactions can be identified and characterised using different techniques, but differential scanning calorimetry (DSC) and rheometry (particularly small-amplitude oscillatory measurements at atmospheric pressure) are preferred most of the times. Order-disorder transitions in materials such as starch, hydrocolloids and proteins result in major rheological changes, which sometimes are better detected than thermal transitions of these materials by DSC. Especially for some biopolymers, the glass transition temperature may be difficult to analyze by DSC and other complementary techniques are necessary or even more adequate to employ. Dielectrical properties and nuclear magnetic resonance (NMR) analysis can be applied. Raman, X-ray diffraction and scanning electron microscopy (SEM) analyses (Rolandelli et al. 2022; Wang et al. 2021) may also complement DSC determinations.

2.9 Overview and Concluding Remarks

During the last years, climate changes, water scarcity, increasing world population, rising of food prices, and other socioeconomic impacts have threatened food security in many populations. These emergencies became even more dramatic in scenarios such as COVID-19 pandemics, wars, and other political conflicts which exposed the need to generate more resilient systems. Thus, conservation of biodiversity, the reversion or detention of climate change and the mitigation of world hunger have been detected as the main challenges facing humanity.

It is important not only to increase the production and efficiency of the major cereals, pseudocereals, legumes and oilseed crops but also avoid wastes and diversify their sources by popularizing and increasing the production of minor crops. The efficient and safe use of these non-conventional resources represent a challenge to scientists both from technological and social fields to investigate the possibilities of producing, processing, and utilizing other potential food sources to end hunger and poverty in a sustainable way. Thus, analysis of compositional data and physicochemical properties of the involved materials are necessary for their sustainable use.

Among the most used cereals for human consumption, rice and corn are known to be gluten-free and thus, safe for coeliacs. Other gluten-free cereals, such as sorghum, millets, teff, and canary seed, are considered "minor" grains for human consumption, although they are important to food security and health in at-risk communities in several parts of the world. The protein balance of cereals meets the FAO nutritional requirements for adults, with a good proportion of essential sulfur containing aminoacids, but it is not complete for infants or children, since they are deficient in the essential amino acid lysine. The lipid profile of cereals also lacks adequate proportion of essential fatty acids. On the other side, the pseudocereals like amaranth, quinoa, and buckwheat, are dicotiledoneous gluten-free grains that provide good quality protein, dietary fibre, and lipids rich in unsaturated fatty acids, besides being important energy sources due to their starch content. In addition, they contain adequate levels of important micronutrients such as minerals and vitamins and significant amounts of other bioactive components such as flavonols, squalene, and phytosterols.

Both minor cereal grains and pseudocereals can grow in arid or semi-arid environments, with lower nutritional and water requirements as compared to main cereals crops, and support high temperatures and have short cultivation periods, which represent several advantages over other traditional cereal crops.

Legume seeds are important sources of protein, dietary fibre and starch, with the advantage of having about two to three times higher protein content with higher lysine values than corn or rice and less starch, and higher fibre amount, being also a good source of essential fatty acids. Moreover, the higher content of resistant starch, in comparison to cereals, acts as dietary fibre. Besides these nutritional characteristics a very important feature of legumes to produce gluten-free products is the presence of hydrocolloids (arabinoxylanes, galactomannans, and other branched polysaccharides) that efficiently contribute to delay starch re-crystallization and also have many other industrial uses as thichener agents, emulsifying or structure-stabilizers.

Regarding oilseeds, their main reserve components are lipids, and they are good source of proteins, with adequate aminoacidic balance. Oilseeds or their by-products have found many uses in the bakery industry to produce gluten-free foods, especially in improving the structural aspects. The presence of mucilage favors the water holding capacity and increased functionality and fibre content. Industrial applications of oilseeds are based on the properties of particular saturated fatty acid components of these oils, while the protein-rich residue remaining after oil extraction, is an important source of nutrients and potentially a source of bioactive compounds. Non-conventional oilseeds, such as wild almond, camelina, grapeseeds, watermelon seeds, have interesting oil and protein quality and are promising for organic and local production systems.

Global climate change may affect the agroecosystems where oilseeds crops are being grown around the world. Many initiatives have been considered to find applications for sustainable uses of underutilized plants, especially in areas in which conventional crops cannot grow due to soil salinity, temperature changes or lack of water. However, there are still many non-conventional sources of food (especially Fabaceae and oilseeds) that are unexplored and have a significant potential to favor non-timber applications of woods resources. Nevertheless, the use of these non-conventional sources of food components should be performed in a comprehensive way, to take advantage of the benefits of its high fibre content and bioactive components such as polyphenolic compounds present in the bran, either in free or complexed form, finding the way to eliminate anti-nutrients or potentially toxic compounds.

Besides the improvement of the nutritional quality, the incorporation of novel ingredients modify physicochemical properties of food. To take full advantage of the functional properties of these non-conventional food ingredients it is of mayor importance to get a deep understanding of their effects. The physical state, water mobility, water-solid interactions, and main components modifications affect storage stability, textural, and functional properties of food. The techniques that allow assessing these properties (water sorption modeling, DSC, NMR, X-ray diffraction, microscopic images, and mechanical analysis, among others) can provide complementary information on components interactions and their effects on product quality. An integral approach that understands ingredients' functionality as an improvement in food nutritional composition, texture, acceptability and preservation would help to develop innovative food products with the incorporation of either traditional or non-traditional raw ingredients on a scientific basis.

Acknowledgments The authors acknowledge funding from University of Buenos Aires (UBACYT Project 20020170100459BA), Agencia Nacional de Promoción Científica y Tecnológica (PICT 2018-01822) and INTA (Instituto Nacional de Tecnología Agropecuaria, project PD-I152) of Argentina.

References

Abdel-Aal ESM (2021) Nutritional and functional attributes of hairless canary seed groats and components and their potential as functional ingredients. Trends Food Sci Technol 111:680–687. https://doi.org/10.1016/j.tifs.2021.03.029

Abdel-Aal ESM, Hucl PJ, Sosulski FW (1997) Structural and compositional characteristics of canaryseed (*Phalaris canariensis* L.). J Agric Food Chem 45:3049–3055. https://doi.org/10.1021/jf970100x

Abdel-Aal ESM, Hucl P, Shea Miller S, Patterson CA, Gray D (2011) Microstructure and nutrient composition of hairless canary seed and its potential as a blending flour for food use. Food Chem 125:410–416. https://doi.org/10.1016/j.foodchem.2010.09.021

Abdel-Aal ESM, Hernandez M, Rabalski I, Hucl P (2020) Composition of hairless canary seed oil and starch-associated lipids and the relationship between starch pasting and thermal properties and its lipids. LWT 125:109257. https://doi.org/10.1016/j.lwt.2020.109257

Acquistucci R, Francisci R, Bucci R, Ritota M, Mazzini F (2009) Nutritional and physicochemical characterization of Italian rice flours and starches. Food Sci Technol 15:507–518. https://doi.org/10.3136/fstr.15.507

Adamu HM, Ushie OA, Elisha B (2013) Chemical and nutrient analysis of raw and fermented seeds of *Cassia tora*. J Phys Sci Innov 5:125–138

Ahmed IAM, Uslu N, Al Juhaimi F, Özcan MM, Osman MA, Alqah HAS, Babiker EE, Ghafoor K (2021) Effect of roasting treatments on total phenol, antioxidant activity, fatty acid compositions, and phenolic compounds of teff grains. Cereal Chem 98:1027–1037. https://doi.org/10.1002/cche.10442

Ai Y, Jane J (2016) Macronutrients in corn and human nutrition. Compr Rev Food Sci Food Saf 15:581–598. https://doi.org/10.1111/1541-4337.12192

Akinfenwa AO, Cheikhyoussef B, Cheikhyoussef N, Hussein AA (2020) Cold pressed chia (*Salvia hispanica* L.) seed oil. In: Ramadan MF (ed) Cold pressed oils. Academic, pp 181–190. https://doi.org/10.1016/B978-0-12-818188-1.00015-3

Al-Bachir M, Sahloul H (2017) Fatty acid profile of olive oil extracted from irradiated and non-irradiated olive fruits. Int J Food Prop 20:2550–2558. https://doi.org/10.1080/10942912.2016.1243557

Alonso-Miravalles L, O'Mahony JA (2018) Composition, protein profile and rheological properties of pseudocereal-based protein-rich ingredients. Foods 7:73. https://doi.org/10.3390/foods7050073

Althwab S, Carr TP, Weller CL, Dweikat IM, Schlegel V (2015) Advances in grain sorghum and its co-products as a human health promoting dietary system. Food Res Int 77:349–359. https://doi.org/10.1016/j.foodres.2015.08.011

Alvarez-Jubete L, Arendt EK, Gallagher E (2009) Nutritive value and chemical composition of pseudocereals as gluten-free ingredients. Int J Food Sci Nutr 60:240–257. https://doi.org/10.1080/09637480902950597

Amagliani L, O'Regan J, Kelly AL, O'Mahony JA (2017) Composition and protein profile analysis of rice protein ingredients. J Food Compos Anal 59:18–26. https://doi.org/10.1016/j.jfca.2016.12.026

Angelova-Romova MY, Simeonova ZB, Petkova ZY, Antova GA, Teneva OT (2019) Lipid composition of watermelon seed oil. Bulg Chem Commun 51:268–272

Arrutia F, Binner E, Williams P, Waldron KW (2020) Oilseeds beyond oil: press cakes and meals supplying global protein requirements. Trends Food Sci Technol 100:88–102. https://doi.org/10.1016/j.tifs.2020.03.044

Asare EK, Jaiswal S, Maley J, Båga M, Sammynaiken R, Rossnagel BG, Chibbar RN (2011) Barley grain constituents, starch composition, and structure affect starch in vitro enzymatic hydrolysis. J Agric Food Chem 59:4743–4754. https://doi.org/10.1021/jf200054e

Awika JM, Rooney LW (2004) Sorghum phytochemicals and their potential impact on human health. Phytochemistry 65:1199–1221. https://doi.org/10.1016/j.phytochem.2004.04.001

Bagul M, Sonawane SK, Arya SS (2015) Tamarind seeds: chemistry, technology, applications and health benefits: a review. Indian Food Ind 34:28–35

Barrera-Arellano D, Badan-Ribeiro AP, Serna-Saldivar SO (2019) Corn oil: composition, processing, and utilization. In: Serna-Saldivar SO (ed) Corn, chemistry and technology. Woodhead Publishing/AACC International Press, Cambridge, pp 593–613. https://doi.org/10.1016/B978-0-12-811971-6.00021-8

Batterman-Azcona SJ, Hamaker BR (1998) Changes occurring in protein body structure and α-zein during cornflake processing. Cereal Chem 75:217–221. https://doi.org/10.1094/CCHEM.1998.75.2.217

Belitz HD, Grosch W, Schieberle P (2009) Legumes. In: Belitz HD, Grosch W, Schieberle P (eds) Food chemistry, 4th edn. Springer, Berlin/Heidelberg, pp 746–769. https://doi.org/10.1007/978-3-540-69934-7_17

Bengoechea C, Arrachid A, Guerrero A, Hill SE, Mitchell JR (2007) Relationship between the glass transition temperature and the melt flow behavior for gluten, casein and soya. J Cereal Sci 45:275–284. https://doi.org/10.1016/j.jcs.2006.08.011

Bernardi C, Sánchez H, Freyre M, Osella C (2010) Gluten-free bread formulated with *Prosopis ruscifolia* (vinal) seed and corn flours. Int J Food Sci Nutr 61:245–255. https://doi.org/10.3109/09637480903373336

Biel W, Bobko K, Maciorowski R (2009) Chemical composition and nutritive value of husked and naked oats grain. J Cereal Sci 49:413–418. https://doi.org/10.1016/j.jcs.2009.01.009

Biswas R, Ghosal S, Chattopadhyay A, Datta S (2017) A comprehensive review on watermelon seed oil – an underutilized product. IOSR J Pharm 7:1–7

Boucheham N, Galet L, Patry S, Zidoune MN (2019) Physicochemical and hydration properties of different cereal and legume gluten-free powders. Food Sci Nutr 7:3081–3092. https://doi.org/10.1002/fsn3.1170

Bressani R, Ligorría LE (1994) Effect of lime cooking of grain amaranth on selected chemical components and on its protein quality. J Agric Food Chem 42:1998–2001. https://doi.org/10.1021/jf00045a031

Buckeridge MS, Dietrich SMC, de Lima DU (2000) Galactomannans as the reserve carbohydrate in legume seeds. Dev Crop Sci 26:283–316. https://doi.org/10.1016/S0378-519X(00)80015-X

Buera MP, Roos YH, Levine H, Slade L, Corti HR, Reid DS, Auffret T, Angell CA (2011) State diagrams for improving processing and storage of foods, biological materials, and pharmaceuticals (IUPAC technical report). Pure Appl Chem 83:1567–1617. https://doi.org/10.1351/PAC-REP-10-07-02

Busch MV, Kolender AA, Santagapita PR, Buera MP (2015) *Vinal* gum, a galactomannan from *Prosopis ruscifolia* seeds: physicochemical characterization. Food Hydrocoll 51:495–502. https://doi.org/10.1016/j.foodhyd.2015.04.035

Călinoiu LV, Vodnar DC (2020) Thermal processing for the release of phenolic compounds from wheat and oat bran. Biomol Ther 10:21. https://doi.org/10.3390/biom10010021

Celdir MG, Jansson-Knodell CL, Hujoel IA, Prokop LJ, Wang Z, Murad MH, Murray JA (2020) Latitude and celiac disease prevalence: a meta-analysis and meta-regression. Clin Gastroenterol Hepatol 20:e1231–e1239. https://doi.org/10.1016/j.cgh.2020.09.052

Chanvrier H, Colonna P, Della Valle G, Lourdin D (2005) Structural and mechanical behavior of corn flour and starch-zein based materials in the glassy state. Carbohydr Polym 59:109–119. https://doi.org/10.1016/j.carbpol.2004.09.005

Chaunier L, Della Valle G, Lourdin D (2007) Relationships between texture, mechanical properties and structure of cornflakes. Food Res Int 40:493–503. https://doi.org/10.1016/j.foodres.2006.07.014

Costamagna MS, Ordoñez RM, Zampini IC, Sayago EJ, Isla MI (2013) Nutritional and antioxidant properties of *Geoffroea decorticans*, an Argentinean fruit, and derived products (flour, arrope, decoction and hydroalcoholic beverage). Food Res Int 54:160–168. https://doi.org/10.1016/j.foodres.2013.05.038

Cova A, Müller AJ, Laredo E, Sandoval AJ (2012) Effect of two different lipid sources on glass transition temperatures and tensile properties of corn semolina. J Food Eng 113:265–274. https://doi.org/10.1016/j.jfoodeng.2012.05.040

Cueto MA (2016) Transformaciones físico-químicas de granos de maíz en la elaboración de laminados y extrudados para el desayuno (Physicochemical transformations of corn grains in the elaboration of flaked and extrudates for breakfast). Buenos Aires, Argentina. https://bibliotecadigital.exactas.uba.ar/collection/tesis/document/tesis_n5964_Cueto

D'Arcy RL, Watt IC (1970) Analysis of sorption isotherms of non-homogeneous sorbents. Trans Faraday Soc 66:1236–1245

Dakia PA, Blecker C, Robert C, Wathelet B, Paquot M (2008) Composition and physicochemical properties of locust bean gum extracted from whole seeds by acid or water dehulling pretreatment. Food Hydrocoll 22:807–818. https://doi.org/10.1016/j.foodhyd.2007.03.007

de Conto LC, Gragnani MAL, Maus D, Ambiel HCI, Chiu MC, Grimaldi R, Guaraldo Gonçalves LA (2011) Characterization of crude watermelon seed oil by two different extractions methods. J Am Oil Chem Soc 88:1709–1714. https://doi.org/10.1007/s11746-011-1850-8

De Lamo B, Gómez M (2018) Bread enrichment with oilseeds. A review. Foods 7:191. https://doi.org/10.3390/foods7110191

Del Re-Jiménez BL, Amado R (1989) Comparative study of the chemical composition of germ meals from carob, guar and tara seeds. Food Hydrocoll 3:149–156. https://doi.org/10.1016/S0268-005X(89)80024-4

Dhital S, Bhattarai RR, Gorham J, Gidley MJ (2016) Intactness of cell wall structure controls the *in vitro* digestion of starch in legumes. Food Funct 7:1367–1379. https://doi.org/10.1039/C5FO01104C

Dias-Martins AM, Pessanha KLF, Pacheco S, Rodrigues JAS, Carvalho CWP (2018) Potential use of pearl millet (*Pennisetum glaucum* (L.) R. Br.) in Brazil: food security, processing, health benefits and nutritional products. Food Res Int 109:175–186. https://doi.org/10.1016/j.foodres.2018.04.023

Difonzo G, de Gennaro G, Pasqualone A, Caponio F (2021) Potential use of plant-based by-products and waste to improve the quality of gluten-free foods. J Sci Food Agric 102:2199–2211. https://doi.org/10.1002/jsfa.11702

Dykes L, Rooney LW (2006) Sorghum and millet phenols and antioxidants. J Cereal Sci 44:236–251. https://doi.org/10.1016/j.jcs.2006.06.007

Erbaş M, Certel M, Uslu MK (2005a) Some chemical properties of white lupin seeds (*Lupinus albus* L.). Food Chem 89:341–345. https://doi.org/10.1016/j.foodchem.2004.02.040

Erbaş M, Ertugay MF, Certel M (2005b) Moisture adsorption behaviour of semolina and farina. J Food Eng 69:191–198. https://doi.org/10.1016/j.jfoodeng.2004.07.017

Fan F, Roos Y (2017) Glass transition-associated structural relaxations and applications of relaxation times in amorphous food solids: a review. Food Eng Rev 9:257–270. https://doi.org/10.1007/s12393-017-9166-6

Farroni A (2011) Transformaciones estructurales y físico-químicas de maíces argentinos en la producción de alimentos obtenidos por procesos de gelatinización-laminación (Structural and physicochemical transformations of Argentinean corns in the production of foods obtained by gelatinization-flaking processes). Buenos Aires, Argentina. https://bibliotecadigital.exactas.uba.ar/collection/tesis/document/tesis_n4896_Farroni

Field FJ, Born E, Mathur SN (2003) Fatty acid flux suppresses fatty acid synthesis in hamster intestine independently of SREBP-1 expression. J Lipid Res 44:1199–1208. https://doi.org/10.1194/jlr.M300013-JLR200

Freyre M, Bernardi CM, Baigorria C, Rozycki V, Piagentini A, Presa M, Taher H (2010) Parámetros de Interés Nutricional en Semillas de Vinal (*Prosopis Ruscifolia*). FAVE Sección Ciencias Agrarias 9:89–96. https://doi.org/10.14409/fa.v9i1/2.1358

Friedman M (2013) Rice brans, rice bran oils, and rice hulls: composition, food and industrial uses, and bioactivities in humans, animals, and cells. J Agric Food Chem 61:10626–10641. https://doi.org/10.1021/jf403635v

Furmaniak S, Terzyk AP, Gołembiewski R, Gauden PA, Czepirski L (2009) Searching the most optimal model of water sorption on foodstuffs in the whole range of relative humidity. Food Res Int 42:1203–1214. https://doi.org/10.1016/j.foodres.2009.06.004

Furmaniak S, Terzyk AP, Gauden PA (2011) Some remarks on the classification of water vapor sorption isotherms and Blahovec and Yanniotis isotherm equation. Dry Technol 29:984–991. https://doi.org/10.1080/07373937.2011.566399

Galante M, Boeris V, Risso PH (2019) Evaluation of the effect of *Gleditsia amorphoides* gum on the properties of rennet-induced milk protein gels. Int Dairy J 97:216–221. https://doi.org/10.1016/j.idairyj.2019.06.008

Gallagher E, Gormley TR, Arendt EK (2004) Recent advances in the formulation of gluten-free cereal-based products. Trends Food Sci Technol 15:143–152. https://doi.org/10.1016/j.tifs.2003.09.012

Garavaglia J, Markoski MM, Oliveira A, Marcadenti A (2016) Grape seed oil compounds: biological and chemical actions for health. Nutr Metab Insights 9:59–64. https://doi.org/10.4137/NMI.S32910

García-Alonso A, Goñi I, Saura-Calixto F (1998) Resistant starch and potential glycaemic index of raw and cooked legumes (lentils, chickpeas and beans). Z Lebensm Unters Forsch 206:284–287. https://doi.org/10.1007/s002170050258

Gebremariam MM, Zarnkow M, Becker T (2014) Teff (*Eragrostis tef*) as a raw material for malting, brewing and manufacturing of gluten-free foods and beverages: a review. J Food Sci Technol 51:2881–2895. https://doi.org/10.1007/s13197-012-0745-5

Genevois CE, de Escalada Pla MF (2021) Soybean by-products and modified cassava starch for improving alveolar structure and quality characteristics of gluten-free bread. Eur Food Res Technol 247:1477–1488. https://doi.org/10.1007/s00217-021-03725-x

Giuberti G, Rocchetti G, Sigolo S, Fortunati P, Lucini L, Gallo A (2018) Exploitation of alfalfa seed (*Medicago sativa* L.) flour into gluten-free rice cookies: nutritional, antioxidant and quality characteristics. Food Chem 239:679–687. https://doi.org/10.1016/j.foodchem.2017.07.004

Givianrad MH, Saber-Tehrani M, Jafari Mohammadi SA (2013) Chemical composition of oils from wild almond (*Prunus scoparia*) and wild pistachio (*Pistacia atlantica*). Grasas Aceites 64:77–84. https://doi.org/10.3989/gya.070312

Goffman FD, Pinson S, Bergman C (2003) Genetic diversity for lipid content and fatty acid profile in rice bran. J Am Oil Chem Soc 80:485–490. https://doi.org/10.1007/s11746-003-0725-x

Gonzales-Barron U, Dijkshoorn R, Maloncy M, Finimundy T, Calhelha RC, Pereira C, Stojković D, Soković M, Ferreira ICFR, Barros L, Cadavez V (2020) Nutritive and bioactive properties of mesquite (*Prosopis pallida*) flour and its technological performance in breadmaking. Foods 9:597. https://doi.org/10.3390/foods9050597

González-Pérez S, Arellano JB (2009) Vegetable protein isolates. In: Phillips GO, Williams PA (eds) Handbook of hydrocolloids, 2nd edn. Woodhead Publishing, pp 383–419. https://doi.org/10.1533/9781845695873.383

Greenspan L (1977) Humidity fixed points of binary saturated aqueous solutions. J Res Natl Bur Stand A Phys Chem 81:89–96

Gulati P, Brahma S, Rose DJ (2020) Impacts of extrusion processing on nutritional components in cereals and legumes: carbohydrates, proteins, lipids, vitamins, and minerals. In: Ganjyal GM (ed) Extrusion cooking. Cereal grains processing. Woodhead Publishing/AACC International Press, pp 415–443. https://doi.org/10.1016/B978-0-12-815360-4.00013-4

Hager AS, Wolter A, Jacob F, Zannini E, Arendt EK (2012) Nutritional properties and ultra-structure of commercial gluten free flours from different botanical sources compared to wheat flours. J Cereal Sci 56:239–247. https://doi.org/10.1016/j.jcs.2012.06.005

Hou D, Yousaf L, Xue Y, Hu J, Wu J, Hu X, Feng N, Shen Q (2019) Mung bean (*Vigna radiata* L.): bioactive olyphenols, polysaccharides, peptides, and health benefits. Nutrients 11:1238. https://doi.org/10.3390/nu11061238

Jaeger W, Siegel R (2008) Economics of oilseed crops and their biodiesel potential in Oregon's Willamette Valley. Oregon State University Extension Service. https://catalog.extension.oregonstate.edu/sites/catalog/files/project/pdf/sr1081.pdf

Jafari M, Koocheki A, Milani E (2017) Effect of extrusion cooking on chemical structure, morphology, crystallinity and thermal properties of sorghum flour extrudates. J Cereal Sci 75:324–331. https://doi.org/10.1016/j.jcs.2017.05.005

Jebalia I, Maigret JE, Réguerre AL, Novales B, Guessasma S, Lourdin D, Della-Valle G, Kristiawan M (2019) Morphology and mechanical behavior of pea-based starch-protein composites obtained by extrusion. Carbohydr Polym 223:115086. https://doi.org/10.1016/j.carbpol.2019.115086

Juliano BO, Hicks PA (1996) Rice functional properties and rice food products. Food Rev Int 12:71–103. https://doi.org/10.1080/87559129609541068

Kapcsándi V, Hanczné Lakatos E, Sik B, Linka LÁ, Székelyhidi (2021) Antioxidant and polyphenol content of different *Vitis vinifera* seed cultivars and two facilities of production of a functional bakery product. Chem Pap 75:5711–5717. https://doi.org/10.1007/s11696-021-01754-0

Khan MA, Ammar MH, Migdadi HM, El-Harty EH, Osman MA, Farooq M, Alghamdi SS (2015) Comparative nutritional profiles of various faba bean and chickpea genotypes. Int J Agric Biol 17:449–457. https://doi.org/10.17957/IJAB/17.3.14.990

Kim SL, Kim SK, Park CH (2004) Introduction and nutritional evaluation of buckwheat sprouts as a new vegetable. Food Res Int 37:319–327. https://doi.org/10.1016/j.foodres.2003.12.008

Kim MY, Yoon N, Lee YJ, Woo KS, Kim HY, Lee J, Jeong HS (2020) Influence of thermal processing on free and bound forms of phenolics and antioxidant capacity of rice hull (*Oryza sativa* L.). Prev Nutr Food Sci 25:310–318. https://doi.org/10.3746/pnf.2020.25.3.310

Kirkhus B, Lundon AR, Haugen JE, Vogt G, Borge GIA, Henriksen BIF (2013) Effects of environmental factors on edible oil quality of organically grown *Camelina sativa*. J Agric Food Chem 61:3179–3185. https://doi.org/10.1021/jf304532u

Kokini J, Cocero MJ, Madeka H (1994) The development of state diagrams for cereal proteins. Trends Food Sci Technol 51:281–288. https://doi.org/10.1016/0924-2244(94)90136-8

Kotecka-Majchrzak K, Sumara A, Fornal E, Montowska M (2020) Oilseed proteins – properties and application as a food ingredient. Trends Food Sci Technol 106:160–170. https://doi.org/10.1016/j.tifs.2020.10.004

Kozioł MJ (1992) Chemical composition and nutritional evaluation of quinoa (*Chenopodium quinoa* Willd.). J Food Compos Anal 5:35–68. https://doi.org/10.1016/0889-1575(92)90006-6

Kupper C (2005) Dietary guidelines and implementation for celiac disease. Gastroenterology 128:S121–S127. https://doi.org/10.1053/j.gastro.2005.02.024

Labeau MP (2012) Guar and Guar derivatives. Poly Sci 10:195–203. https://doi.org/10.1016/B978-0-444-53349-4.00256-9

Labuza TP, Dugan LR (1971) Kinetics of lipid oxidation in foods. CRC Crit Rev Food Technol 2:355–405. https://doi.org/10.1080/10408397109527127

Lamarque AL, Maestri DM, Zygadlo JA, Guzmán CA (2000) Chemical evaluation of *Geoffroea decorticans* seeds as source of oil and protein. Grasas Aceites 51:241–243. https://doi.org/10.3989/gya.2000.v51.i4.418

Lazouk MA, Savoire R, Kaddour A, Castello J, Lanoisellé JL, Van-Hecke E, Thomasset B (2014) Oilseeds sorption isoterms, mechanical properties and pressing: global view of water impact. J Food Eng 153:73–80. https://doi.org/10.1016/j.jfoodeng.2014.12.008

Levent H, Sayaslan A, Yeşil S (2020) Physicochemical and sensory quality of gluten-free cakes supplemented with grape seed, pomegranate seed, poppy seed, flaxseed, and turmeric. J Food Process Preserv 45:e15148. https://doi.org/10.1111/jfpp.15148

Li W, Beta T (2012) An evaluation of carotenoid levels and composition of glabrous canaryseed. Food Chem 133:782–786. https://doi.org/10.1016/j.foodchem.2012.01.092

Li SQ, Zhang QH (2001) Advances in the development of functional foods from buckwheat. Crit Rev Food Sci Nutr 41:451–464. https://doi.org/10.1080/20014091091887

Li W, Qiu Y, Patterson CA, Beta T (2011) The analysis of phenolic constituents in glabrous canary-seed groats. Food Chem 127:10–20. https://doi.org/10.1016/j.foodchem.2010.12.033

Li X, Han X, Tao L, Jiang P, Qin W (2021) Sorption equilibrium moisture and isosteric heat of Chinese wheat bran products added to rice to increase its dietary fibre content. Grain Oil Sci Technol 4:149–164. https://doi.org/10.1016/j.gaost.2021.09.001

Madeka H, Kokini JL (1996) Effects of glass transition and cross-linking on rheological properties of zein: development of a preliminary state diagram. Cereal Chem 73:433–438

Magnuson BA, Patterson CA, Hucl P, Newkirk RW, Ram JI, Classen HL (2014) Safety assessment of consumption of glabrous canary seed (*Phalaris canariensis* L.) in rats. Food Chem Toxicol 63:91–103. https://doi.org/10.1016/j.fct.2013.10.041

Mahajan P, Bera MB, Panesar PS, Chauhan A (2021) Millet starch: a review. Int J Biol Macromol 180:61–79. https://doi.org/10.1016/j.ijbiomac.2021.03.063

Mason E, L'Hocine L, Achouri A, Karboune S (2018) Hairless canaryseed: a novel cereal with health promoting potential. Nutrients 10:1–16. https://doi.org/10.3390/nu10091327

Mathur V, Mathur NK (2005) Fenugreek and other less known legume galactomannan-polysaccharides: scope for development. J Sci Ind Res 64:475–481

Matiacevich SB, Castelli6n ML, Maldonado SB, Buera MP (2006) Water-dependent thermal transitions in quinoa embryos. Thermochim Acta 448:117–122. https://doi.org/10.1016/j.tca.2006.06.016

Matthaus B, Özcan MM, Al Juhaimi F (2016) Some rape/canola seed oils: fatty acid composition and tocopherols. Z Naturforsch C J Biosci 71:73–77. https://doi.org/10.1515/znc-2016-0003

Mehmood S, Orhan I, Ahsan Z, Aslan S, Gulfraz M (2008) Fatty acid composition of seed oil of different *Sorghum bicolor* varieties. Food Chem 109:855–859. https://doi.org/10.1016/j.foodchem.2008.01.014

Mestres C, Colonna P, Buleon A (1988) Gelation and crystallization of maize starch after pasting, drum-drying or extrusion cooking. J Cereal Sci 7:123–134. https://doi.org/10.1016/S0733-5210(88)80014-6

Mir SA, Bosco SJD, Bashir M, Shah MA, Mir MM (2016) Physicochemical and structural properties of starches isolated from corn cultivars grown in Indian temperate climate. Int J Food Prop 20:821–832. https://doi.org/10.1080/10942912.2016.1184274

Moaddabdoost Baboli Z, Safe Kordi AA (2010) Characteristics and composition of watermelon seed oil and solvent extraction parameters effects. J Am Oil Chem Soc 87:667–671. https://doi.org/10.1007/s11746-010-1546-5

Monnet AF, Laleg K, Michon C, Micard V (2019) Legume enriched cereal products: a generic approach derived from material science to predict their structuring by the process and their final properties. Trends Food Sci Technol 86:131–143. https://doi.org/10.1016/j.tifs.2019.02.027

Moore MM, Schober TJ, Dockery P, Arendt EK (2004) Textural comparisons of gluten-free and wheat-based doughs, batters, and breads. Cereal Chem 81:567–575. https://doi.org/10.1094/CCHEM.2004.81.5.567

Morales A, Kokini JL (1998) Phase transitions of soy globulins and the development of state diagrams. In: Tunick MH, Palumbo SA, Fratamico PM (eds) New techniques in the analysis of foods. Springer, Boston, pp 69–77. https://doi.org/10.1007/978-1-4757-5995-2_6

Morrison WR (1994) Wheat lipids: structure and functionality. In: Bushuk W, Rasper VF (eds) Wheat. Springer, Boston, pp 128–142. https://doi.org/10.1007/978-1-4615-2672-8_9

Mua JP, Jackson DS (1997) Relationships between functional attributes and molecular structure of amylose and amylopectin fractions from corn starch. J Agric Food Chem 45:3848–3854. https://doi.org/10.1021/jf9608783

Navruz-Varli S, Sanlier N (2016) Nutritional and health benefits of quinoa (*Chenopodium quinoa* Willd.). J Cereal Sci 69:371–376. https://doi.org/10.1016/j.jcs.2016.05.004

Nickel J, Spanier LP, Botelho FT, Gularte MA, Helbig E (2016) Effect of different types of processing on the total phenolic compound content, antioxidant capacity, and saponin content of *Chenopodium quinoa* Willd grains. Food Chem 209:139–143. https://doi.org/10.1016/j.foodchem.2016.04.031

Nomura K, Sakai M, Ohboshi H, Nakamura A (2021) Extraction of a water-soluble polysaccharide fraction from lentils and its potential application in acidified protein dispersions. Food Hydrocoll 117:106740. https://doi.org/10.1016/j.foodhyd.2021.106740

Nowak V, Du J, Charrondière UR (2016) Assessment of the nutritional composition of quinoa (*Chenopodium quinoa* Willd.). Food Chem 193:47–54. https://doi.org/10.1016/j.foodchem.2015.02.111

Nyström L, Lampi AM, Andersson AAM, Kamal-Eldin A, Gebruers K, Courtin CM, Delcour JA, Li L, Ward JL, Fraś A, Boros D, Rakszegi M, Bedo Z, Shewry PR, Piironen V (2008) Phytochemicals and dietary fiber components in rye varieties in the healthgrain diversity screen. J Agric Food Chem 56:9758–9766. https://doi.org/10.1021/jf801065r

Ortak M, Caltinoglu C, Sensoy I, Karakaya S, Mert B (2017) Changes in functional properties and *in vitro* bioaccessibilities of β-carotene and lutein after extrusion processing. J Food Sci Technol 54:3543–3551. https://doi.org/10.1007/s13197-017-2812-4

Patterson CA, Malcolmson L, Lukie C, Young G, Hucl P, Abdel-Aal ESM (2018) Glabrous canary seed: a novel food ingredient. Cereal Foods World 63:194–200. https://doi.org/10.1094/CFW-63-5-0194

Pavón YL, Lazzaroni SM, Sabbag NG, Rozycki SD (2014) Simultaneous effects of gelatin and espina corona gum on rheological, physical and sensory properties of cholesterol-reduced probiotic yoghurts. Int J Food Sci Technol 49:2245–2251. https://doi.org/10.1111/ijfs.12538

Pelgrom PJM, Schutyser MAI, Boom RM (2013) Thermomechanical morphology of peas and its relation to fracture behaviour. Food Bioprocess Technol 6:3317–3325. https://doi.org/10.1007/s11947-012-1031-2

Perumalla AVS, Hettiarachchy NS (2011) Green tea and grape seed extracts – potential applications in food safety and quality. Food Res Int 44:827–839. https://doi.org/10.1016/j.foodres.2011.01.022

Petrović M, Dajić-Stevanović Z, Sokolović D, Radović J, Milenković K, Marković J (2014) Study of red clover wild populations from the territory of Serbia for the purpose of pre-selection. Genetika 46:471–484. https://doi.org/10.2298/GENSR1402471P

Przbylski R, Lee YC, Eskin NAM (1998) Antioxidant and radical-scavenging activities of buckwheat seed components. J Am Oil Chem Soc 75:1595–1601. https://doi.org/10.1007/s11746-998-0099-3

Rahman M, de Jiménez MM (2016) Designer oil crops. In: Gupta SK (ed) Breeding oilseed crops for sustainable production. Academic, pp 361–376. https://doi.org/10.1016/B978-0-12-801309-0.00015-X

Raji AO, Ojediran JO (2011) Moisture sorption isotherms of two varieties of millet. Food Bioprod Process 89:178–184. https://doi.org/10.1016/j.fbp.2010.06.001

Rashwan AK, Yones HA, Karim N, Taha EM, Chen W (2021) Potential processing technologies for developing sorghum-based food products: un update and comprehensive review. Trends Food Sci Technol 110:168–182. https://doi.org/10.1016/j.tifs.2021.01.087

Repo-Carrasco-Valencia R, Hellström JK, Pihlava JM, Mattila PH (2010) Flavonoids and other phenolic compounds in Andean indigenous grains: quinoa (*Chenopodium quinoa*), kañiwa (*Chenopodium pallidicaule*) and kiwicha (*Amaranthus caudatus*). Food Chem 120:128–133. https://doi.org/10.1016/j.foodchem.2009.09.087

Ring SG, Colonna P, I'Anson KJ, Kalichevsky MT, Miles MJ, Morris VJ, Orford PD (1987) The gelation and crystallization of amylopectin. Carbohydr Res 162:277–293. https://doi.org/10.1016/0008-6215(87)80223-9

Roberts SE, Morrison-Rees S, Thapar N, Benninga MA, Borrelli O, Broekaert I, Dolinsek J, Martin-De-Carpi J, Mas E, Miele E, Pienar C, Ribes-Koninckx C, Thomassen RA, Thomson M, Tzivinikos C, Thorne K, John A, Williams JG (2021) Systematic review and meta-analysis: the incidence and prevalence of paediatric coeliac disease across Europe. Aliment Pharmacol Ther 54:109–128. https://doi.org/10.1111/apt.16337

Rolandelli G, Farroni AE, Buera MP (2022) Analysis of molecular mobility in corn and quinoa flours through ^{1}H-NMR and its relationships with water distribution, glass transition and enthalpy relaxation. Food Chem 373:131422. https://doi.org/10.1016/j.foodchem.2021.131422

Rombaut N, Savoire R, Thomasset B, Castello J, Van Hecke E, Lanoisellé JL (2015) Optimization of oil yield and oil total phenolic content during grape seed cold screw pressing. Ind Crop Prod 63:26–33. https://doi.org/10.1016/j.indcrop.2014.10.001

Roos YH (2010) Glass transition temperature and its relevance in food processing. Annu Rev Food Sci Technol 1:469–496. https://doi.org/10.1146/annurev.food.102308.124139

Roos YH (2020) State and supplemented phase diagrams for the characterization of food. In: Barbosa-Cánovas GV, Fontana AJ Jr, Schmidt SJ, Labuza TP (eds) Water activity in foods. Fundamentals and applications. Wiley, pp 45–60. https://doi.org/10.1002/9781118765982.ch4

Rosell CM, Barro F, Sousa C, Mena MC (2014) Cereals for developing gluten-free products and analytical tools for gluten detection. J Cereal Sci 59:354–364. https://doi.org/10.1016/j.jcs.2013.10.001

Rouf Shah T, Prasad K, Kumar P (2016) Maize – a potential source of human nutrition and health: a review. Cogent Food Agric 2:1166995. https://doi.org/10.1080/23311932.2016.1166995

Salarbashi D, Bazeli J, Fahmideh-Rad E (2019) Fenugreek seed gum: biological properties, chemical modifications, and structural analysis – a review. Int J Biol Macromol 138:386–393. https://doi.org/10.1016/j.ijbiomac.2019.07.006

Salinas F, Vardanega N, Espinosa-Álvarez C, Jimenéz D, Bugueño Muñoz W, Ruiz-Domínguez MC, Meireles MA, Cerezal-Mezquita P (2020) Supercritical fluid extraction of chañar (*Geoffroea decorticans*) almond oil: global yield, kinetics and oil characterization. J Supercrit Fluids 161:104824. https://doi.org/10.1016/j.supflu.2020.104824

Satheesh N, Fanta SW (2018) Review on structural, nutritional and anti-nutritional composition of teff (*Eragrostis tef*) in comparison with quinoa (*Chenopodium quinoa* Willd.). Cogent Food Agric 4:1546942. https://doi.org/10.1080/23311932.2018.1546942

Scanlin L, Lewis KA (2017) Quinoa as a sustainable protein source: production, nutrition, and processing. In: Nadathur SR, Scanlin L, Wanasundara JPD (eds) Sustainable protein sources. Academic, pp 223–238. https://doi.org/10.1016/B978-0-12-802778-3.00014-7

Schober TJ, Messerschmidt M, Bean SR, Park SH, Arendt EK (2005) Gluten-free bread from sorghum: quality differences among hybrids. Cereal Chem 82:394–404. https://doi.org/10.1094/CC-82-0394

Schoenlechner R, Siebenhandl S, Berghofer E (2008) Pseudocereals. In: Arendt EK, Dal Bello F (eds) Gluten-free cereal products and beverages. Academic, pp 149–190. https://doi.org/10.1016/B978-012373739-7.50009-5

Sciammaro L, Ferrero C, Puppo MC (2016) Chemical and nutritional properties of different fractions of *Prosopis alba* pods and seeds. J Food Meas Charact 10(1):103–112. https://doi.org/10.1007/s11694-015-9282-z

Sharma P, Kaur A, Aggarwal P (2016) Physicochemical, thermal, rheological, and morphological properties of flour from different guar seed (*Cyamopsis tetragonoloba*) cultivars. Int J Food Prop 20:1280–1289. https://doi.org/10.1080/10942912.2016.1207663

Sheng S, Li T, Liu R (2018) Corn phytochemicals and their health benefits. Food Sci Human Wellness 7:185–195. https://doi.org/10.1016/j.fshw.2018.09.003

Silva KS, Romero JT, Mauro MA (2015) Sorption isotherms and thermodynamic analysis ofseed fruits used to obtain vegetable oil. Lat Am Appl Res 45:21–26. https://doi.org/10.52292/j.laar.2015.361

Simopoulos AP (2001) n-3 faaty acids and human health: defining strategies for public policy. Lipids 36:S83–S89. https://doi.org/10.1007/s11745-001-0687-7

Singh N, Singh J, Kaur L, Sodhi NS, Gill BS (2003) Morphological, thermal and rheological properties of starches from different botanical sources. Food Chem 81:219–231. https://doi.org/10.1016/S0308-8146(02)00416-8

Singh N, Nakaura Y, Inouchi N, Nishinari K (2008) Structure and viscoelastic properties of starches separated from different legumes. Starch 60:349–357. https://doi.org/10.1002/star.200800689

Singh A, Raina SN, Sharma M, Chaudhary M, Sharma S, Rajpal VR (2021) Functional uses of peanut (*Arachis hypogaea* L.) seed storage proteins. In: Jimenez-Lopez JC (ed) Grain and seed proteins functionality. IntechOpen. https://doi.org/10.5772/intechopen.96871

Slade L, Levine H (1991) A food polymer science approach to structure-property relationships in aqueous food systems: non-equilibrium behavior of carbohydrate-water systems. In: Levine H, Slade L (eds) Water relationships in foods. Springer, New York, pp 29–101. https://doi.org/10.1007/978-1-4899-0664-9_3

Socorro A, Vega M, Calderón S (2010) Seed equilibrium moisture curves, water binding and its relationship with thermodynamic magnitudes. Int Agrophys 24:313–320

Song Y, He L, Wang XD, Smith N, Wheeler S, Garg ML, Rose RJ (2017) Regulation of carbon partitioning in the seed of the model legume *Medicago truncatula* and *Medicago orbicularis*: a comparative approach. Front Plant Sci. https://doi.org/10.3389/fpls.2017.02070

Sorkheh K, Kiani S, Sofo A (2016) Wild almond (*Prunus scoparia* L.) as potential oilseed resource for the future: studies on the variability of its oil content and composition. Food Chem 212:58–64. https://doi.org/10.1016/j.foodchem.2016.05.160

Srivastava M, Kapoor VP (2005) Seed galactomannans: an overview. Chem Biodivers 2:295–317. https://doi.org/10.1002/cbdv.200590013

Strocchi A (1982) Fatty acid composition and triglyceride structure of corn oil, hydrogenated corn oil, and corn oil margarine. J Food Sci 47:36–39. https://doi.org/10.1111/j.1365-2621.1982.tb11021.x

Sun WQ, Davidson P, Chan HSO (1998) Protein stability in the amorphous carbohydrate matrix: relevance to anhydrobiosis. Biochim Biophys Acta Gen Subj 1425:245–254. https://doi.org/10.1016/S0304-4165(98)00077-4

Suriano S, Balconi C, Valoti P, Redaelli R (2021) Comparison of total polyphenols, profile anthocyanins, color analysis, carotenoids and tocols in pigmented maize. LWT 144:111257. https://doi.org/10.1016/j.lwt.2021.111257

Tayade R, Kulkarni KP, Jo H, Song JT, Lee JD (2019) Insight into the prospects for the improvement of seed starch in legume – a review. Front Plant Sci 10:1213. https://doi.org/10.3389/fpls.2019.01213

Taylor JRN, Emmambux MN (2008) Products containing other speciality grains: sorghum, the millets and pseudocereals. In: Hamaker BR (ed) Technology of functional cereal products. CRC Press/Woodhead Publishing Limited, Cambridge, pp 281–335. https://doi.org/10.1533/9781845693886.2.281

Taylor JRN, Belton PS, Beta T, Duodu KG (2014) Increasing the utilization of sorghum, millets and pseudocereals: developments in the science of their phenolic phytochemicals, biofortification and protein functionality. J Cereal Sci 59:257–275. https://doi.org/10.1016/j.jcs.2013.10.009

Thakur P, Kumar K, Dhaliwal HS (2021) Nutritional facts, bio-active components and processing aspects of pseudocereals: a comprehensive review. Food Biosci 42:101170. https://doi.org/10.1016/j.fbio.2021.101170

Thompson T, Dennis M, Higgins LA, Lee AR, Sharrett MK (2005) Gluten-free diet survey: are Americans with coeliac disease consuming recommended amounts of fibre, iron, calcium and grain foods? J Hum Nutr Diet 18:163–169. https://doi.org/10.1111/j.1365-277X.2005.00607.x

Toğrul H, Arslan N (2006) Moisture sorption behaviour and thermodynamic characteristics of rice stored in a chamber under controlled humidity. Biosyst Eng 95:181–195. https://doi.org/10.1016/j.biosystemseng.2006.06.011

Torbica A, Belović M, Popović L, Čakarević J, Jovičić M, Pavličević J (2021) Comparative study of nutritional and technological quality aspects of minor cereals. J Food Sci Technol 58:311–322. https://doi.org/10.1007/s13197-020-04544-w

Ubwa ST, Abah J, Asemave K, Shambe T (2012) Studies on the gelatinization temperature of some cereal starches. Int J Chem 4:22–28. https://doi.org/10.5539/ijc.v4n6p22

Ullah F, Ahmad S, Wahab S, Zeb A, Khan Khattak M, Khan S, Kang M (2016) Quality evaluation of biscuits supplemented with alfalfa seed flour. Foods 5:68. https://doi.org/10.3390/foods5040068

United States Department of Agriculture – Natural Resources Conservation Service (USDA-NRCS) (2022) Plants database. https://plants.sc.egov.usda.gov/. Accessed 8 June 2022

Urbizo-Reyes UC, Aguilar-Toalá JE, Liceaga AM (2021) Hairless canary seeds (*Phalaris canariensis* L.) as a potential source of antioxidant, antihypertensive, antidiabetic, and antiobesity biopeptides. Food Prod Process Nutr 3:6. https://doi.org/10.1186/s43014-020-00050-w

Van Den Berg C, Bruin S (1981) Water activity and its estimation in food systems: theoretical aspects. In: Rockland L, Stewart G (eds) Water activity: influence on food quality. Academic, New York, pp 1–61

Vázquez G, Chenlo F, Moreira R (2003) Sorption isotherms of lupine at different temperatures. J Food Eng 60:449–452. https://doi.org/10.1016/S0260-8774(03)00068-2

Vertucci CW, Leopold AC (1986) Physiological activities associated with hydration level in seeds. In: Leopold AC (ed) Membranes, metabolism and dry organisms. Cornell University Press, Ithaca, pp 35–49

Vilcacundo R, Hernández-Ledesma B (2017) Nutritional and biological value of quinoa (*Chenopodium quinoa* Willd.). Curr Opin Food Sci 14:1–6. https://doi.org/10.1016/j.cofs.2016.11.007

Wang Y, Chen L, Yang T, Ma Y, McClements DJ, Ren F, Tian Y, Jin Z (2021) A review of structural transformations and properties changes in starch during thermal processing of foods. Food Hydrocoll 113:106543. https://doi.org/10.1016/j.foodhyd.2020.106543

Wijngaard HH, Arendt EK (2006) Buckwheat. Cereal Chem 83:231–401. https://doi.org/10.1094/CC-83-0391

Wilson LA, Birmingham VA, Moon DP, Snyder HE (1978) Isolation and characterization of starch from mature soybeans. Cerel Chem 55:661–670

Yang C, Shang K, Lin C, Wang C, Shi X, Wang H, Li H (2021) Processing technologies, phytochemical constituents, and biological activities of grape seed oil (GSO): a review. Trends Food Sci Technol 116:1074–1083. https://doi.org/10.1016/j.tifs.2021.09.011

Yousaf L, Hou D, Liaqat H, Shen Q (2021) Millet: a review of its nutritional and functional changes during processing. Food Res Int 142:110197. https://doi.org/10.1016/j.foodres.2021.110197

Zampronio Zorzi C, Garske RP, Flôres SH, Silveira Thys RC (2020) Sunflower protein concentrate: a possible and beneficial ingredient for gluten-free bread. Innov Food Sci Emerg Technol 66:102539. https://doi.org/10.1016/j.ifset.2020.102539

Zanetti F, Alberghini B, Marjanović Jeromela A, Grahovac N, Rajković D, Kiprovski B, Monti A (2021) Camelina, an ancient oilseed crop actively contributing to the rural renaissance in Europe. A review. Agron Sustain Dev 41:2. https://doi.org/10.1007/s13593-020-00663-y

Zhang W, Li S, Zhang B, Drago SR, Zhang J (2015) Relationships between the gelatinization of starches and the textural properties of extruded texturized soybean protein-starch systems. J Food Eng 174:29–36. https://doi.org/10.1016/j.jfoodeng.2015.11.011

Zhang H, Bai Y, Zhao X, Duan R (2016) Probing water desorption mechanism of glutinous rice flour with four theoretical isotherm models: a comparative study. Am J Food Technol 11:264–272. https://doi.org/10.3923/ajft.2016.264.272

Zhu F (2018) Chemical composition and food uses of teff (*Eragrostis tef*). Food Chem 239:402–415. https://doi.org/10.1016/j.foodchem.2017.06.101

Zobel HF (1988) Starch crystal transformations and their industrial importance. Starch 40:1–7. https://doi.org/10.1002/star.19880400102

Chapter 3
Non-cereals Starch Resources

Cecilia Dini, Silvia Flores, María Gabriela Kupervaser, Carola Sosa, Maria Victoria Traffano-Schiffo, and Sonia Zulma Viña

Abbreviations

CS	cassava starch
DHT	dry heat treatment
DSC	scanning differential calorimetry
FTIR	fourier transform infrared
GF	gluten-free
GI	glycaemic index
HMT	heat-moisture treated
HPMC	hydroxypropyl methylcellulose
PS	potato starch

C. Dini · S. Z. Viña
Centro de Investigación y Desarrollo en Criotecnología de Alimentos (CIDCA), UNLP-CONICET-CICPBA, La Plata, Argentina
e-mail: cdini@biol.unlp.edu.ar; soniavia@quimica.unlp.edu.ar

S. Flores (✉)
Universidad de Buenos Aires (UBA), Facultad de Ciencias Exactas y Naturales (FCEN), Departamento de Industrias, Intendente Güiraldes 2160 (1428), Ciudad Autónoma de Buenos Aires, Argentina

CONICET – Universidad de Buenos Aires, Instituto de Tecnología de Alimentos y Procesos Químicos (ITAPROQ), Buenos Aires, Argentina
e-mail: sflores@di.fcen.uba.ar

M. G. Kupervaser · C. Sosa
Grupo de Investigación en Biotecnología y Alimentos (BIOTEC), Universidad Tecnológica Nacional. Facultad Regional Resistencia, Resistencia, Chaco, Argentina
e-mail: g_kupervaser@ca.frre.utn.edu.ar; departamentoiq@frre.utn.edu.ar

M. V. Traffano-Schiffo
Instituto de Química Básica y Aplicada del Nordeste Argentino, IQUIBA-NEA, UNNE-CONICET, Corrientes, Argentina
e-mail: m.traffanoschiffo@conicet.gov.ar

M. F. de Escalada Pla, C. E. Genevois (eds.), *Designing Gluten Free Bakery and Pasta Products*, https://doi.org/10.1007/978-3-031-28344-4_3

R&T	roots and tubers
RS	resistant starch
RVA	rapid visco analyser
RVU	rapid visco units
SEF	soybean extruded–expelled meal
SEM	scanning electron microscopy
WS	waxy starches
XG	xanthan gum

3.1 Introduction

To produce bakery goods, the gluten protein is the key factor due to its contribution to water absorption capacity and because it provides extensibility, elasticity and cohesiveness to bread dough. This allows the fermentation gas remains occluded and maintained in the liquid phase during dough development, leading to obtain high-grade breads (Wieser 2007). However, gluten has been identified as the responsible of celiac disease (Ronda et al. 2009), and the only effective treatment for patients is to follow strictly a gluten-free (GF) diet (Witczak et al. 2016). It has been observed that, if formulation is not properly adjusted, baked products without gluten could result in lower quality attributes, reduced nutritional characteristics and consumer acceptance (Naqash et al. 2017). Therefore, the development of GF products appropriate for consumers with disorders related to gluten intake was growing in importance (Zhang et al. 2017).

Formerly, hydrocolloids and starch were the major ingredients in GF diets (Shi and Bemiller 2002). From last decades, the demand of new food ingredients suitable for GF products is expanding in order to obtain more foods for a wider diet without potentially allergenic proteins. Among those ingredients, alternative starches resources are intensely searching. Starch is one of the most abundant and consumed natural polysaccharide in human diet. It is a biopolymer composed of glucose and it is obtained from plants such as grains, legumes, and tubers (Karmakar et al. 2014). Despite its high abundance, commercially sustainable sources of starch are limited to corn, wheat, cassava, potato and rice. With respect to corn, the global market reached 78 million tons (Mt) in 2020, being mainly produced in the United States, Europe and China (70–80%), whereas wheat is produced (6.3 Mt) mostly in Europe China and India (98%). The cassava starch (CS) production (6.9 Mt) comes from Asian Pacific region (Thailand, China and Indonesia) and Brazil (75%). Finally, potato starch (PS) which global market attained 3.4 Mt, accounting the highest productions from China, India, United States and Europe (80%); while rice is produced particularly in Asia (Expert Market Research 2020; Murphy 2000). Each region has a more convenient source of starch production mostly determined by climatic and logistic requirements (Semeijn and Buwalda 2018).

For food production (noodles, baked goods, etc.), starch is widely used as a gelling, thickening, and/or stabilizing agent (Fonseca et al. 2021; Rożnowski et al. 2014), besides being processed and used as binder, sweetener and as emulsifier (Mahmood et al. 2017; Bello-Pérez et al. 2006).

In particular, natural starches with low or without gluten are intensely requested because of their possibility to be used in the formulation of GF bakery products. In this context, corn and potato are the most commonly used starches, together with cassava and rice (Masure et al. 2016), due to their beneficial characteristics, such as neutral taste, soft texture, and high digestibility. They are frequently used in combination with proteins and hydrocolloids to counter their minimal structure-building potential, contributing to the structure, texture and stability of food through their thickening or gelling behaviour and surface properties (Capriles and Arêas 2014; Doublier et al. 2000). Other cereals, like minor or pseudo-cereals, like sorghum, millet, quinoa, amaranths and buckwheat, are being tested as alternative ingredientes tolerated by celiac patients (Comino et al. 2013). In addition, new sources of non-cereal starch are being explored including beans (pea, chickpea), sweet potato and other ethnical tubers, carrots, nuts and some fruits as banana or mango (unripe pulp and kernel) (Witczak et al. 2016; Punia Bangar et al. 2021; Lagunes-Delgado et al. 2022). Till the moment, many reports are found describing general properties of such novel starches but there are not clear applications yet.

To better understanding the functionality of starch in food production, some general aspects about structure, functional, nutritional properties and a brief mention to available techniques to modify starches is described in the following sections. A special description and some applications of potato, cassava and others non-conventional resources starches is also exposed.

3.2 Native Starch

3.2.1 Morphology and Chemical Structure

Starch is usually stored during photosynthesis in the amyloplasts of tubers, seeds of cereals and legume crops, rhizomes and other reserve organs of some plants (Emmambux and Taylor 2013).

Regarding to the morphology and surface properties (smooth or dented) of starch granules (different shapes such as spherical, polygonal to splits or lenticular), depends on the starch source and the lipid, protein and phosphorus contents, which influence the behaviour in terms of functional characteristics such as pasting properties and water binding capacity. For example, smaller and angular starch granules, show higher resistance to amylolysis and to gelatinization than large and spherical granules (Przetaczek-Rożnowska et al. 2018; Malumba et al. 2017). Additionally, starch granules can present different types of size distribution (unimodal, bimodal, or trimodal) (Schmiele and Sampaio 2019). As it can be observed in Fig. 3.1, rice

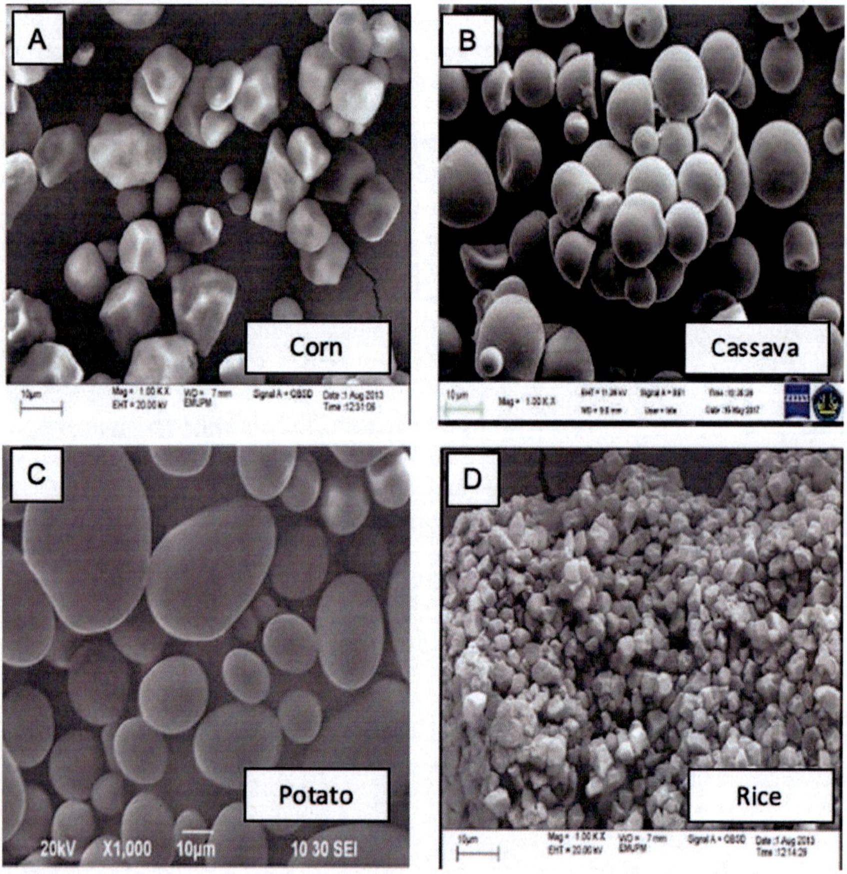

Fig. 3.1 Scanning electron microscopy (SEM) of starch granules (**a**) corn, (**b**) cassava, (**c**) potato and (**d**) rice with × 1000 magnification at 20 kV. (Reprinted with permission from: (**a**) and (**d**) Aghazadeh et al. 2017; (**b**) Yulianto et al. 2020, Copyright © 2020 by the authors. This is an open access article distributed under the Creative Commons Attribution License which permits unrestricted use, distribution, and reproduction in any medium, provided the original work is properly cited; (**c**) Liu et al. 2016)

starch granules (3–8 μm, are very small polygonal) are considerably smaller than those of potato (20–50 μm large, are round or oval), cassava (8–20 μm, are round or truncated) and corn (10–15 μm, are polygonal) (Semeijn and Buwalda 2018; Waterschoot et al. 2014).

There is a consensus regarding starch granule structure, however researchers are continuously proposing more suitable models. The most consolidated structure suggests a multiscale granule organization (Fig. 3.2).

From the highest to lowest scale, the whole granule (2–100 μm) is composed by amorphous and semi-crystalline growth rings (120–500 nm thick) which are built for ovoid blocklets (20–50 nm). They support nanometric crystalline regions

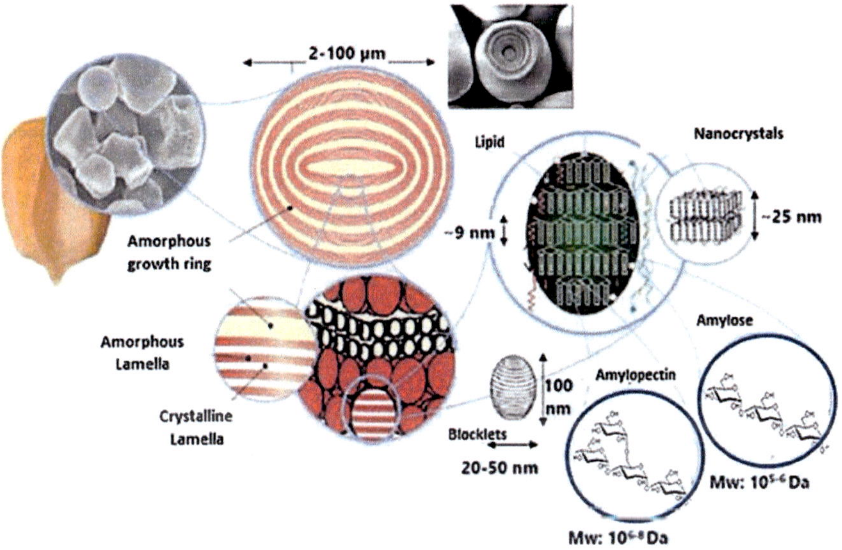

Fig. 3.2 Starch granule and its hierarchical structure. (Adapted with permission from Le Corre et al. 2010; Copyright 2010. American Chemical Society)

disposed as lamella, called starch nanocrystals. Both amorphous and ordered zones are conforming by two main biopolymers, amylopectin and amylose in different arranges (Lu and Tian 2021; Yu et al. 2021a; Goren et al. 2018). Amylose and amylopectin chains occupy approximately 98% granule dry matter and the content of each one depends on the botanical source of starch (Tester et al. 2004). The ratio of amylose and amylopectin can vary between 20–30% and 70–80%, respectively (Jane 2009). Moreover, although they are composed of the same glycosidic monomer (glucose), linked by hydrogen bonding which maintains the integrity of the granule, they exhibit totally different characteristics (solubility and paste formation-gel) and are radially arranged with their terminal reducing groups oriented toward the centre or hilum, point of origin of the ring structure (Swinkels 1985; Pérez and Bertoft 2010). Amylose is conformed by D-glucose units linked by α-(1→4) glycosidic linkage, resulting in a long chain linear polymer, whereas amylopectin also present α-(1→4) D-glucose linked units but branched with numerous short chains which are linked through α-(1→6) glycosidic linkage to the linear parts of the macromolecule (Fan and Picchioni 2020). Both are deposited to form the starch granule, defining a semi-crystalline structure made up of alternating amorphous (amylose) and crystalline (amylopectin) shells, which are called "growth rings" as was previously described (Fig. 3.1) (Jane 2009; Donald et al. 2001).

The genetic modification into the plant can generate starches with high amount of amylopectin, called starches (WS) (brittle, above 85% amylopectin) and also starches with high amylose content (resistant to amylases activity, difficult to gelatinize- above 40% amylose) (Jane 2009; Tester et al. 2004). Physical and chemical characteristics of both structures vary considerably due to their conformational space, while the functionality is significantly dependent on its fraction. Pure amylose is insoluble in cold water and contributes to increase the gelatinisation capacity of starch, while not degraded amylopectin is water soluble; and contributes to increase the adhesion characteristics of starch (Hernández-Carmona et al. 2017).

3.2.2 *Extraction, Functional Properties and General Characterisation*

Starch can be extracted from various parts of plants such as fruits, leaves, seeds, and roots (Makroo et al. 2021). Conventionally, extraction methods can be classified as wet and dry milling, being the last one the most appropriate technically, but the extract obtained showed weaker functional properties compared to the first one (Lee et al. 2007). Once vegetable raw material was milled, starch extraction usually consists of four main steps: washing, cleaning from fat and protein, centrifugation and drying, producing a large amount of waste, which could contain high quality compounds (Moorthy 2002; Bernardo et al. 2018). In order to overcome the shortcomings of traditional methods, novel technologies have been employed such as enzyme and carbon dioxide assisted extraction (Buksa 2018), high hydrostatic pressure, ultrasound, and moderate electric field for the extraction (Makroo et al. 2021).

The extracted and dried starch granules are highly robust and impermeable to water at ambient temperature, preventing the interaction between starch and water molecules and, therefore, avoiding swelling and caking. When aqueous suspension of granules is heated, at above the melting point of starch crystalline structure (≥60 °C), granules can absorb water and gelatinise through an endothermic and irreversible process (Tester et al. 2004). Gelatinisation generates the swelling of particles, water absorption, loss of crystallinity, leaching of amylose and solubilisation of granular content resulting in viscosity development (Sciarini et al. 2015; Silva Nykänen et al. 2014). Furthermore, the gelatinisation process is not only influenced by starch source characteristics, such as the growing conditions, cultivar, maturity and amylose-amylopectin ratio, but also, processing conditions and the amount of water used (Brunt et al. 2002). For instance, when starch is cooked in a given process and leaves behind remnants of the parent starch granules it is defined as ¨ghosts¨, leading to a product with less surface shine, affecting the final starch-based products characteristics (Li and Wei 2020; Debet and Gidley 2007). After cooling and storage, the viscosity increases dramatically as starch undergoes gelation and molecular re-crystallisation being undesirable in some gels and bakery products as it causes texture hardness and moisture loss, known as staling. In bakery products, it is defined as "retrogradation process" (Šmídová and Rysová 2022). Pasting characteristics are important quality parameters (texture, hardness and taste) in starch further processing.

On the other hand, besides food formulation, starch is being profusely studied as one of the most convenient biopolymer matrix to constitute edible coatings to be applied on food surface and also to generate self-supporting biodegradable packaging materials. The starch matrix can provide an effective barrier against hazards by reducing moisture migration, gas exchange (mainly O_2 and CO_2), respiration and oxidative reaction rates; suppressing physiological disorders; delaying changes in textural properties; and improving mechanical integrity or food handling characteristics (Versino et al. 2016). The edible matrix can be added with other compounds such as plasticizers (glycerol, propylene glycol, etc.) to obtain a flexible film, or active agents (antimicrobial, antioxidants, colourants, etc.) to become the film or coating in functional, with the aim to extend food shelf-life (Díaz-Montes and Castro-Muñoz 2021; Campos et al. 2011). Chapter 7 gives a deeper insight about this important filmogenic property of the starch.

Regarding to the methodology to characterize starch morphology, structure, physical, chemical, or functional properties, there is a wide range of methods that have been used. Once starch granules were separated and purified, their size distribution can be determined using sieving, light or SEM, laser light scattering, among other techniques (Lindeboom et al. 2004). Colour is usually determined by reflectance spectrophotometers (Soison et al. 2015), while shape and surface morphology can be analysed by SEM or atomic force microscopies, with the properly sample preparation (Chakraborty et al. 2020). Information about strength of granules can be obtained through a compression test (Molenda et al. 2006). Since granules present an anisotropic character, it can be observed the birefringence phenomenon using a polarization microscope showing the characteristic Maltese cross and the hilum position (Chakraborty et al. 2020). More information about long-range ordered structure or repetitive crystalline and amorphous lamellae fraction are obtained by wide angle X-ray diffraction or small angle X-ray scattering respectively (Wang et al. 2015). Other basic assays used to describe starch functionality are swelling, solubility, water retention or holding capacity tests (Ačkar et al. 2010). The molecular weight of amylose and amylopectin can be determined by high-performance size-exclusion chromatography (Kobayashi et al. 1985) and by field-flow fractionation coupled to multi-angle light scattering (Rübsam et al. 2012). Amylose content is determined by a colorimetric method using standards of amylose and amylopectin after association with I_3^- to form the known amylose/iodine recognized for the typical blue colour of the solution (Alzate et al. 2020). The presence of chemical groups, their connectivity and spin–spin relaxation time has been studied with spectroscopic techniques such as Fourier transformed infra-red, near-infrared reflectance, Raman and H^1 and C^{13} nuclear magnetic resonance spectroscopies (Wang et al. 2015). The thermal characterisation involves the determination of the gelatinisation temperature in presence of water, loss mass during heating and decomposition temperature, are commonly performing by scanning differential calorimetry (DSC) and thermogravimetric analysis (Wu et al. 2019). The viscous capacity of starch is one of the most important properties that must be exploited. The pasting viscosity profiles of starch solutions when are submitted to a standardised heating and cooling cycles under stirring can be performed in Rapid Visco Analyser (RVA) instrument (pasting test) (Gupta et al. 2009). Once gelatinised, the rheological characteristics of the starch slurries, which are strongly dependent on concentration and storage time, can be performed under large deformations applying tangential forces (flow behaviour) in a viscometer or uniaxial compression in a texture-meter or press device. On the contrary, assays using small perturbations have been developed to determine the viscoelastic properties of starchy systems using a dynamic rheometer. In general, oscillatory test are carried out to describe gelation mechanisms, molecular interactions, and starch retrogradation (González et al. 2021; Li et al. 2020; Gupta et al. 2009). Moreover, when starch is used to prepare dough, the properties such as resistance, extensibility, consistency, viscosity, mixing time and tolerance are usually studied by extensigraph, farinograph, alveograph and development time tests (Rasper 1993), in addition to DSC and dynamic rheology studies (Witczak et al. 2012). Several freezing-thermal cycles to observe the water presence (syneresis) and compression of the gelling system are used to test retrogradation level (Karim 2000). It is important to remark that no single method can provide a complete information about starch structure and the changes during gelatinisation or retrogradation at both macroscopic and molecular level, being necessary to perform parallel some of the mentioned tests (Wang et al. 2015).

Other important aspect of starch that must be analysed is the amount of resistant starch (RS) because of the nutritional implications (Bojarczuk et al. 2022). The RS is defined as a portion of starch that cannot be digested by human amylases in the small intestine and passes to the colon to be fermented by the microbiota (Nugent 2005). Although the cooked raw material is highly digestible by healthy humans, after cooking and under certain conditions, part of the starch may not be digested. Some possible causes be the retrogradation due to re-association of amylose chains in double helices, the lipid-amylose interaction forming inclusion complexes and the chemical modification of starches (Birt et al. 2013). Due to the recent recognition of incomplete digestion and absorption of starch in the small intestine as a normal phenomenon, interest in RS has increased. Several studies have shown that RS has physiological functions similar to those of dietary fibre (Sajilata et al. 2006). Regarding methodology to determine RS, it can be classified as *in vivo* and *in vitro* methods. The most used *in vivo* methodology consists of evaluating undigested starch at the end of the ileum in healthy human models with ileostomy (McCleary 2013). However, this method is difficult, laborious, expensive and ethically controversial (Iacovou et al. 2017). More practical are the *in vitro* tests that attempt to simulate gastrointestinal digestion, but results depend on the types of enzymes and the experimental conditions used (Li and Hu 2022; Maningat and Seib 2013; Perera et al. 2010).

3.3 Methods for Modifying Starch Structure

It was observed that performance of native starch in food-industry processing is often limited by some of its physical and chemical properties. Viscosity of cooked native starch is often relatively high or unstable to be used in certain products. In addition, low mechanical, acid, and thermal resistance, as well as high tendency toward retrogradation are the main limitations of native starches. In such sense, rheological properties of some starch dispersions such as potato, tapioca, and maize WS affect the final product characteristics, providing a gummy, stiff structure thus deteriorating their sensory properties. Therefore, starches need to be modified to enhance their properties and make them more functional in wider applications (Punia Bangar et al. 2022a). Aforementioned drawbacks can be overcome by starch modification through different methods as chemical, enzymatic, physical, and a combination of them, in order to improve its functional characteristics. According to the changes introduced in starch structure, it is possible to decrease the viscosity, increase the stability in dispersions and hot paste stability, decrease gelatinisation temperature and breakdown viscosity, improve cold-water dispersibility and contribute to new starch characteristics by substituting the molecule with different functional groups (Gilet et al. 2018; Hadnađev et al. 2018; Molavi et al. 2018; Lacerda et al. 2019).

Chemical methods are the most used for starch modification and can be grouped as: conversion, cross-linking, and substitution (including esterification and etherification) (Cui 2005). Starch conversion treatment and final properties can be described as: (a) acid converted (thin-boiling starches), the granular starches that are partially acid hydrolysed, reduce hot-paste viscosity forming strong gels upon cooling due to shortening of starch macromolecules; (b) oxidised (bleached starches) treated with sodium hypochlorite and yielding high paste clarity, low paste viscosity, short and good paste stability; and (c) pyroconverted (dry heating treatment, 140–200 °C, with or without acid), as pyrodextrins (white and yellow dextrins, British gums), giving low viscosity, good film-forming ability, high solubility, good hot-paste stability.

In the other group are cross-linked starches: (a) di-starch phosphates by sodium trimetaphosphate or phosphorus oxychloride treatment; (b) di-starch adipate using adipic anhydride; both with the same final desirable properties, high stability, and resistance to processing conditions (increased temperature, shear, low pH stability).

Finally, stabilised starches obtained by esterification or etherification. These can be: (a) acetylated starch (esterified with acetic anhydride) resulting in increased paste clarity and stability, reduced starch retrogradation, lower gelatinization temperature; (b) monostarch phosphated starch (esterified with *ortho*-phosphoric acid, sodium/potassium *ortho*-phosphate, or sodium tripolyphosphate) obtaining higher paste viscosity and stability, improved clarity, cohesive texture, high resistance to retrogradation, lower gelatinization temperature, high freeze–thaw stability; (c) sodium octenyl succinate starch (esterified with octenylsuccinic anhydride and octenylsuccinate) and (d) hydroxypropylated starch (etherified with propylene oxide) causing in both cases, increased peak viscosity, lower gelatinisation temperature, good freeze–thaw stability, film-forming ability and emulsifying properties (Semeijn and Buwalda 2018; Hadnađev et al. 2018).

On the other hand, physical modification consists of the application of mechanical friction to change starch granules size or temperature/moisture, pressure, shearing, milling, UV-radiation, and some novel techniques, such as ultrasound (Alzate et al. 2020), pulsed electric fields, superheating, iterated syneresis and instantaneous controlled pressure drop process (Kaur et al. 2012). To obtain pre-gelatinised (instant cold-water swelling) starches, suspension is treated by drum drying, spray cooking, or extrusion. Heat/moisture treatment consists of applying heat to starch at a temperature above their gelatinisation point with insufficient moisture to cause gelatinisation, in contrast annealed starches heat at a temperature below from gelatinisation point for prolonged periods of time (Singh et al. 2007). Continuously, alternative, sustainable and eco-friendly techniques are investigated to replace traditional and polluting methodology to obtain modified starches. In this sense, the use of microwave radiation, cold plasma, ultrasonication, supercritical CO_2, ionic liquids, mechano-chemistry, etc., were reported as unconventional and green technologies (Otálora González et al. 2020; Gilet et al. 2018).

Another green approach to produce starch with altered molecular mass, branch chain-length distribution and amylose/amylopectin ratio is the employment of hydrolytic enzymes (α-amylase, pullulanase, glucoamylase and, less frequently, transferases). The modification can be performed in a single, dual, triple, and quadruple enzymatic reaction using combinations of several enzymes. As a result of the enzymatic modification, freeze-thaw stability and retrogradation effects on gels were improved during storage. In addition, cyclodextrin glycosyltransferases have been used to obtain cyclodextrins. Despite the benefits obtained by enzymatic modification, the technology is quite expensive and new sources of safe enzyme should be provided (Punia Bangar et al. 2022b).

Chemical modified starch production is regulated by the American Food and Drug Administration. Backwards, physically modified starches are not considered food additives and therefore, they could be used to develop "clean label" products, which are highly demanded by the consumers nowadays. Locally, the Argentine Food Code rules in relation to levels and labelling of native and modified starches (Argentine Food Code 2021). In Table 3.1. it is described recent developments of modified starches for food application.

3.4 Native and Modified Potato Starch – Different Alternatives and Applications

Potato (*Solanum tuberosum*) is a rich source of starch (79 % dry base) among other nutritional components such as protein, dietary fibre, vitamins and minerals, being the fourth most well-known food crop after rice, wheat and corn worldwide (Gui et al. 2022). There are thousands of potato varieties that grow in temperate, tropical, and sub-tropical regions. The world production (359 Mt, 2020 data) is shared among Asia (48%), Europe (32%), Americas (17%) and Africa (7%) (FAOSTAT 2021). The potatoes are milled to extract the starch granules from the cellulose cell wall compartments (amyloplasts) (Fig. 3.3, panel a). After removing the protein and the fibre subsequent washing and drying steps yields to the starch as final product (Semeijn and Buwalda 2018). Starch from potatoes is a very significant commodity that has a wide inclusion in food and non-food industry and a high economical

Table 3.1 Recent developments of modified starches for food application

Starch modification method	Food application	Benefit in functionality/ physicochemical characteristic	Reference
Sour/fermented starches physical modification	Bread, noodles.	Improve swelling and solubility. Less susceptible to hydrolysis and thermally stable. Increase gelling potential. Decrease aging ability. Adjuvant or as a main ingredient in GF foods	Punia Bangar et al. (2022a)
Instant starches/ cold-water swelling starch	Desserts, cake or muffin batters with particles, puddings, sauces, salad dressings, dry soups, baby foods, pie fillings, jellies. Foods with bioactive materials, heat-sensitive colourants, cold desserts and microwavable.	Increase viscosity and produce a soft paste without heating. Prevent sinking to the bottom during baking of particles (chocolate chips or fruit pieces). Reduce or eliminate cooking time and act as thickening agent, stabiliser and emulsifier in instant foods and non-thermal processing. Used as encapsulating material for the encapsulation of bioactive materials and nutrients. Improved freeze-thaw stability.	Majzoobi and Farahnaky (2020)
Degraded starches	Confections, cheese analogues, surimi, glazing, toppings, drinks, soups.	Gelling agents.	Semeijn and Buwalda (2018)
Enzyme-treated starches	Bread, low fat yogurt.	Fat replacer, mouthfeel enhancer, fillers, and in co-spray drying of flavours. Emulsifier. Gelling agent.	Punia Bangar et al. (2022b)
Acid-degraded	Gum candies, jellies, pastilles baked goods. Confections, Cheese analogues.	Reduce gelatinisation temperature and increase the solubility. Loss of swelling capacity and viscosity. Improve gelling or gel strength. Favour the retrogradation that leads to slowly digestible and RS formation. Reduces the tolerance to refrigeration, storage and freeze-thaw cycles.	Semeijn and Buwalda (2018) and Wang et al. (2022)

(continued)

Table 3.1 (continued)

Starch modification method	Food application	Benefit in functionality/ physicochemical characteristic	Reference
Oxidised starches	Coating, sealing, batter binding, emulsification, and dough conditioning in baking. Clear drinks, soups. Battered meat and breading, film former. Crispy coating in fried foods and texturizer in dairy products.	Low viscosity, high stability, clarity, film-forming, and binding properties. Reduce retrogradation of the cooked paste, enhanced stability at low temperature. Higher adhesion and improved film-forming properties	Chakraborty et al. (2022)
Cross-linked starches/ inhibited starches.	Snacks, sauces, food coatings, mashed potatoes, GF breads.	Prevention of full disintegration of the starch during gelatinisation. Form strong and stable gels with limited susceptibility to staling and retrogradation	Roman et al. (2020) and Witczak et al. (2012)
Acetate starches	Meat, oriental noodles, ready meals Pulping pies, gravy, salad dressing and pies.	For extended shelf-life and refrigeration are required. Better freeze-thaw stability, expansion, and dissolution characteristics. Have no heat and shear stability.	Lin et al. (2019)
Octenylsuccinate starches	Drinks (clouding agent), salad dressing, creams, mayonnaise style products, butter, margarine.	Emulsifier: adjust viscosity levels for products and processes. Encapsulating agent for enzymes, fatty acids, salt, fragrances, and flavours. Biodegradable edible packaging. Fat replacer or flour substitute for bread dough formulation.	Altuna et al. (2018)
High Hydrostatic Pressure (HHP) treated sweet potato starch	Doughs	Higher water absorption, dough development time, and stability with the increase of HHP The dough height, maximum gaseous height, total gas production, and retention capacity were significantly increased for at 500 MPa. More consistent and uniformed network structure.	Rahman et al. (2022)
Heat-Moisture-treated sweet potato starch	Noodles	Similar acceptability scores for raw starch noodles, plain boiled, comparing to the commercials.	Collado et al. (2001)

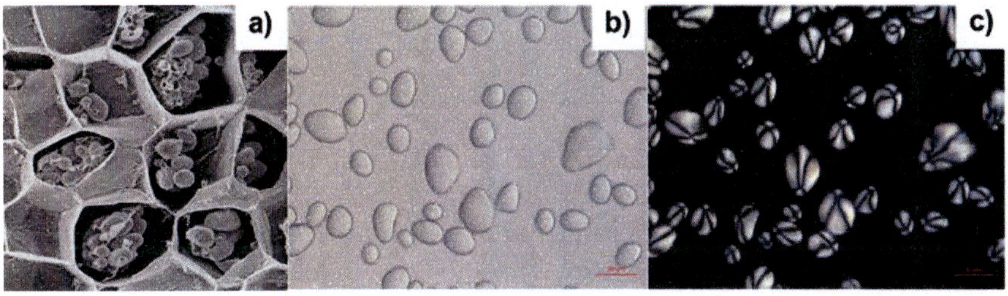

Fig. 3.3 PS granules: (**a**) SEM of potato cells (magnification: 50x), (**b**) bright field microscopy (scale bar: 50 μm) and (**c**) polarized light microscopy (scale bar: 50 μm). (Image (**a**) is from https://render.fineartamerica.com/images/rendered/share/24341696&domainId=1 which property release is not required. Images (**b**) and (**c**) are reprinted with permission from Dupuis and Liu 2019; Springer Nature)

Table 3.2 Characteristics, composition and pasting properties of starch granules

Starch source	Shape	Diameter (mm)	Amylose (%)	Lipids (%)	Proteins (%)	Phosphate (nmol/mg)	T_m[a] (°C)	Peak Viscosity (RVU)[b]
Potato	Round, oval	5–100	18–29	0.02–0.2	0.1–0.4	23.2	62.6	510
Maize	Round, polygonal	2–30	23–32	0.6–0.8	0.3–0.4	0.11	68.9	250
Wheat	Round, lenticular	1–40	23–29	0.3–0.8	0.3	0.20	61.6	230
Barley	Round, lenticular	2–40	22–27	0.6–0.9	0.1	0.12	58.0	100
Tapioca	Oval, truncated	4–45	17–33	0.03–0.1	0.2	1.11	67.5	220
Rice	Polygonal	3–8	14–29	0.6–1.4	0.1–0.5	~1[c]	70.1	239[d]

[a]T_m is the mid-point temperatures measured by DSC, [b]RVU are Rapid Visco Units measured in a Rapid Visco Analyser (RVA) instrument. Reprinted with permission from Vamadevan and Bertoft (2015) (John Wiley and Sons), [c]Chen et al. (2017b); [d]Baxter et al. (2004)

relevance. From human nutrition point of view, its main role is to provide the metabolic energy for a large portion of the world's population. Native potato starch is quite resistant to digestion, but it becomes digestible after cooking, resulting food products with a high glycaemic index (GI). There is an interest in elucidating how nutritional properties of starch could be modified under specific conditions of composition, structure, or processing of food stuff (Dupuis and Liu 2019). Table 3.2. summarises some properties and components of several starch granules sources for comparison reasons. Potato starch (PS) is one of the biggest in size (Fig. 3.3, panels b and c). Regarding PS composition, it has a very low amount of lipids and proteins as many others starch sources. However, the high number endogenous phosphate in PS is another distinctive characteristic. The principal constituents of PS are amylose (18–29%) and amylopectin (Vamadevan and Bertoft 2015). In addition, PS pastes show low temperature of gelatinisation, better transparency and very high viscosity compared to other sources. Such properties have been related to the phosphate groups esterified to the amylopectin fraction and the superior granule integrity (Xu et al. 2017).

PS is commonly used as a thickener, colloidal stabilizer, gelling, bulking and water-retention agents (Li et al. 2021). These properties are adequate for food formulation such as clear soups, meat (Joly and Anderstein 2009), Asian style noodles (Chen et al. 2003), confections (Buwalda et al. 2014; Woltjes et al. 2004), fillings and snacks. Regarding the latter, PS is responsible for the balance between crunchy and crispy characteristics (van der Sman and Broeze 2013). On the other hand, PS is naturally GF, satisfying consumers with gluten-related disorders and people searching for non-allergenic ingredients, contributing to the growing GF market (Villanueva et al. 2018). Normally, PS is used in GF pasta production since its addition could increase the overall quality (including appearance, colour, odour, and hardness) of GF pasta made from corn, rice, and sorghum flours (Rodrigues Ferreira et al. 2016). In addition, the incorporation of different GF ingredients such potato flours can simulate the viscoelastic properties of gluten, retain gas, and improve the maintenance of structure, texture and shelf life of bakery products (Gallagher et al. 2004; Arendt et al. 2002).

It is known that the larger size of the native PS granules and their high swelling capacity lead to extremely bulky swollen granules, which result in a high viscosity but also in a less smooth texture. Despite native PS can meet several requirements in food applications (particularly high viscosity, low off-taste and clarity), starches with modified properties are highly required because processes and storage conditions become more demanding on characteristics of final product (Semeijn and Buwalda 2018). Due to the higher fragility of the swollen PS granules, their pastes are prone to disperse or solubilize on heating and shearing, giving a weak-bodied, stringy, and cohesive slurries (Singh et al. 2016). As other native starches, PS can be modified using a chemical, physical or enzymatic method, single or combined, as was previously described (Morikawa and Nishinari 2000). In addition, modification of PS could increase their resistance to enzymatic hydrolysis rendering in a novel and high RS content product (Dupuis and Liu 2019). Therefore, different kinds of PS are successfully used in a broad range of food products. Table 3.3. describes some examples where the incorporation of native and modified PS was performed to obtain GF bakery products.

3.5 Native and Modified Cassava Starch – Different Alternatives and Applications

Cassava (*Manihot esculenta* Crantz) also known as tapioca or yucca, is a tuberous root vegetable of the Euphorbiaceae family. Although cassava is a crop native to Latin America (mainly Brazil, Paraguay and Colombia) and the Caribbean, this region contributes only 11% (2010–2020 average) of world production (251–303 Mt,

Table 3.3 Formulation of GF bakery and pasta goods with native and modified potato starch (PS)

Native or modified PS inclusion in formulation	Food	Main findings	Reference
High protein brown rice flour + tapioca starch + PS	Cupcake	PS increased cupcakes specific volume and decreased hardness	Aleman et al. (2021)
PS + Hydroxypropyl methylcellulose (HPMC)/ Carboxymethylcellulose, xanthan gum (XG) /apple pectin.	Bread	Hydrocolloids increased the gelatinization temperature and water absorption capacity of potato dough. Bread had higher specific volume, lower hardness and rapidly digestible starch.	Liu et al. (2018)
Modified PS (acidification acetic and lactic acid) + caseinate or soy-protein isolate + HPMC.	Dough	Proteins structured and strengthened the protein isolate-PS dough. Increased pasting viscosities with protein addition. Acidification of protein-enriched starch matrices modulates dough rheological properties.	Villanueva et al. (2018)
PS	Bread	Decreased protein levels, an increased moisture content (about 2%) and carbohydrates levels due to the composition of potato. Sensory analysis (80% PS) bread with better characteristics: taste, colour and odour.	Nemar et al. (2015)
PS + powdered sugar + artificial colour + vanilla flavour	Pudding	Sensory evaluation showed non-significant difference between non cereal pudding mix and control (corn starch). PS-based pudding mix can be stored for 12 months without impacting quality.	Singh et al. (2021)
PS + Potato protein + Potato fibre + Potato flour + Fresh tube	Bread	By balancing the strong swelling power of PS, was resolved the cracks on the crust. The breads showed a typical appearance, loaf size, low porosity but high cell density crumb structure and unique favourable sensory qualities (2% potato fibre or 30% fresh tuber). Breads staled quickly during storage.	Lu et al. (2021)
Corn/PS mix + Waxy corn/ waxy PS mix	Bread	WS increased the storage and loss moduli due to the increased swelling capacity. The presence of WS (10–15%) reduced the hardness and chewiness of crumb, limiting the increase of these parameters during storage and reducing staling.	Witczak et al. (2019)

(continued)

Table 3.3 (continued)

Native or modified PS inclusion in formulation	Food	Main findings	Reference
Heat-Moisture Treated (HMT) PS + Sodium Chloride as a binder paste.	Noodles	Dough owned higher hardness and noodles exhibited less solid loss and broken noodles, firmer texture, and better elasticity.	Yang et al. (2022)
Rice flour, Corn starch and PS blends + XG or Guar gum	Flat bread	Gums improved the weight and roundness. Formulations Rice flour:Corn starch:PS 40%:20%:40% and 40%:40%:20% with 3% XG showed higher moisture retention, lower hardness and remained softer up to 72 h.	Mahmoud et al. (2013)
Sorghum, rice, Corn flours and PS mix + egg + oil	Pasta	Sorghum, rice flours and PS (40:20:40) showed the best cooking quality, density, yield, weight increase and the lowest solids loss.	Rodrigues Ferreira et al. (2016)

2010–2020 data). Africa (mainly Nigeria, Congo) and Asia (mostly Thailand, Indonesia) share almost all the world cassava production with of 60% and 30%, respectively (FAOSTAT 2021). Cassava represents the third most important source of calories in the tropics, after rice and maize (Zhu 2015a) and continues its transition towards a market oriented to products and raw materials for the processed food industry. Mature roots have an average composition of 60–70% water, 30–35% carbohydrate, 1–2% fat, 1–2% fibre and 1–2% protein, with trace quantities of vitamins and minerals. Cassava also contains different amounts of cyanogenic glucosides depending on varieties. Proper processing of roots can eliminate such toxic compound (Wang and Guo 2020). Starch content in mature cassava parenchyma (Fig. 3.4a, b) ranges from 15% to 33% (up to approximately 80% of dried weight of tuber), depending on the climate and harvest time. For starch extraction, roots must be firstly washed, chopped and grated in sulfur-containing water to separate starch from pulp. Then, the separated starch fraction is reduced in water content by centrifugation or filtration, before final drying (flash dryer) and packaging (Breuninger et al. 2009). Typically, cassava starch (CS) present granules with a medium size and contains 17–33% amylose and minimal amounts of proteins, lipids, ashes and phosphates (Fig. 3.4 and Table 3.2).

In addition, amylose from cassava has a higher molecular weight than other starches. The swelling power of CS is moderate compared to potato and cereal starches but has a higher solubility, which can be attributed partially to the high swelling power. Regarding, gelatinisation properties, CS has low gelatinisation temperature and higher water-binding capacity, viscosity and shear resistance making it a suitable option in food, feed, chemicals and pharmaceutical products (Wang et al. 2022). The CS gels trend to be more stable than starch gels from cereals, which is of importance in food applications (Wang and Guo 2020). The mentioned characteristics of CS (low content of amylose, lipids and proteins, high molecular weight

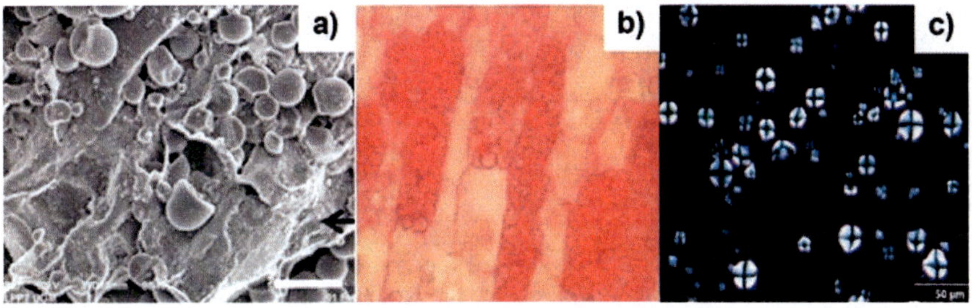

Fig. 3.4 CS granules: (**a**) SEM of cassava parenchyma (scale bar: 10 μm), (**b**) light microscopy (Objective: 40X) and (**c**) polarized light microscopy (scale bar: 50 μm). (Images (**a**) and (**b**) from Maherawati et al. (2017); Asian Network for Scientific Information. Copyright ©2017: Maherawati et al. This is an open access article distributed under the terms of the creative commons attribution License, which permits unrestricted use, distribution and reproduction in any medium, provided the original author and source are credited. Image (**c**) is reprinted from Grace and Henry (2020). Copyright © 2020 by the authors. Licensee MDPI, Basel, Switzerland. This article is an open access article distributed under the terms and conditions of the Creative Commons Attribution (CC BY) license (http://creativecommons.org/licenses/by/4.0/))

amylose), make it a unique native starch for direct use. The CS is also distinguished by its gel-forming ability and bland taste (Breuninger et al. 2009). Concerning nutritional aspects, CS has high digestion rate and, consequently, a rapid increase of glucose in blood is observed. There is a great interest to increase the RS content in CS to develop improved functional foods for particular health requirements (type 2 diabetes, obesity, etc.).

Native CS is used in many applications in food industry such as row material for sweeteners production (high-fructose syrup, glucose, dextrin and monosodium glutamate), for obtaining bakery and pastry products, noodles, soups, soft drinks, ice creams, and yoghurts as well as feedstock for microbial fermentation in the bioethanol, butanol, L-lactic acid and trehalose production. As other starches, technological limitations of CS include low cold solubility, freeze-thaw stability, shear and thermal resistance, poor enzymatic hydrolysis, high syneresis, high tendency towards retrogradation and high digestibility. Particularly, chemical modification can convert CS into a rich RS starch with many health benefits (Wang et al. 2022). Table 3.4 summarises some applications of native and modified CS to produce GF products.

3.6 Native and Modified Non-conventional Starches. Different Alternatives and Applications

Added to conventional starch sources such as cereal grains, potato tubers and cassava roots, starches from minor or geographically circumscribed crops, with diverse functional properties, are becoming relevant in food manufacturing. One of the significant characteristics of these raw materials is their natural lack of gluten proteins and, therefore, their suitability to be used in GF products.

Table 3.4 Formulation of GF bakery and pasta goods with native and modified cassava starch (CS)

Native or modified CS inclusion in formulation	Food	Major Findings	Reference
Sorghum starch + gelatinised CS + cellulose derivatives + emulsifiers + egg white powder	Bread	Emulsifiers strengthened the doughs (increased elastic recovery) and decreased crumb firmness and staling rate when compared to the control (without emulsifiers and cellulose derivatives). Particularly, at 2.4% w/w emulsifiers. The effect of cellulose derivatives on dough strength was influenced by the type, concentration and ionic character.	Onyango et al. (2009)
CS + corn flour (80:20) + vegetable fat + hen egg + soybean flour	Bread	The optimum bread (highest levels of fat and soybean flour and one egg), presented low values of firmness (≤100 N) and elasticity (>65%) and the lowest variation of these parameters with storage. Overall acceptability was 84% for habitual consumers and 100% by celiac people. Bread was enriched in proteins due to soybean flour.	Milde et al. (2012)
Cassava (flour, native and sour starch) + maize starch/rice flour	Bread	CS and, to a lesser extent, flour can help to improve the quality of GF breads. The addition of CS in small percentages (10%) can help to improve its texture and mouth feel, as well as its specific volume. Sour CS give slightly affect taste and texture in the mouth.	Sigüenza-Andrés et al. (2021)
Flour, coarse and bran rice + Pre-gelatinised CS + hydroxypropyl methylcellulose (HPMC) + soybean extruded–expelled meal (SEF) + sucrose + salt	Bread	Lower pre-gelatinised CS and SEF levels presented loaves with higher specific volume, softer crumb with faster recuperation of springiness and less susceptibility to being disintegrated during chewiness. SEF decreased lightness, increased the colour intensity and gave a more uniform microstructure. Optimal formulation was: Pre-gelatinised CS 15 g/100 g, SEF 6 g/100 g and water 160 g/100 g. SEF addition would increase the intake of dietary fibre and proteins in 1.4 and 3.7fold, respectively.	Genevois and de Escalada Pla (2021)

(continued)

Table 3.4 (continued)

Native or modified CS inclusion in formulation	Food	Major Findings	Reference
Cassava flour + Sucrose + NaCl + Extra-virgin olive oil + Egg white	Bread	Baking trials were carried out by using egg white or/and olive oil, due to their high nutritional value. Significant improvements of loaf specific volume (from 2.24 to 3.93 mL/g) and crumb firmness (from 9.14 to 4.67 N) were achieved by contemporarily including egg white and olive oil. Cassava breads containing both these ingredients obtained the best scores from panellists and resulted attractive as the wheat bread.	Pasqualone et al. (2010)
Heat-moisture-treated CS, sorghum flour, amaranth flour (50:40:10) + sugar + baker's fat + salt + amaranth malt	Bread	Heat-moisture-treated CS had higher crystallinity, onset pasting temperature and water absorption index; and lower swelling power, water solubility index and peak viscosity, affecting properties and crumb texture of GF batter and bread, respectively. Batter consistency increased but crumb hardness and chewiness decreased with increasing moisture content and incubation time of starch modification and increasing amaranth malt content.	Onyango et al. (2013)
Bread: maize starch + rice flour + CS + sugar + salt + yeast + ice cream neutral mixture (guar gum, Carboxymethylcellulose, emulsifiers) + soybean extract powder + margarine + emulsifier + eggs Muffin: idem bread (maize starch) but using brown sugar + baking powder + cinnamon + chocolate	Breads and muffins	A comparative analysis of specific volume, elasticity, firmness, and triangular test was performed with pre-baked, baked, and frozen bread. From sensory analysis of acceptance, it was concluded that the formulation relating to the optimal simultaneous point between instrumental measurements (20% rice flour + 30% CS + 50% maize starch) obtained the best results. The sensory evaluation of the muffin conducted by common and celiac consumers showed good acceptability and buy intention. The addition of the soybean extract powder enriched in protein both products.	Schamne et al. (2010)

(continued)

Table 3.4 (continued)

Native or modified CS inclusion in formulation	Food	Major Findings	Reference
Modified CS (oxidised, modified, sour) + cheese + corn starch + pre-cooked corn flour + whole milk	Cheese bread	All doughs were prepared and frozen previous elaboration. The chemically modified starches had higher resistance to freezing and resulted with lower hardness and number of pores than sour CS. A better overall appearance, higher softness but higher compaction and hardness, and less salty in taste were observed for samples with oxidised CS, detectable by panellists in comparison with fresh dough.	Mesa et al. (2019)
Damaged cassava + sugar + peanut oil + salt	Crackers	The increase in damage level led to a slight increase in amylose content and reduction in crystallinity. Also exerted a major influence on the pasting properties and interaction between damaged cassava and water. Damage (>11.5%) rendered texture properties similar with those of wheat flour. Cracker made with damaged cassava had acceptable sensory qualities comparable to control.	Liu et al. (2019)
Cassava WS + wild-type CS fermented for up to 30 days and oven or sun dried + cheese + sunflower oil	Baked or fried expanded products.	The specific volume after baking for cassava WS was 3.5 times higher than that in wild-type starches. There was a synergistic combination of fermentation (10–14 days) and sun-drying. Fermentation reduced viscosities and the weight average molar mass led to denser macro-molecules and increased branching degree, which were linked to a high loaf volume. Cassava WS can emerge as a cheaper, GF, clean label, and neutral taste alternative.	Dufour et al. (2022)

(continued)

Table 3.4 (continued)

Native or modified CS inclusion in formulation	Food	Major Findings	Reference
Defated marama flour + CS	Bread-type dough	Defated marama flour and CS (33:67) can produce a dough of similar strength but less stability to wheat flour dough, but which can produce an alveograph dough bubble and has good gas-holding capacity during proofing. The presence of the dietary fibre in the defated marama flour and the inclusion CS appear to favourably modify the marama protein rheological properties. Defated marama flour have considerable potential as a functional gluten replacement.	Nyembwe et al. (2018)
Pre gelatinized cassava flour + CS and amaranth flour	Pasta	The use of pre-gelatinized cassava flour, native CS and amaranth flour (10:60:30), allowed a pasta similar in quality as commercial wheat products: light yellowish colour, fibre rich [9.37 g (100 g)$^{-1}$], source of protein [10.41 g (100 g)$^{-1}$], adequate firmness (43.6 N) and low stickiness (3.2 N). In addition, the use of cassava bagasse improved the fibre content.	Fiorda et al. (2013)
CS and corn flour (80:20) + Whole milk powder + Vegetable fat + Whole egg fresh + XG	Pasta	0.6% XG concentration developed the highest potential to improve the pasta capacity to prevent structure disintegration with the lowest cooking loss and the lowest values for firmness, cohesiveness, chewiness, springiness and cutting force.	Milde et al. (2020)
CS and corn flour (80:20) + Whole milk powder + Vegetable fat + Whole egg fresh + XG + Salt + Egg albumen	Pasta	Egg albumen was used to fortify dry GF pasta. 1.5 g egg albumen/100 g showed great potential in prospective for industrial development, with intermediate cooking time, low cooking loss, firm texture, low adhesiveness and good sensory evaluation. Also it increased protein and fibre content, and maintained high protein digestibility. In addition, shelf life was determined of up to 8 months.	Milde et al. (2021)

(continued)

Yields higher than 30% are expected for these unconventional sources to be considered for commercial purposes (Tagliapietra et al. 2021). Applied extraction methods depend on the complexity of the matrix, including solvents, acid/base reagents, enzymes or physical treatments such as ultrasound, shear forces, etc., and could lead to modifications of the starch granules and the rheological properties of their pastes.

Considering the growing consumer demand for food products made with natural, unmodified ingredients, the starches obtained from these sources may allow to bypass or reduce the use of chemically modified starches in several industries. Chemical modifications are usually designed for the increasing of starch shear resistance, the reduction of retrogradation and syneresis and the stabilization of the macromolecules during heating, shearing, freezing and/or storage (Mason 2009). These features might be at least partially achieved by little-explored natural sources which could, in consequence, boost the production worldwide of such alternative native starches. These starches could also serve as new starting points to attain technological properties different from those of traditional sources (mainly cereal starches) upon chemical or physical modifications. Diverse gel strengths, gelatinisation temperatures or swelling degrees are demanded by the food industry depending on the process and the desired characteristics of the final product but, as a general rule, starches with high whiteness index and low retrogradation tendency are sought.

Non-cereal GF starch sources include fruits, seeds, roots and tubers, and pulses, from which starch can be readily extracted with acceptable yield and purity. Among them, some extraction paths are sheared for matrices with similar characteristics, which may include processing steps such as pericarp removal, dehulling, wet or dry milling, or grinding in water. Some examples are discussed in more detail below.

3.6.1 Non-traditional Root and Tuber Starches

Starchy roots and tubers (R&T) are excellent alternatives to cereal crops. These are high in water and usually contain low quantity of proteins and lipids compared to cereals, which eases starch extraction and enables R&T to be directly crushed in water without the need for a pre-soaking, turning the milling and the beginning of the extraction into a single step. Furthermore, the negligible content of lipids (<0.1%) in starches from R&T leads to a tasteless product compared to those from cereals, which is desirable for food applications (Moorthy et al. 2018).

Among the R&T, only potato and starch have a worldwide commercial distribution. However, non-traditional R&T starches are gaining increasing attention related to production sustainability, use of by-products, its regional availability which derives in foods typical of each local gastronomy, as well as the diverse technological properties that can distinguish them from common starches (Tagliapietra et al. 2021). Some of these starch-rich non-traditional crops are listed in Table 3.5.

Due to the high moisture content of starchy R&T, processing installations for starch extraction must be close to cropping areas, as described for cassava, to avoid

Table 3.5 Content and characteristics of starches from non-traditional sources

Common name	Scientific name	Starch content (% db)	Starch characteristics: Lightness (L*)	Granule size (μm)	Granule morphology	Crystallinity degree	Amylose content (%)	Resistant starch (%)	Gelatinisation temperature (°C)	References
Arracacha	*Arracacia xanthorrhiza*	46–64	86	7–23	Round, polygonal, irregular and elliptical	24.0–31.5	3–39	10.1–15.3	57.8–61.2	Salazar et al. (2021), Castanha et al. (2018), López Calderón (2017), Pinzon et al. (2020), Santacruz et al. (2002).
Taro	*Colocasia esculenta*	64–85	88–96	3–6	Round irregular and polygonal	23.9–45.1	2.5–35.9	10.3–23.7	54.4–107	Wongsagonsup et al. (2021), Singla et al. (2020), Salazar et al. (2021), Martins et al. (2020), Nagar et al. (2021), Setiarto et al. (2020)
Achira	*Canna indica C. edulis*	55–80	95–96	20–100	Round, oval and elliptical	23.4–36.6	24.8–31.5	20–26.7	63.4–67.9	Salazar et al. (2021), Fuentes et al. (2019), Zhang et al. (2018), Lan et al. (2016a, b), Cabrera-Canales et al. (2021), Vamadevan et al. (2018), Wu et al. (2020), Mendez-Montealvo et al. (2022)

(continued)

Table 3.5 (continued)

Common name	Scientific name	Starch content (% db)	Starch characteristics							References
			Lightness (L*)	Granule size (µm)	Granule morphology	Crystallinity degree	Amylose content (%)	Resistant starch (%)	Gelatinisation temperature (°C)	
Kudzu or kuzu	*Pueraria spp.*	30–80	94	2–20	Spherical and polygonal	34.8–48.2	20.0–24.3	24.1–68.5	65.6–83.7	Zhao et al. (2017, 2021), Guo et al. (2016), Li et al. (2019a), Chen et al. (2017a), Liu et al. (2021), Reddy et al. (2017), Guo et al. (2021)
Sweet potato	*Ipomoea batatas*	38–80	91–97	16–24	Spherical, oval, irregular and polygonal	32.8–39.6	17.7–34.2	1.4–49.9	68.3–79.3	Guo et al. (2020), Wang et al. (2020b), Na et al. (2021), Bajaj et al. (2021), Sun et al. (2022)
Yam	*Dioscorea spp.*	20–85	97	1–90	Round, oval, polygonal and irregular	25.1–53.0	10–36	15.6–55.8	66.0–85.1	Zhu (2015b), Lovera et al. (2017), Chen et al., (2019), Liu et al. (2020), Ribeiro Oliveira et al. (2021), Yu et al. (2021b)
Andean yam bean, ajipa or asipa	*Pachyrhizus ahipa*	43.7–65	93–96	2–20	Spherical and polygonal	41.9–44.5	11.6–16.8	N/D	64.8–67.2	Dini et al. (2013), López et al. (2010), Díaz et al. (2016), Doporto et al. (2012, 2014), Forsyth and Shewry (2002)
Jícama or Mexican yam bean	*Pachyrhizus erosus*	83	N/D	5–35	Spherical and poligonal	34.3	16.9–25.1	N/D	61.7	Stevenson et al. (2007), Forsyth and Shewry (2002)

Sago starch	*Metroxylon sagu*	79–88	55.2–93.3	10–50	Polygonal or oval, some truncated oval	23.0–50.4	21.4–30.0	62.61	69.5–72.5	Karim et al. (2008), Abdorreza et al. (2012), Othman et al. (2015), Azfaralariff et al. (2020), Arshad et al. (2018), Ahmad et al. (1999), Grace and Henry (2020), Mustafa Kamal et al. (2017), Zhu (2019)
Bean/ Common Bean	*Phaseolus vulgaris*	36.8–40.3	85.4–87.7[a]	24–47 length; 23–32 width	Round to oval, with smooth surface	27.7–30.3	38.0–41.5	32.4–36.0	73.7–74.5	Chung et al. (2008), Shimelis et al. (2006)
Pea/Field pea/ Dry pea	*Pisum sativum*	27.22–57.53[b]	N/D	3–20	Oval or kidney-like, round, spherical, irregular or polygonal	25.1–30.0	40.7–82.6	35.5–37.9	63.5–79.8	Li et al. (2019b), Shen et al. (2016)
Lentil	*Lens culinaris*	35–53	N/D	6–37 length; 6–32 width	Oval, round, elliptical	26.2–30.6	23.5–38.0	41.3	65.2–76.1	Hoover et al. (2010), Keskin et al. (2022), Li et al. (2019b), Romano et al. (2021)

(continued)

Table 3.5 (continued)

Common name	Scientific name	Starch content (% db)	Starch characteristics							References
			Lightness (L*)	Granule size (μm)	Granule morphology	Crystallinity degree	Amylose content (%)	Resistant starch (%)	Gelatinisation temperature (°C)	
Chickpea	*Cicer arietinum*	29.1–46.0	N/D	14–30 length; 9–30 width	Oval, spherical	23.0–27.6	23.0–35.2	N/D	63.5–77.3	Hoover et al. (2010), Keskin et al. (2022), Tan et al. (2021)
Acorn	*Quercus spp.*	50–60	83–91	2.5–126.2	Spherical and elliptical	22–28	16–39	31–41	59–88	Taib and Bouyazza (2021), Correia et al. (2021), Yoo et al. (2012)
Chestnuts	*Castanea spp.*	42–82	>93	10.8–111.7	Spherical, elliptical and irregular	9–51	17–57	4–85	61–69	Guo et al. (2019), de La Montaña Míguelez et al. (2004), Liu et al. (2015), Correia and Beirão-da-Costa (2012), Cruz et al. (2013), Yoo et al. (2012), Zhang et al. (2011), Yang et al. (2010)

starch degradation due to enzymatic processes and root rotting (Manthey 2016). With some modifications, starch extraction from non-traditional R&T at laboratory scale was successfully applied in similar way to that used for industrial starch extraction. The process mostly consists in washing, peeling, chopping and crushing the roots with water, alkali or other aqueous solutions (e.g., sodium bisulfite) in a blender, and then washing the slurry on screens where fibre bagasse is retained and the starch slurry passes through (Manthey 2016; Zhao et al. 2021; Zhu 2015b). After separation of the fibre fraction, other steps for removing small non-starch material can be required.

According to Opara (2003) R&T can be divided into three groups (a) those that are grown worldwide and used in large quantities, such as potatoes; (b) tropical crops that are staple foods in developing countries: e.g. cassava, aroids (such as taro), and yams; and (c) lesser-known crops such as the Andean R&T (like some from the *Pachyrhizus, Canna* and *Arracacia* genera) or certain specialty vegetables (e.g. Chinese water chestnut and Kudzu). Except for potatoes, R&T are grown in warmer areas of the world (Opara 2003; Dini et al. 2012).

Among the second group, sweet potato (*Ipomoea batatas*) is one of the most widespread crops, grown in many tropical and subtropical countries in Asia, Africa, and Latin America (Tong et al. 2020), being China the world's biggest producer and consumer (FAOSTAT 2021). Flour is the mostly used ingredient derived from sweet potato roots. Starch separation carries a difficulty due to the presence of fibrous material and latex, which prevents easy settling of the granules, and the high amount of sugars in the slurry which makes it susceptible to fermentation (Moorthy et al. 2018). Also, if not properly processed, starch may have an off-colour due to the phenolic compounds present, mainly in exocarp, which diminishes its lightness value (L*). Sweet potato starch has lipid and phosphorus content similar to cassava starch, and hence exhibits similar properties (Moorthy et al. 2018).

Taro (*Colocasia esculenta*) also known as pituca or Malanga, is widely cultivated in Asia, India and other tropical and subtropical regions. Taro flour is scarcely available on the international market while starch is almost non-existent. Nip et al. (2007) used taro flour as major component to formulate snap and drop cookies, tested different ratios of ingredients and reached a highly acceptable formulation as indicated by a taste test. Analogous to the difficulty that latex provides to sweet potato starch extraction is that produced by mucilage in taro. The strong binding of starch with protein in mucilage may produce loss of starch granules during the filtration step and results in lower yields of taro starch (Wongsagonsup et al. 2021). Taro starch is distinctive from other R&T starches in its small granule size, which derives in enhanced emulsion stabilizing properties and a good performance as a filler in edible films (Singla et al. 2020). Taro starch was also assayed to improve textural properties in yogurt and ketchup, and α-amylase treated starch was successfully applied as stabilizer in ice cream (Singla et al. 2020).

Yam is a root vegetable and comprises several species of the genus *Dioscorea*. The most commonly cultivated species include *D. alata* (water yam), *D. cayenensis* (yellow yam), *D. esculenta* (lesser yam), *D. opposita* (Chinese yam), *D. rotundata* (white yam), and *D. trifida* (cush-cush yam) (Zhu 2015b). Starch yield at lab scale has been reported to reach up to 88% (db) (Zhu 2015b). Starch is almost unavailable in the global market, but some studies assayed the incorporation of yam starch in pasta and bread (Zhu 2015b), the latter exhibiting good quality attributes by 30% wheat flour replacement with yam starch (Zhu 2015b; Nindjin et al. 2011).

The group of lesser-known crops include Andean R&T such as arracacha, achira, and the Andean yam bean. Arracacha (*Arracacia xanthorrhiza*) is a tuberous root popular in several South American countries (Bolivia, Brazil, Colombia, Peru, Ecuador, and Venezuela), and traditionally used for the preparation of soups, stews and purees, and for making bread, cakes and drinks (Leidi et al. 2018). Starch is the main carbohydrate present in arracacha, with high resistant starch and significant FOS contents reported for these roots (Lovera et al. 2017; Sancho et al. 2017); thus, arracacha could provide suitable ingredients for low glycaemic index foods with potential prebiotic properties (Leidi et al. 2018). Arracacha roots may be used for starch extraction and because of its properties (low gelatinisation temperature and low retrogradation and syneresis) may have specific uses in the food industry (e.g., milk-based drinks or soups). The industrial use of arracacha starch has led to a complete characterisation of its physicochemical and rheological properties (Leidi et al. 2018).

Pachyrhizus ahipa (Andean yam bean) from the Andean region and its closely related Mesoamerican species P. erosus (jicama) are another tuberous-root producing crops. The starch content in ahipa roots reaches 44–65% (Dini et al. 2013) while P. erosus has more than 80% db of this carbohydrate (Stevenson et al. 2007). Starches from both sources exhibit similar morphological and physicochemical properties (Table 3.5). Jicama is a popular dietary staple in Mexico, Central and South America (Stevenson et al. 2007) while ahipa is only consumed locally in some Andean regions of Bolivia, and the north of Argentina (Dini et al. 2012). This crop has higher crude protein content than other R&T (6.5–9.4%) (Dini et al. 2021), and these are non-prolamins thus ahipa is suitable for GF products (Doporto et al. 2011). Ahipa proteins are highly hydrosoluble and have low molecular weight thus most of them are removed during the starch extraction process (Dini et al. 2012). Similar to Ipomoea batatas, some P. ahipa accessions have anthocyanin pigments which provide a dark layer of a protein and anthocyanins mixture over the sedimented starch cake (Dini et al. 2021), which is reflected in a lower L* value of the starch powder compared to P. erosus (Table 3.5), the latter being non-pigmented roots. Native ahipa starch exhibits better expansion properties during baking than native CS (Díaz et al. 2019). Modifications such as natural fermentation and protein enrichment were assayed in this starch, which provided mainly modifications in the rheological properties (fermentation) (Díaz et al. 2019) and in the texture and crumb alveolar distribution of GF baked products (Malgor et al. 2019).

Pueraria (kudzu) root starch is only popular in China, Japan and other East Asian countries. Starch is an important component of kudzu root, accounting for ~50% of its dry weight, and can be extracted in high purity (up to 99%) (Zhao et al. 2021). Industrial root processing is established in these countries and starch is commercially available. Furthermore, kudzu starch can be purchased as a specialty in western countries. In artisanal produced starches, relatively high isoflavones levels can be detected, which are stated to enhance its nutritional value (Zhao et al. 2021). Native kudzu starch has some intrinsic limitations such as low solubility, thus, various physical, chemical, and enzymatic modifications have been assayed, attempting to improve and broaden its food applications, such as emulsification properties and film forming capacity (Zhao et al. 2021).

3.6.2 *Legume Starches*

Legume dicotyledonous seeds (Fabaceae botanical family) such as beans, peas, chickpeas, cowpeas, and lentils are a good source of total carbohydrates, which represents 65–72% of the weight of dried legumes. This fraction comprises starch (about 85%) and dietary fibre (between 10 and 20%) (Fabbri and Crosby 2016). Oligosaccharides (α-galactosides) are also present (Carpenter et al. 2017). Galacto-oligosaccharides were held as flatulence-causing compounds, so that soaking, and processing treatments have been suggested to remove them or significantly reduce their content. Recently, these kinds of carbohydrates have been recognized as prebiotics and promoters of beneficial intestinal bacteria (Affrifah et al. 2021).

Although starch is the major component of legume seeds, its content varies significantly depending on species and cultivars, from 35% to 60% of the total mass of pulses (Kringel et al. 2020). Likewise, the starch yield could reach 84.7% as reported for faba bean, or be relatively low as informed for black bean (16.4–22.2%) (Ashogbon et al. 2021) depending on the different methods of dehulling, the seed coat hardness, soaking procedures, etc.

The fact that most of legume total carbohydrates is represented by starch and, at the same time, legumes are good sources of dietary fibre can be explained by the relatively high proportion of resistant starch in these seeds.

Starch extraction processes are generally classified into wet and dry milling (Fig. 3.5). The isolation of proteins from defatted legume flours also yields starch as a by-product (Wani et al. 2016). Dry milling is principally used for industrial processing and wet milling is commonly applied at the laboratory, allowing the isolation of purer pulse starches (Hoover et al. 2010).

The obtaining of starch from legume seeds performed by wet milling method implies the co-decantation of proteins, small fibre components and the starch granules (Wani et al. 2016). Thus, starch isolation from legume grains is challenging because of the insoluble accompanying macromolecules that interfere in the sedimentation and co-settles with the starch to form a brownish cake (Hoover et al. 2010).

The main steps for isolating starch from legumes by wet milling (Fig. 3.5) are soaking, dehulling, washing, blending, screening, centrifugation or sedimentation, to end with the drying, grinding up and sieving of the obtained starch (Hoover et al. 2010; Lawal and Adebowale 2005). Wet milling is performed in alkaline conditions, being the pH used for the extraction in the range 8.5–10. In some cases, dehulled seeds are soaked in water with the addition of sodium chloride (6 g L^{-1}; solid to liquid ratio 1:5) for the extraction of salt soluble proteins (Abu et al. 2006) or

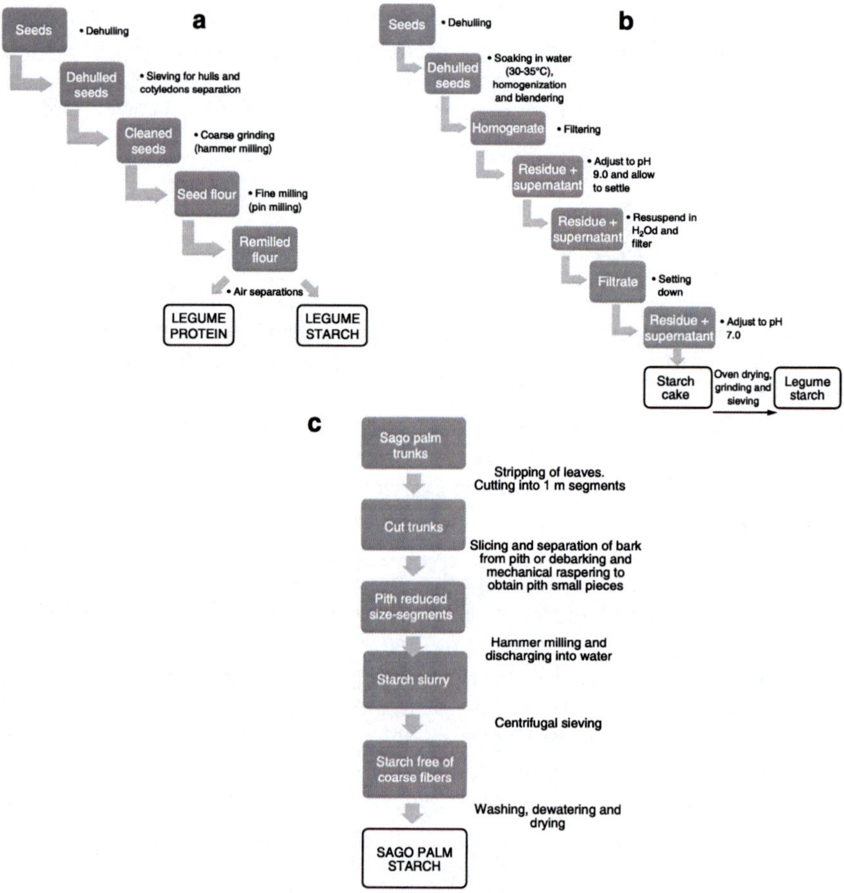

Fig. 3.5. Dry (**a**) and wet milling (**b**) processes for obtaining legume starches and sago starch extraction process (**c**). (Flow diagrams were adapted from Hoover et al. 2010 and Kringel et al. 2020)

potassium metabisulfite, to avoid occurrence of browning phenomena (Aggarwal et al. 2004).

Hoover et al. (2010) have pointed out that the starches of several pulses such as smooth and wrinkled peas (*Pisum sativum* subsp. arvense), faba bean (*Vicia faba*), mung bean (*Vigna radiata*), lentil (*Lens culinaris*), navy bean (Phaseolus vulgaris), lima bean (*Phaseolus lunatus*) and cowpea (*Vigna unguiculata*) have been obtained by dry milling, using hammer and/or pin mills and air sorting. A high degree of particle size reduction is demanded to separate the starch granules from the protein matrix and, as it was previously mentioned, air separation does not allow to achieve a complete fractionation of these components. Even after repetitive milling and air classification, the starch obtained by this method shows lower purity than that coming from wet milling process, and a water washing step must be implemented to reduce the remnant attached protein to approximately 0.25% in the separated starch.

Table 3.5 shows the main morphological and physicochemical characteristics of the starches obtained from bean, pea, chickpea and lentil grains.

Most pulse starch granules are oval, although spherical, round, elliptical and irregularly shaped granules were also described (Hoover et al. 2010). Based on its X-ray diffraction pattern, legume starches are often classified into the C-crystalline-type, which indicates that the granules contain both A-crystalline structures forming the outer layers, and B-crystalline types found in the centre of the granules (Manthey 2016). Some pulse starches, such as pea, lentil and bean starches, are typically rich in amylose, show relatively low swelling power, deficient dispersibility in water, and tend to retrograde. These starches possess strongly bonded chains, which is reflected in their high gelatinisation transition temperatures and enthalpies (Ashogbon et al. 2021).

Total amylose content of legume grain starches has been reported to be in the range 14–88% (Tayade et al. 2019). These wide differences are generally related to inter and intra specific genetic variability, climate and soil growing conditions, physiological status of the plants, and analytical methods. In this sense, amylose content can be determined spectrophotometrically and, sometimes, under or overestimated if defatting is not previously carried out, and/or the iodine complexing phenomena of long external amylopectin chains are not considered.

Pulse starches present a relatively high proportion of resistant and slowly digestible starch fractions, which are the preferable forms of dietary starch due to their slow glycaemic response and relative control of the plasma insulin levels (Keskin et al. 2022). Thus, functional and healthier food products can be developed using legume starches as ingredients.

On the other hand, the relatively high amylose content of some legume starches usually causes detriment to desired functional properties in many food applications as compared to prevalent cereal and root starch sources. Nevertheless, with the development of starch modification agents and techniques, it is possible to restructure practically all starches to meet targeted uses. γ-Irradiation is an alternative to preserve and functionally modify the starches obtained from different sources. Abu et al. (2006) analysed the physicochemical and thermal properties of the starch isolated from 2, 10 and 50 kGy irradiated cowpea flours and pastes. The authors reported that pasting and swelling properties were significantly decreased in a γ-irradiation dose-dependent way. Differential scanning calorimetry of cowpea starch showed increments in peak gelatinisation temperature with higher irradiation doses. On the other hand, scanning electron microscopy and Fourier transform infrared (FTIR) spectroscopy revealed that, up to a 50 kGy dose, irradiation did not cause visible physical effects on cowpea starch granule surface.

3.6.3 Palm Starch

Sago palm (*Metroxylon sagu* Rottb.) is a tropical plant species belonging to the *Arecaceae* botanical family, grown in Southeast Asia and Oceania (Malaysia, Indonesia, Papua New Guinea, Philippines, Thailand and the Solomon Islands) (Chua et al. 2021). The plant produces an upright trunk ~10 m high and 0.75 m in diameter. During the vegetative phase (10–15 years), the stem stores starch to a maximum level up to the development of a huge inflorescence at its top. This energy and carbon storage is then consumed during fruiting, and the plant dies after mature fruit falls from the palm (Manthey 2016). Although the long harvesting time of sago palm discourages its cultivation, this crop presents high-starch producing capability: 25 tons per hectare per year (i.e., amongst 4–5 times that of rice, corn and wheat, and about 17 times that of cassava) (Chua et al. 2021).

The storage parenchyma of the trunk pith contains simple, 10–50 μm in size, oval or polygonal shaped starch granules in its cells. Sago palm starch comprises about 27% amylose and its gelatinisation temperature varies from 69.5 to 70.2 °C (Karim et al. 2008). Abdorreza et al. (2012) have shown that hydrolysing sago starch with hydrochloric acid at 50 °C for 6, 12, 18, and 24 h significantly augmented gelatinisation temperature and enthalpy with increasing degree of hydrolysis.

Othman et al. (2015) applied γ-irradiation (6, 10 and 25 kGy) to sago starch and observed that the apparent amylose content and swelling power of irradiated-sago starch was significantly reduced, while the starch solubility increased due to degradation. Although there was no physical damage to sago starch even at the highest dose assayed, the treatments induced a decrease in the relative crystallinity, but did not alter the crystalline type.

Recently, Azfaralariff et al. (2020) analysed the physicochemical properties of starch nanocrystals extracted from sago starch and their performance as a Pickering emulsifier agent. The authors concluded that significant differences in morphological, thermal and pasting properties were derived from the conventional acid hydrolysis method applied for obtaining de starch nanocrystals (3.16 M H_2SO_4 at 40 °C for 5 days, then rinsing with distilled water until pH 7). Nevertheless, no major chemical changes were identified by FTIR analysis when compared to the native sago starch. Required sago starch nanocrystals concentration was at least 3.5% (w/v) to produce Pickering emulsions that showed good stability and no sign of creaming during 2 months of storage at room temperature (Azfaralariff et al. 2020).

To improve starch functionality for the formulation of food products, Zailani et al. (2022) exposed previously washed or cold-soaked sago starch to microwave heat treatment and found that the modified starches exhibit better solubility in hot water, oil and water binding capacity, and higher resistant starch content of cooked samples compared to the control. The authors also reported an increase in amylose content as well as morphological changes on the previously washed starch granules.

3.6.4 Nut Starches

Among starchy nuts, acorns and chestnuts stand out in their high proportion of this carbohydrate. Acorns is the general name given to the nuts from oak trees (Quercus spp.), being starch the main component of its kernels (Taib and Bouyazza 2021). Among the available commercial products made from acorn starch or flour, are snacks, noodles, breads, cakes, soups, and jelly. Particularly, a traditional jelly product made from acorn starch known as *mook* is a highly popular food in Korea (Kim and Yoo 2011).

Chestnuts are the fruits of trees of the genus *Castanea*, from the *Fagaceae* family. These are widely consumed in many countries, especially from Asia, Europe and America (Guo et al. 2019), toasted (as snack) or included in food preparations. Starch is the main component of chestnuts, with percentages up to ~80% depending on the variety and genotype (de La Montaña Míguelez et al. 2004; Liu et al. 2015). Commercial availability of chestnut starch is rather scarce while the flour is a little more easily found.

Starch extraction from these sources is similar to that of pulses, involving dehulling and wet or dry milling of the kernels (Fig. 3.5), but includes as a preliminary step the removal of the outer shell (pericarp). At laboratory scale, kernels are grinded into a flour which is then suspended in an alkaline (NaOH) or enzymatic (protease) solution, screened and/or centrifuged, rinsed with distilled water and dried (Correia et al. 2021; Deng et al. 2020; Zarroug et al. 2020), reaching yields up to 88.5% and 83.9% for acorns and chestnuts, respectively, and high purity (>96%) (Correia and Beirão-Da-Costa 2012).Cruz et al. (2013) proposed the use of sodium bisulfite solution for chestnuts starch extraction, and purification by sedimentation. Authors reported yields of 94% and high purity (93%) and stated that granules integrity was more preserved this way than using alkali as extractant (Cruz et al. 2013).

Chestnut starch has acceptable whiteness, showing lightness (L*) values above 92 (Guo et al. 2019; Cruz et al. 2013), while acorn starch exhibit average L* values around 88 (Correia et al. 2021; Deng et al. 2020) leading to a more grayish product (Table 3.5).

Starch granules are predominantly spherical and elliptical for both nuts, but in the case of chestnuts, some authors also observed irregular and triangular forms (Guo et al. 2019; Liu et al. 2015; Cruz et al. 2013; Moreira et al. 2015; Yoo et al. 2012).

Acorn starch granules size ranged from 2.5 to 126.2 μm, depending on the genotype and the extraction method used (Taib and Bouyazza 2021; Correia et al. 2021), while for chestnuts starch, mean sizes ranged between 10.8 and 18.1 μm (Liu et al. 2015; Cruz et al. 2013). Particularly, starches from 21 cultivars of *C. mollisima* Blume from different regions of China showed a bimodal distribution, with mean particle sizes ranging from 21.5 to 111.7 μm (Guo et al. 2019).

According to Cruz et al. (2013) the crystallinity degree of chestnut starch is directly related to the moisture content, varying from 9% to 51% for moisture contents rising from 5% to 29%. Likewise, amylose content of chestnut starch varies greatly among species and extraction methods, with high (~41–57%) (Guo et al. 2019; Correia and Beirão-Da-Costa 2012) and intermediate (17–30%) (Liu et al. 2015; Cruz et al. 2013; Yoo et al. 2012; Zhang et al. 2011) values reported. Acorns starch crystallinity degree and amylose values were reported in a narrower range (Table 3.5).

Chestnuts resistant starch percentage is also strongly dependent on the species and the extraction method, for which values from extremely high (84.9%) (Liu et al. 2015) to extremely low (4.3%) (Zhang et al. 2011) were informed.

Acorn flour has low digestibility, partially attributed to its tannin content (approx. 6%) (Soni et al. 1993) which can act as endogenous starch hydrolysing enzyme inhibitors (Lin et al. 2018). Additionally, acorn starch has a high proportion of resistant starch (30.8–41.4%) (Taib and Bouyazza 2021). This may position acorn flour and starch as promising ingredients for the formulation of low-glycaemic index foods.

When used as an additive, it has been reported that native acorn starch in concentrations lower than 1%, can provide improved functional properties, enhanced viscosity and reduced syneresis in a fermented dairy product (Zarroug et al. 2020).

Kim and Yoo (2011) studied the effect of the addition of guar gum and locust bean gum in the rheological and thermal properties of acorn starch and found that galactomannans increased the viscoelastic properties, lowered the gelatinisation enthalpy and raised the gelatinisation temperature compared to the native starch, attributed to a phase separation due to a low interaction between different polymers. Increased gel strength and decreased freeze-thaw stability were reported for the mixture of acorn starch with other hydrocolloids (e.g., carrageenan, xanthan gum) (Saleh et al. 2016).

Regarding starch modifications, physical treatments such as heat moisture treatment (HMT, heating starch at low moisture values) and annealing (heating a starch slurry below the gelatinization temperature) were assayed, individually and combined, on native Persian acorn starch (Molavi et al. 2018). More noticeable changes were produced by individual HMT treatment. Changes included increasing starch solubility, decreasing swelling power and amylose leaching, raising the gelatinisation temperature and lowering the gelatinisation range and enthalpy. Particularly, the changes produced by HMT in the pasting properties of starch could provide increased resistance to conditions such as prolonged heating and/or acidic medium. Furthermore, starch retrogradation was also limited on HMT starches (Molavi et al. 2018).

In the case of chestnuts starch, physical modifications such as dry heat treatment (DHT), addition of XG (Liu et al. 2022), and ultrasonic and microwaves treatments (Wang et al. 2020a) were assayed separately and combined. The DHT plus XG increased in 2% the amount of resistant starch compared to the native sample (Liu et al. 2022), and the microwave treatment followed by ultrasonication increased the freeze-thaw stability of chestnut starch pastes, which could be useful in frozen foods (Wang et al. 2020a). Likewise, chemical modifications such as acetylation and hydroxypropylation also provided increased freeze-thaw stability to chestnut starch, while crosslinking showed better performance in reducing the retrogradation tendency of the starch pastes (Oh et al. 2019).

3.6.5 *Some GF Food Application*

As was expressed in previous sections, much research was made to obtain new and GF resources of starches. A complete physical and chemical characterisation of granules from non-conventional resources has been reported and is available. However, studies related to applications as food ingredient are scarce, particularly to demonstrate the suitability of new starches or for production of GF items. Table 3.6 shows some developments where non-conventional resources were used to produce bakery and pasta items.

Table 3.6 Some non-conventional starch resources used in bakery and pasta production

Starch resource	Food application	Main findings	Reference
Native or hydrothermally modified bean starch	GF bread	Modified starch reduced the hardness and the retrogradation enthalpy. Improved the chemical composition and quality of fresh bread but did not extend its freshness during storage.	Krupa et al. (2010)
Pea starch	Noodles	Noodles prepared by twin-screw extrusion exhibited similar brightness in colour and cooking time to, but firmer texture. The conventional starch noodle-making procedures was simplified.	Wang et al. (2012)
Lentil starch	Noodles	Noodles were less bright in colour, but had superior texture when cooked as compared to commercial mung bean starch noodles	Wang et al. (2014)
Chestnut flour	GF bread, cakes, snacks	In addition with structuring agents, various quality attributes of the bread including hardness, specific volume, colour and sensory scores were improved.	Zhu (2017)
Sweet potato	GF noodles	Fortification with protein and/or another starches enhanced the acceptability as well as functional value. Reduced starch digestibility and enhanced protein content.	Menon et al. (2016)
Sweet potato	Noodles	Addition of hydrocolloids with high water binding capacity was necessary to control the degree of swelling of starch granules.	Silva et al. (2013)

(continued)

Table 3.6 (continued)

Starch resource	Food application	Main findings	Reference
Sweet-potato Starches	Noodle	Starch with high firmness and elasticity of its gel, result in good quality starch noodle. Suitability of sweet-potato for starch noodle making depends on variety.	Chen et al. (2002)
Sweet-potato	GF model doughs	In combination with HPMC reduced the dough development time, strength against mixing but increased gelatinisation temperature.	Zhang et al. (2017)
Green banana flour	Pasta	Greater acceptance and similar appearance, aroma, flavour and over-all quality than whole-wheat flour pasta. Modified pasta had ~98% less lipids.	Zandonadi et al. (2012)
Banana starch	GF sugar-snap cookies	30% replacement of rice flour improved starch digestion rate and consumer's acceptance. RS was increased. Gelatinised starch inclusion increased the water fraction that shifted cookie from brittle to soggy.	Roman et al. (2019a)
Green banana flour	GF muffins	Muffins were rich in minerals, less firm, had more volume and overall acceptability. Physicochemical, baking, texture and sensory evaluation showed that the use of 100% GBF had a favourable effect on muffin quality.	Kaur et al. (2017)
Pre-gelatinized unripe banana flour	GF bread	Volume and specific volume increased with the addition of HPMC and flour, while the hardness decreased. The addition of flour and water increased the number and size of alveoli and affected their distribution in crumbs.	Hernández-Aguirre et al. (2019)
Ripe banana flour	GF bread	The highest specific volume was obtained with 2-week ripening and 70% water. The flour was shown to have good potential as a substitute for gluten. The swelling ability on GF breadmaking was achieved with 10% flour.	Hosokawa et al. (2020)
Banana starch	GF bread	Slowed down the starch digestibility of bread crumb and crust	Roman et al. (2019b)
Banana flour and starch	GF cookies	Sensory profiling of cookies meet consumer requirement but also compared favourably with conventional cookies.	Olawoye and Gbadamosi (2020)

3.7 Conclusions

Starch is a substantial ingredient for the development of GF foods. Depending on the physical and chemical properties of starch, baking products and pasta will have characteristics. Amylose content and minor compounds, such as lipid, protein and phosphorus modulate the suitability of the starch in bread or pasta making. The pasting, gelatinisation, swelling and solubility behaviour of starch affect the development of volume and texture integrity in the GF breads and pasta. It is also important, the response of starch to fermentation process in which amylase enzyme must reach the starchy substrate. In these sense, physically damaged starches improve the rate of the fermentation process under amylase action. Resistant starch (RS) amount is an important nutritional aspect to take into account. It is considered that RS enhance the nutritional properties of GF breads by reducing the digestion rate of starch and, consequently, glycaemic index. Upon modification, the physicochemical and functional properties of starch could be adjusted in order to obtain improved foods with better texture and more stable products, since most of the modified starches reduce the retrogradation rate and the staling. When gluten is take off from formulation, natural GF non-cereal starches can be used as gelling, thickening, adhesion, moisture-retention, stabilizing, film forming, texturizing, and antistaling ingredients. However, other compounds may be added to achieve optimal expansion, integrity and stability of GF breads and pasta. Although many different sources of starch have been studied, as an alternative to cereal ones, the reports give information about properties of granules and scarce results were found in relation to accessibility and application as ingredient for GF products. Therefore, much more efforts must be done to elucidate the suitability of the new starches for GF food production.

References

Abdorreza MN, Robal M, Cheng LH, Tajula AY, Karima AA (2012) Physicochemical, thermal, and rheological properties of acid-hydrolyzed sago (*Metroxylon sagu*) starch. LWT 46:135–141. https://doi.org/10.1016/J.LWT.2011.10.015

Abu JO, Duodu KG, Minnaar A (2006) Effect of γ-irradiation on some physicochemical and thermal properties of cowpea (*Vigna unguiculata* L. Walp) starch. Food Chem 95:386–393. https://doi.org/10.1016/J.FOODCHEM.2005.01.008

Ačkar Đ, Babić J, Šubarić D, Kopjar M, Miličević B (2010) Isolation of starch from two wheat varieties and their modification with epichlorohydrin. Carbohydr Polym 81(1):76–82. https://doi.org/10.1016/j.carbpol.2010.01.058

Affrifah NS, Phillips RD, Saalia FK (2021) Cowpeas: nutritional profile, processing methods and products – a review. Legume Sci 4(3):e131. https://doi.org/10.1002/leg3.131

Aggarwal V, Singh N, Kamboj SS, Brar PS (2004) Some properties of seeds and starches separated from different Indian pea cultivars. Food Chem 85:585–590. https://doi.org/10.1016/J.FOODCHEM.2003.07.036

Aghazadeh M, Karim R, Sultan MT, Paykary M, Johnson SK, Shekarforoush E (2017) Comparison of starch films and effect of different rice starch-based coating formulations on physical properties of walnut during storage time at accelerated temperature. J Food Process Eng 41:e12607. https://doi.org/10.1111/jfpe.12607

Ahmad FB, Williams PA, Doublier JL, Durand S, Buleon A (1999) Physico-chemical characterisation of sago starch. Carbohydr Polym 38:361–370. https://doi.org/10.1016/S0144-8617(98)00123-4

Aleman RS, Paz G, Morris A, Prinyawiwatkul W, Moncada M, King JM (2021) High protein brown rice flour, tapioca starch & potato starch in the development of gluten-free cupcakes. LWT 152:112326. https://doi.org/10.1016/j.lwt.2021.112326

Altuna L, Herrera ML, Foresti ML (2018) Synthesis and characterization of octenyl succinic anhydride modified starches for food applications. A review of recent literature. Food Hydrocoll 80:97–110. https://doi.org/10.1016/j.foodhyd.2018.01.032

Alzate P, Gerschenson L, Flores S (2020) Ultrasound application for production of nano-structured particles from esterified starches to retain potassium sorbate. Carbohydr Polym 247:116759. https://doi.org/10.1016/j.carbpol.2020.116759

Arendt EK, O'Brien CM, Schober T, Gormley TR, Gallagher E (2002) Development of gluten-free cereal products. Farm and Food 12:21–27

Argentine Food Code (2021) Cap XVIII https://www.argentina.gob.ar/anmat/codigoalimentario. Accessed 20 Oct 2022

Arshad NH, Zaman SA, Rawi MH, Sarbini SR (2018) Resistant starch evaluation and in vitro fermentation of lemantak (native sago starch), for prebiotic assessment. Int Food Res J 25:951–957

Ashogbon AO, Akintayo ET, Oladebeye AO, Oluwafemi AD, Akinsola AF, Imanah OE (2021) Developments in the isolation, composition, and physicochemical properties of legume starches. Crit Rev Food Sci 61:2938–2959. https://doi.org/10.1080/10408398.2020.1791048

Azfaralariff A, Fazial FF, Sontanosamy RS, Nazar MF, Lazim AM (2020) Food-grade particle stabilized pickering emulsion using modified sago (*Metroxylon sagu*) starch nanocrystal. J Food Eng 280:109974. https://doi.org/10.1016/J.JFOODENG.2020.109974

Bajaj R, Singh N, Ghumman A, Kaur A, Mishra HN (2021) Effect of high pressure treatment on structural, functional, and *In-Vitro* digestibility of starches from tubers, cereals, and beans. Starch/Staerke. https://doi.org/10.1002/star.202100096

Baxter G, Blanchard C, Zhao J (2004) Effects of prolamin on the textural and pasting properties of rice flour and starch. J Cereal Sci 40(3):205–211. https://doi.org/10.1016/j.jcs.2004.07.004

Bello-Pérez LA, González-Soto RA, Sánchez-Rivero MM, Gutiérrez-Meraz F, Vargas-Torres A (2006) Extrusión de almidones de fuentes no convencionales para la producción de almidón resistente. Agrociencia 40(4):441–448

Bernardo CO, Ascheri JLR, Chávez DWH, Carvalho CWP (2018) Ultrasound assisted extraction of yam (Dioscorea bulbífera) starch: effect on morphology and functional properties. Starch/Stärke 70(5–6):1700185. https://doi.org/10.1002/star.201700185

Birt DF, Boylston T, Hendrich S, Jane JL, Hollis J, Li L, McClelland J, Moore S, Phillips GJ, Rowling M, Schalinske K, Scott MP, Whitley EM (2013) Resistant starch: promise for improving human health. Adv Nutr 4(6):587–601. https://doi.org/10.3945/an.113.004325

Bojarczuk A, Skąpska S, Khaneghah AM, Marszałek K (2022) Health benefits of resistant starch: a review of the literature. J Funct Foods 93:105094. https://doi.org/10.1016/j.jff.2022.105094

Breuninger WF, Piyachomkwan K, Sriroth K (2009) Chapter 12 - Tapioca/Cassava Starch: Production and Use, Editor(s): James BeMiller, Roy Whistler, In Food Science and Technology, Starch (Third Edition), Academic Press, 541–568. ISBN 9780127462752. https://doi.org/10.1016/B978-0-12-746275-2.00012-4

Brunt K, Keizer-Zinsmeester J, Cazemier J, Yntema P (2002) Potato and starch quality in relation to variety, growing location and year. In: *Papers and posters of the 15th Triennial conference of the EAPR*, Hamburg, p. 58.

Buksa K (2018) Extraction and characterization of rye grain starch and its susceptibility to resistant starch formation. Carbohydr Polym 194:184–192. https://doi.org/10.1016/j.carbpol.2018.04.024

Buwalda SJ, Boere KW, Dijkstra PJ, Feijen J, Vermonden T, Hennink WE (2014) Hydrogels in a historical perspective: from simple networks to smart materials. J control release 190:254–273. https://doi.org/10.1016/j.jconrel.2014.03.052

Cabrera-Canales ZE, Velazquez G, Rodríguez-Marín ML, Méndez-Montealvo G, Hernández-Ávila J, Morales-Sánchez E, Gómez-Aldapa CA (2021) Dual modification of achira (Canna indica L) starch and the effect on its physicochemical properties for possible food applications. J Food Sci Technol 58:952–961. https://doi.org/10.1007/s13197-020-04609-w

Campos CA, Gerschenson LN, Flores SK (2011) Development of Edible Films and Coatings with Antimicrobial Activity. Food Bioproc Tech 4(6):849–875. https://doi.org/10.1007/s11947-010-0434-1

Capriles VD, Arêas JAG (2014) Novel approaches in gluten-free breadmaking: interface between food science, nutrition, and health. Compr Rev Food Sci Food Saf 13(5):871–890. https://doi.org/10.1111/1541-4337.12091

Carpenter MA, Shaw M, Cooper RD, Frew TJ, Butler RC, Murray SR, Moya L, Coyne CJ, Timmerman-Vaughan GM (2017) Association mapping of starch chain length distribution and amylose content in pea (*Pisum sativum* L.) using carbohydrate metabolism candidate genes. BMC plant biology 17:1–23. https://doi.org/10.1186/s12870-017-1080-9

Castanha N, Villar J, da Matta Junior MD, dos Anjos CBP, Duarte Augusto PE (2018) Structure and properties of starches from Arracacha (*Arracacia xanthorrhiza*) roots. Int J Biol Macromol 117:1029–1038. https://doi.org/10.1016/j.ijbiomac.2018.06.015

Chakraborty I, Pallen S, Shetty Y, Roy N, Mazumder N (2020) Advanced microscopy techniques for revealing molecular structure of starch granules. Biophys Rev 12(1):105–122. https://doi.org/10.1007/s12551-020-00614-7

Chakraborty I, Mal SS, Paul UC, Rahman M, Mazumder N (2022) An insight into the gelatinization properties influencing the modified starches used in food industry: a review. Food Bioproc Tech 15:1195–1223. https://doi.org/10.1007/s11947-022-02761-z

Chen Z, Sagis L, Legger A, Linssen JPH, Schols HA, Voragen AGJ (2002) Evaluation of Starch Noodles Made from Three Typical Chinese Sweet-potato Starches. J Food Sci 67(9):3342–3347. https://doi.org/10.1111/j.1365-2621.2002.tb09589.x

Chen Z, Schols HA, Voragen AGJ (2003) The use of potato and sweet potato starches affects white salted noodle quality. J Food Sci 68(9):2630–2637. https://doi.org/10.1111/j.1365-2621.2003.tb05781.x

Chen B, Dang L, Zhang X, Fang W, Hou M, Liu T, Wang Z (2017a) Physicochemical properties and micro-structural characteristics in starch from kudzu root as affected by cross-linking. Food Chem 219:93–101. https://doi.org/10.1016/j.foodchem.2016.09.128

Chen Y, Sun X, Zhou X, Hebelstrup KH, Blennow A, Bao J (2017b) Highly phosphorylated functionalized rice starch produced by transgenic rice expressing the potato GWD1 gene. Sci Rep 7:3339. https://doi.org/10.1038/s41598-017-03637-5

Chen H, Hu Z, Liu D, Li C, Liu S (2019) Composition and physicochemical properties of three Chinese Yam (Dioscorea opposita Thunb.) starches: a comparison study. Molecules 24:2973. https://doi.org/10.3390/molecules24162973

Chua SND, Kho EP, Lim SF, Hussain MH (2021) Sago palm (M *etroxylon sagu*) starch yield, influencing factors and estimation from morphological traits. Adv Mater Process Technol:1–23. https://doi.org/10.1080/2374068X.2021.1878702

Chung HJ, Liu Q, Peter Pauls K, Fan MZ, Yada R (2008) *In vitro* starch digestibility, expected glycemic index and some physicochemical properties of starch and flour from common bean (*Phaseolus vulgaris* L.) varieties grown in Canada. Food Res Int 41:869–875. https://doi.org/10.1016/J.FOODRES.2008.03.013

Collado LS, Mabesa LB, Oates CG, Corke H (2001) Bihon-Type Noodles from Heat-Moisture-Treated Sweet Potato Starch. J Food Sci 66(4):604–609. https://doi.org/10.1111/j.1365-2621.2001.tb04608.x

Comino I, de Lourdes MM, Real A, Rodríguez-Herrera A, Barro F, Sousa C (2013) The gluten-free diet: testing alternative cereals tolerated by celiac patients. Nutrients 5(10):4250–4268. https://doi.org/10.3390/nu5104250

Correia PR, Beirão-Da-Costa ML (2012) Starch isolation from chestnut and acorn flours through alkaline and enzymatic methods. Food Bioprod Process 90:309–316. https://doi.org/10.1016/j.fbp.2011.06.005

Correia PMR, Cruz-Lopes L, Beirão-Da-Costa L (2021) Morphology and structure of acorn starches isolated by enzymatic and alkaline methods. Open Agric 6:37–46. https://doi.org/10.1515/opag-2021-0214

Cruz BR, Abraão AS, Lemos AM, Nunes FM (2013) Chemical composition and functional properties of native chestnut starch (*Castanea sativa* Mill). Carbohydr Polym 94:594–602. https://doi.org/10.1016/j.carbpol.2012.12.060

Cui SW (2005) Food carbohydrates: chemistry, physical properties, and applications. CRC press, Boca Raton

de La Montaña Míguelez J, Míguez Bernárdez M, García Queijeiro JM (2004) Composition of varieties of chestnuts from Galicia (Spain). Food Chem 84:401–404. https://doi.org/10.1016/S0308-8146(03)00249-8

Debet MR, Gidley MJ (2007) Why do gelatinized starch granules not dissolve completely? Roles for amylose, protein, and lipid in granule "ghost" integrity. J Agric Food Chem 55:4752–4760. https://doi.org/10.1021/jf070004o

Deng M, Reddy CK, Xu B (2020) Morphological, physico-chemical and functional properties of underutilized starches in China. Int J Biol Macromol 158:648–655. https://doi.org/10.1016/j.ijbiomac.2020.05.031

Díaz A, Dini C, Viña SZ, García MA (2016) Starch extraction process coupled to protein recovery from leguminous tuberous roots (Pachyrhizus ahipa). Carbohydr Polym 152. https://doi.org/10.1016/j.carbpol.2016.07.004

Díaz A, Dini C, Viña SZ, García MA (2019) Fermentation and drying effects on bread-making potential of sour cassava and ahipa starches. Food Res Int 116:620–627. https://doi.org/10.1016/j.foodres.2018.08.081

Díaz-Montes E, Castro-Muñoz R (2021) Edible films and coatings as food-quality preservers: an overview. Foods 10(2):249. https://doi.org/10.3390/foods10020249

Dini C, García MA, Viña SZ (2012) Non-traditional flours: Frontiers between ancestral heritage and innovation. Food Funct 3:606–620. https://doi.org/10.1039/C2FO30036B

Dini C, Doporto MC, García MA, Viña SZ (2013) Nutritional profile and anti-nutrient analyses of Pachyrhizus ahipa roots from different accessions. Food Res Int 54:255–261. https://doi.org/10.1016/j.foodres.2013.07.027

Dini C, Quiroga A, Viña SZ, García MA (2021) Extraction and characterization of proteins from *Pachyrhizus ahipa* roots: an unexploited protein-rich crop. Plant Foods Hum Nutr 76:179–188. https://doi.org/10.1007/s11130-021-00890-y/Published

Donald AM, Kato KL, Perry PA, Waigh TA (2001) Scattering studies of the internal structure of starch granules. Starch/Stärke 53(10):504. https://doi.org/10.1002/1521-379x(200110)53:10<504::aid-star504>3.0.co;2-5

Doporto MC, Mugridge A, García MA, Viña SZ (2011) *Pachyrhizus ahipa* (Wedd.) Parodi roots and flour: biochemical and functional characteristics. Food Chem 126:1670–1678. https://doi.org/10.1016/J.FOODCHEM.2010.12.053

Doporto MC, Dini C, Mugridge A, Viña SZ, García MA (2012) Physicochemical, thermal and sorption properties of nutritionally differentiated flours and starches. J Food Eng 113:569–576. https://doi.org/10.1016/j.jfoodeng.2012.07.021

Doporto MC, Dini C, Viña SZ, García MA (2014) *Pachyrhizus ahipa* roots and starches: composition and functional properties related to their food uses. Starch/Staerke 66:539–548. https://doi.org/10.1002/star.201300196

Doublier JL, Garnier C, Renard D, Sanchez C (2000) Protein–polysaccharide interactions. Curr Opin Colloid Interface Sci 5(3–4):202–214. https://doi.org/10.1016/S1359-0294(00)00054-6

Dufour D, Rolland-Sabaté A, Mina Cordoba HÁ, Luna Melendez JL, Moreno Alzate JL, Pizzaro M, Guilois Dubois S, Sánchez T, Eiver Belalcazar J, Morante N, Tran T, Moreno-Santander M, Vélez-Hernández G, Ceballos H (2022) Native and fermented waxy cassava starch as a novel gluten-free and clean label ingredient for baking and expanded product development. Food Funct 13:9254–9267. https://doi.org/10.1039/D2FO00048B

Dupuis JH, Liu Q (2019) Potato starch: a review of physicochemical, functional and nutritional properties. Am J Potato Res 96:127–138. https://doi.org/10.1007/s12230-018-09696-2

Emmambux MN, Taylor JR (2013) Morphology, physical, chemical, and functional properties of starches from cereals, legumes, and tubers cultivated in Africa: a review. Starch-Stärke 65(9-10):715–729. https://doi.org/10.1002/star.201200263

Expert Market Research (2020). www.expertmarketresearch.com. Accessed 20 Oct 2022

Fabbri ADT, Crosby GA (2016) A review of the impact of preparation and cooking on the nutritional quality of vegetables and legumes. Int J Gastron Food Sci 3:2–11. https://doi.org/10.1016/J.IJGFS.2015.11.001

Fan Y, Picchioni F (2020) Modification of starch: a review on the application of "green" solvents and controlled functionalization. Carbohydr Polym 241:116350. https://doi.org/10.1016/j.carbpol.2020.116350

FAOSTAT (2021) Food and Agriculture Organization of the United Nations (FAO). Statistics division. https://www.fao.org/faostat/en/#data/QCL/visualize. Accessed 20 Oct 2022

Fiorda FA, Soares Jr. MS, da Silva FA, Grosmann MVE, Souto Luciana RF (2013) Microestructure texture and colour of gluten-free pasta made with amaranth flour cassava starch and cassava bagasse LWT - Food Science and Technology 54(1):132–138. https://doi.org/10.1016/j.lwt.2013.04.020

Fonseca LM, Halal SLME, Dias ARG, da Rosa Zavareze E (2021) Physical modification of starch by heat-moisture treatment and annealing and their applications: a review. Carbohydr Polym 274:118665. https://doi.org/10.1016/j.carbpol.2021.118665

Forsyth JL, Shewry PR (2002) Characterization of the major proteins of tubers of yam bean (*Pachyrhizus ahipa*). J Agric Food Chem 50:1939–1944. https://doi.org/10.1021/jf011017j

Fuentes C, Perez-Rea D, Bergenståhl B, Carballo S, Sjöö M, Nilsson L (2019) Physicochemical and structural properties of starch from five Andean crops grown in Bolivia. Int J Biol Macromol 125:829–838. https://doi.org/10.1016/j.ijbiomac.2018.12.120

Gallagher E, Gormley TR, Arendt EK (2004) Recent advances in the formulation of gluten-free cereal-based products. Trends Food Sci Tech 15:143–152. https://doi.org/10.1016/j.tifs.2003.09.012

Genevois CE, de Escalada Pla MF (2021) Soybean by-products and modified cassava starch for improving alveolar structure and quality characteristics of gluten-free bread. Eur Food Res Technol 247:1477–1488. https://doi.org/10.1007/s00217-021-03725-x

Gilet A, Quettier C, Wiatz V, Bricout H, Ferreira M, Rousseau C, Monflier E, Tilloy S (2018) Unconventional media and technologies for starch etherification and esterification. Green Chem 20:1152–1168. https://doi.org/10.1039/C7GC03135A

González LC, Loubes MA, Bertotto MM, Baeza RI, Tolaba MP (2021) Flow behavior and syneresis of ball milled rice starch and their correlations with starch structure. Carbohydr Polym Technol Appl 2:100168. https://doi.org/10.1016/j.carpta.2021.100168

Goren A, Ashlock D, Tetlow IJ (2018) Starch formation inside plastids of higher plants. Protoplasma 255:1855–1876. https://doi.org/10.1007/s00709-018-1259-4

Grace NCF, Henry CJ (2020) The physicochemical characterization of unconventional starches and flours used in Asia. Foods 9:182. https://doi.org/10.3390/foods9020182

Gui Y, Zou F, Zhu Y, Li J, Wang N, Guo L, Cui B (2022) The structural thermal pasting and gel properties of the mixtures of enzyme-treated potato protein and potato starch. LWT 154112882. https://doi.org/10.1016/j.lwt.2021.112882

Guo L, Hu J, Zhou X, Li X, Du X (2016) In vitro digestibility of kudzu starch by using α-amylase and glucoamylase. Starch/Staerke 68:140–150. https://doi.org/10.1002/star.201500213

Guo J, Kong L, Du B, Xu B (2019) Morphological and physicochemical characterization of starches isolated from chestnuts cultivated in different regions of China. Int J Biol Macromol 130:357–368. https://doi.org/10.1016/j.ijbiomac.2019.02.126

Guo K, Bian X, Jia Z, Zhang L, Wei C (2020) Effects of nitrogen level on structural and functional properties of starches from different colored-fleshed root tubers of sweet potato. Int J Biol Macromol 164:3235–3242. https://doi.org/10.1016/j.ijbiomac.2020.08.199

Guo L, Li J, Yuan Y, Gui Y, Zou F, Lu L, Cui B (2021) Structural and functional modification of kudzu starch using α-amylase and transglucosidase. Int J Biol Macromol 169:67–74. https://doi.org/10.1016/j.ijbiomac.2020.12.099

Gupta M, Bawa AS, Semwal AD (2009) Morphological, thermal, pasting, and rheological properties of barley starch and their blends. Int J Food Prop 12(3):587–604. https://doi.org/10.1080/10942910801947763

Hadnađev M, Dapčević-Hadnađev T, Dokić L (2018) Chapter 9 – Functionality of Starch Derivatives in Bakery and Confectionery Products. In: Grumezescu AM, Holban AM (eds) Handbook of food bioengineering, biopolymers for food design. Academic Press, Cambridge, MA, pp 279–311. https://doi.org/10.1016/b978-0-12-811449-0.00009-8

Hernández-Aguirre MA, Islas-Hernández JJ, Sánchez-Pardo ME, Rodríguez-Ambriz SL, Osorio-Díaz P (2019) Response surface methodology for optimization of gluten-free bread made with unripe banana flour. J Food Meas Charact 13(3):1652–1660. https://doi.org/10.1007/s11694-019-00082-y

Hernández-Carmona F, Morales-Matos Y, Lambis-Miranda H, Pasqualino J (2017) Starch extraction potential from plantain peel wastes. J Environ Chem Eng 5(5):4980–4985. https://doi.org/10.1016/j.jece.2017.09.034

Hoover R, Hughes T, Chung HJ, Liu Q (2010) Composition, molecular structure, properties, and modification of pulse starches: a review. Food Res Int 43:399–413. https://doi.org/10.1016/J.FOODRES.2009.09.001

Hosokawa K, Ohishi K, Ikeda T, Inagaki K (2020) Properties of ripe banana flour and application to gluten-free breadmaking. J Food Process Preserv 44(10):e14789. https://doi.org/10.1111/jfpp.14789

Iacovou M, Lim J, Maningat CC, Bogatyrev A, Ly E, Dhital S, Gidley MJ, Shi YC, Muir J, Seib PA (2017) *In vivo* digestibility of cross-linked phosphorylated (RS4) wheat starch in ileostomy subjects. Bioact Carbohydr Diet Fibre 12:25–36. https://doi.org/10.1016/j.bcdf.2017.08.002

Jane J (2009) Chapter 6 – Structural features of starch granules II. In: BeMiller J, Whistler R (eds) Starch: chemistry and technology, 3rd edn. Academic Press, Cambridge, MA, pp 193–237. https://doi.org/10.1016/B978-0-12-746275-2.00006-9

Joly G, Anderstein B (2009) Starches. In: Tarté R (ed) Ingredients in meat products. Springer, New York, pp 25–55. https://doi.org/10.1007/978-0-387-71327-4_2

Karim A (2000) Methods for the study of starch retrogradation. Food Chem 71(1):9–36. https://doi.org/10.1016/s0308-8146(00)00130-8

Karim AA, Tie P-L, Manan DMA, Zaidul ISM (2008) Starch from the sago (*Metroxylon sagu*) palm tree-properties, prospects, and challenges as a new industrial source for food and other uses. Compr Rev Food Sci Food Saf 7:215–228. https://doi.org/10.1111/j.1541-4337.2008.00042.x

Karmakar R, Ban DK, Ghosh U (2014) Comparative study of native and modified starches isolated from conventional and nonconventional sources. Int Food Res J 21(2):597

Kaur B, Ariffin F, Bhat R, Karim AA (2012) Progress in starch modification in the last decade. Food Hydrocoll 26:398–404. https://doi.org/10.1016/j.foodhyd.2011.02.016

Kaur K, Singh G, Singh N (2017) Development and evaluation of gluten free muffins utilizing green banana flour. Bioved 28(2):359–365

Keskin SO, Ali TM, Ahmed J, Shaikh M, Siddiq M, Uebersax MA (2022) Physico-chemical and functional properties of legume protein, starch, and dietary fiber – a review. Legume Sci 4(1):e117. https://doi.org/10.1002/leg3.117

Kim WW, Yoo B (2011) Rheological and thermal effects of galactomannan addition to acorn starch paste. LWT 44:759–764. https://doi.org/10.1016/j.lwt.2010.11.009

Kobayashi S, Schwartz SJ, Lineback DR (1985) Rapid analysis of starch, amylose and amylopectin by high-performance size-exclusion chromatography. J Chromatogr A 319:205–214. https://doi.org/10.1016/s0021-9673(01)90555-2

Kringel DH, el Halal SLM, da Rosa Zavareze E, Dias ARG (2020) Methods for the extraction of roots, tubers, pulses, pseudocereals, and other unconventional starches sources: a review. Starch/Staerke 72:1900234. https://doi.org/10.1002/star.201900234

Krupa U, Rosell CM, Sadowska J, Soral-Śmietana M (2010) Bean starch as ingredient for gluten-free bread. J Food Process Preserv 34:501–518. https://doi.org/10.1111/j.1745-4549.2009.00366.x

Lacerda LD, Leitea DC, da Silveira NP (2019) Relationships between enzymatic hydrolysis conditions and properties ofrice porous starches. J Cereal Sci 89:102819. https://doi.org/10.1016/j.jcs.2019.102819

Lagunes-Delgado C, Agama-Acevedo E, Patiño-Rodríguez O, Martinez MM, Bello-Pérez LA (2022) Recovery of mango starch from unripe mango juice. LWT 153:112514. https://doi.org/10.1016/j.lwt.2021.112514

Lan X, Xie S, Xie F, Liu X, Wu J, Wang Z (2016a) The effect of thermal and enzymatic degradation on the physicochemical properties and in vitro digestibility of canna starch. Starch/Staerke 68:389–398. https://doi.org/10.1002/star.201500118

Lan X, Xie S, Wu J, Xie F, Liu X, Wanga Z (2016b) Thermal and enzymatic degradation induced ultrastructure changes in canna starch: Further insights into short-range and long-range structural orders. Food Hydrocoll 58:335–342. https://doi.org/10.1016/j.foodhyd.2016.02.018

Lawal OS, Adebowale KO (2005) Physicochemical characteristics and thermal properties of chemically modified jack bean (*Canavalia ensiformis*) starch. Carbohydr Polym 60:331–341. https://doi.org/10.1016/J.CARBPOL.2005.01.011

Le Corre D, Bras J, Dufresne A (2010) Starch nanoparticles: a review. Biomacromolecules 11(5):1139–1153. https://doi.org/10.1021/bm901428y

Lee HC, Htoon AK, Paterson JL (2007) Alkaline extraction of starch from Australian lentil cultivars Matilda and Digger optimised for starch yield and starch and protein quality. Food Chem *102*:551–559. https://doi.org/10.1016/j.foodchem.2006.03.042

Leidi EO, Altamirano AM, Mercado G, Rodriguez JP, Ramos A, Alandia G, Sørensen M, Jacobsen S-E (2018) Andean roots and tubers crops as sources of functional foods. J Funct Foods 51:86–93. https://doi.org/10.1016/J.JFF.2018.10.007

Li C, Hu Y (2022) *In vitro* and animal models to predict the glycemic index value of carbohydrate-containing foods. Trends Food Sci Technol 120:16–24. https://doi.org/10.1016/j.tifs.2021.12.031

Li Z, Wei C (2020) Morphology, structure, properties and applications of starch ghost: a review. Int J Biol Macromol. https://doi.org/10.1016/j.ijbiomac.2020.09.077

Li H, Cui B, Janaswamy S, Guo L (2019a) Structural and functional modifications of kudzu starch modified by branching enzyme. Int J Food Prop 22:952–966. https://doi.org/10.1080/10942912.2019.1619576

Li L, Yuan TZ, Setia R, Bharathi Raja R, Zhang B, Ai Y (2019b) Characteristics of pea, lentil and faba bean starches isolated from air-classified flours in comparison with commercial starches. Food Chem 276:599–607. https://doi.org/10.1016/J.FOODCHEM.2018.10.064

Li Y, Shabani KI, Liu H, Guo Q, Liu X (2020) Structural, physicochemical and rheological properties of a novel native starch obtained from Rhizoma Gastrodiae. Food Struct 25:100148. https://doi.org/10.1016/j.foostr.2020.100148

Li D, Fu X, Mu S, Fei T, Zhao Y, Fu J, Li Z (2021) Potato starch modified by Streptococcus thermophilus GtfB enzyme has low viscoelastic and slowly digestible properties. Int J Biol Macromol 183:1248–1256. https://doi.org/10.1016/j.ijbiomac.2021.05.032

Lin Y, Lu Y, Song Z, Huang D (2018) Characterizations of the endogenous starch hydrolase inhibitors in acorns of Quercus fabri Hance. Food Chem 258:111–117. https://doi.org/10.1016/j.foodchem.2018.03.001

Lin D, Zhou W, Yang Z, Zhong Y, Xing B, Wu Z, Li S (2019) Study on physicochemical properties, digestive properties and application of acetylated starch in noodles. Int J Biol Macromol 128:948–956. https://doi.org/10.1016/j.ijbiomac.2019.01.176

Lindeboom N, Chang PR, Tyler RT (2004) Analytical, biochemical and physicochemical aspects of starch granule size, with emphasis on small granule starches: a review. Starch/Stärke 56(34):89–99. https://doi.org/10.1002/star.200300218

Liu C, Wang S, Chang X, Wang S (2015) Structural and functional properties of starches from Chinese chestnuts. Food Hydrocoll 43:568–576. https://doi.org/10.1016/j.foodhyd.2014.07.014

Liu Y, Xie H, Shi M (2016) Effect of ethanol–water solution on the crystallization of short chain amylose from potato starch. Starch/Stärke 68:683–690. https://doi.org/10.1002/star.201500300

Liu X, Mu T, Sun H, Zhang M, Chen J, Fauconnier ML (2018) Influence of different hydrocolloids on dough thermo-mechanical properties and in vitro starch digestibility of gluten-free steamed bread based on potato flour. Food Chem 239:1064–1074. https://doi.org/10.1016/j.foodchem.2017.07

Liu R, Sun W, Zhang Y, Huang Z, Hu H, Zhao M (2019) Preparation of starch dough using damaged cassava starch induced by mechanical activation to develop staple foods: application in crackers. Food Chem 271:284–290. https://doi.org/10.1016/j.foodchem.2018.07.202

Liu XX, Liu HM, Fan LY, Qin GY, Wang XD (2020) Effect of various drying pretreatments on the structural and functional properties of starch isolated from Chinese yam (*Dioscorea opposita* Thumb.). Int J Biol Macromol 153:1299–1309. https://doi.org/10.1016/j.ijbiomac.2019.10.265

Liu D, Ma L, Zhou Z, Liang Q, Xie Q, Ou K, Liu Y, Su Y (2021) Starch and mineral element accumulation during root tuber expansion period of Pueraria thomsonii Benth. Food Chem 343:128445. https://doi.org/10.1016/j.foodchem.2020.128445

Liu W, Zhang Y, Wang R, Li J, Pana W, Zhang X, Xiao W, Wen H, Xie J (2022) Chestnut starch modification with dry heat treatment and addition of xanthan gum: gelatinization, structural and functional properties. Food Hydrocoll 124. https://doi.org/10.1016/j.foodhyd.2021.107205

López Calderón R (2017) Physicochemical characterization of starch from sweet potato (*ipomea batatas*), arracacha (*Arracacia xanthorriza* Bancroft.) and oca (*Oxalis tuberosa*). Agroindustrial Engineering Thesis. National University of Trujillo. http://dspace.unitru.edu.pe/handle/UNITRU/9774

López OV, Viña SZ, Pachas ANA, Sisterna MN, Rohatsch PH, Mugridge A, Fassola HE, García MA (2010) Composition and food properties of *Pachyrhizus ahipa* roots and starch. Int J Food Sci Technol 45:223–233. https://doi.org/10.1111/j.1365-2621.2009.02125.x

Lovera M, Pérez E, Laurentin A (2017) Digestibility of starches isolated from stem and root tubers of arracacha, cassava, cush–cush yam, potato and taro. Carbohydr Polym 176:50–55. https://doi.org/10.1016/j.carbpol.2017.08.049

Lu H, Tian Y (2021) Nanostarch: preparation, modification, and application in pickering emulsions. J Agric Food Chem 69(25):6929–6942. https://doi.org/10.1021/acs.jafc.1c01244

Lu Z, Donner E, Liu Q (2021) Development and characterisation of gluten-free potato bread. Int J Food Sci 56(6):3085–3098. https://doi.org/10.1111/ijfs.14952

Maherawati, Cahyanto MN, Pranoto Y, Utami T (2017) Effect of Cellulase Addition on Linamarin Hydrolysis in Cassava (*Manihot esculenta*) Slurry. Pak J Nutr 16:914–920. https://doi.org/10.3923/pjn.2017.914.920

Mahmood K, Kamilah H, Shang PL, Sulaiman S, Ariffin F, Alias AK (2017) A review: Interaction of starch/non-starch hydrocolloid blending and the recent food applications. Food Biosci 19(1):110–120. https://doi.org/10.1016/j.fbio.2017.05.006

Mahmoud RM, Yousif EI, Gadallah MGE, Alawneh AR (2013) Formulations and quality characterization of gluten-free Egyptian balady flat bread. Ann Agric Sci 58(1):19–25. https://doi.org/10.1016/j.aoas.2013.01.004

Majzoobi M, Farahnaky A (2020) Granular cold-water swelling starch; properties, preparation and applications, a review. Food Hydrocoll 106393. https://doi.org/10.1016/j.foodhyd.2020.106393

Makroo HA, Naqash S, Saxena J, Sharma S, Majid D, Dar BN (2021) Recovery and characteristics of starches from unconventional sources and their potential applications: a review. Appl Food Biotechnol 1(1):100001. https://doi.org/10.1016/j.afres.2021.100001

Malgor M, Viña SZ, Dini C (2019) Root starches enriched with proteins and phenolics from *Pachyrhizus ahipa* roots as gluten-free ingredients for baked goods. Int J Food Sci Tech 55:1763–1772. https://doi.org/10.1111/ijfs.14457

Malumba P, Doran L, Zanmenou W, Odjo S, Katanga J, Blecker C, Béra F (2017) Morphological, structural and functional properties of starch granules extracted from the tubers and seeds of Sphenostylis stenocarpa. Carbohydr Polym 178:286–294. https://doi.org/10.1016/j.carbpol.2017.09.013

Maningat CC, Seib PA (2013) RS4-type resistant starch: chemistry, functionality and health benefits. In: Shi YC, Maningat CC (eds) Resistant starch: sources, applications and health benefits, 1st edn. Wiley, New York, pp 43–77. https://doi.org/10.1002/9781118528723.ch03

Manthey FA (2016) Starch: sources and processing. Encycl Food Health:160–164. https://doi.org/10.1016/B978-0-12-384947-2.00658-9

Martins A, Beninca C, Bet CD et al (2020) Ultrasonic modification of purple taro starch (*Colocasia esculenta* B. Tini): structural, psychochemical and thermal properties. J Therm Anal Calorim 142:819–828. https://doi.org/10.1007/s10973-020-09298-3

Mason WR (2009) Starch use in foods. Starch. https://doi.org/10.1016/B978-0-12-746275-2.00020-3

Masure HG, Fierens E, Delcour JA (2016) Current and forward looking experimental approaches in gluten-free bread making research. J Cereal Sci 67:92–111. https://doi.org/10.1016/j.jcs.2015.09.009

McCleary BV (2013) Measurement of resistant starch and incorporation of resistant starch into dietary fibre measurements. In: Shi YC, Maningat CC (eds) Resistant starch: sources, applications and health benefits, 1st edn. Wiley, New York, pp 131–144. https://doi.org/10.1002/9781118528723.ch07

Mendez-Montealvo G, Velazquez G, Fonseca-Florido HA, Morales-Sanchez E, Solera A (2022) Insights on the acid hydrolysis of achira (Canna edulis) starch: crystalline and double-helical structure changes impacting functionality. LWT 153:112509. https://doi.org/10.1016/j.lwt.2021.112509

Menon R, Padmaja G, Jyothi AN, Asha V, Sajeev MS (2016) Gluten-free starch noodles from sweet potato with reduced starch digestibility and enhanced protein content. J Food Sci Technol 53(9):3532–3542. https://doi.org/10.1007/s13197-016-2330-9

Mesa E, Manjarres-Pinzon K, Rodriguez-Sandoval E (2019) Gluten-free cheese bread from frozen dough: effect of modified cassava starch. Food Sci Technol 39(Suppl. 2):654–661. https://doi.org/10.1590/fst.30118

Milde LB, Ramallo LA, Puppo MC (2012) Gluten-free bread based on tapioca starch: texture and sensory studies. Food Bioprocess Technol 5:888–896. https://doi.org/10.1007/s11947-010-0381-x

Milde LB, Chigal PS, Olivera JE, González KG (2020) Incorporation of xanthan gum to gluten-free pasta with cassava starch. Physical, textural and sensory attributes. LWT 131:109674. https://doi.org/10.1016/j.lwt.2020.109674

Milde LB, Rivero DA, Chigal PS, Zubreski E, Chade M, Brumovsky LA (2021) Changes in the physical, textural and chemical properties of the enriched pasta elaborated with cassava starch. Int J Gastron Food Sci 25:100396. https://doi.org/10.1016/j.ijgfs.2021.100396

Molavi H, Razavi SMA, Farhoosh R (2018) Impact of hydrothermal modifications on the physicochemical, morphology, crystallinity, pasting and thermal properties of acorn starch. Food Chem 245:385–393. https://doi.org/10.1016/j.foodchem.2017.10.117

Molenda M, Stasiak M, Horabik J, Fornal J, Blaszczak W, Ornowski A (2006) Microstructure and mechanical parameters of five types of starch. Pol J Food Nutr Sci 15(2):161–168

Moorthy SN (2002) Physicochemical and functional properties of tropical tuber starches: a review. Starch/Stärke 54(12):559–592. https://doi.org/10.1002/1521-379x(200212)54:12<559::aid-star2222559>3.0.co;2-f

Moorthy SN, Sajeev MS, Anish RJ (2018) Functionality of tuber starches. In: Starch in food: structure, function and applications, 2nd edn. Elsevier Inc., pp 421–508

Moreira R, Chenlo F, Arufe S (2015) Starch transitions of different gluten free flour doughs determined by dynamic thermal mechanical analysis and differential scanning calorimetry. Carbohydr Polym 127:160–167. https://doi.org/10.1016/j.carbpol.2015.03.062

Morikawa K, Nishinari K (2000) Effects of concentration dependence of retrogradation behaviour of dispersions for native and chemically modified potato starch. Food Hydrocoll 14:395–401. https://doi.org/10.1016/S0268-005X(00)00021-7

Murphy P (2000) Starch. In: Phillips GO, Williams PA (eds) Handbook of hydrocolloids. CRC Press, Boca Raton, pp 41–46

Mustafa Kamal M, Baini R, Mohamaddan S, Selaman OS, Ahmad Zauzi N, Rahman MR, Abdul Rahman N, Chong KH, Atan MF, Abdul Samat NAS, Taib SNL, Othman AK (2017) Effect of temperature to the properties of sago starch. IOP Conf Ser Mater Sci Eng 206:012039. https://doi.org/10.1088/1757-899X/206/1/012039

Na JH, Jeong GA, Park HJ, Lee CJ (2021) Impact of esterification with malic acid on the structural characteristics and in vitro digestibilities of different starches. Int J Biol Macromol 174:540–548. https://doi.org/10.1016/j.ijbiomac.2021.01.220

Nagar CK, Dash SK, Rayaguru K, Pal US, Nedunchezhiyan M (2021) Isolation, characterization, modification and uses of taro starch: a review. Int J Biol Macromol 192:574–589. https://doi.org/10.1016/j.ijbiomac.2021.10.041

Naqash F, Gani A, Gani A, Masoodi FA (2017) Gluten-free baking: combating the challenges – a review. Trends Food Sci Technol 66:98–107. https://doi.org/10.1016/j.tifs.2017.06.004

Nemar F, Dilmi Bouras A, Koiche M, Assal N-E, Mezaini A, Prodhomme J (2015) Bread quality substituted by potato starch instead of wheat flour. Ital J Food Sci 27:345–350. https://doi.org/10.14674/1120-1770/ijfs.v277

Nindjin C, Amani GN, Sindic M (2011) Effect of blend levels on composite wheat doughs performance made from yam and cassava native starches and bread quality. Carbohydr Polym 86:1637–1645. https://doi.org/10.1016/J.CARBPOL.2011.06.076

Nip WK, Whitaker CS, Vargo D (2007) Application of taro flour in cookie formulations. Int J Food Sci Technol 29(4):463–468. https://doi.org/10.1111/j.1365-2621.1994.tb02088.x

Nugent AP (2005) Health properties of resistant starch. Nutrition Bulletin 30:27–54. https://doi.org/10.1111/j.1467-3010.2005.00481.x

Nyembwe PM, de Kock HL, Taylor JRN (2018) Potential of defatted marama flour-cassava starch composites to produce functional gluten-free bread-type dough. LWT 92:429–434. https://doi.org/10.1016/j.lwt.2018.02.062

Oh SM, Hy K, Bae JE, Ye S-J, Kim B-Y, Choi HD, Choi H-W, Baik M-Y (2019) Physicochemical and retrogradation properties of modified chestnut starches. Food Sci Biotechnol 28:1723–1731. https://doi.org/10.1007/s10068-019-00622-8

Olawoye B, Gbadamosi SO (2020) Sensory profiling and mapping of gluten-free cookies made from blends Cardaba banana flour and starch. J Food Process Preserv 44(9):e14643. https://doi.org/10.1111/jfpp.14643

Onyango C, Unbehend G, Lindhauer MG (2009) Effect of cellulose-derivatives and emulsifiers on creep-recovery and crumb properties of gluten-free bread prepared from sorghum and gelatinised cassava starch. Food Res Int 42:949–955. https://doi.org/10.1016/j.foodres.2009.04.011

Onyango C, Mewa EA, Mutahi AW, Okoth MW (2013) Effect of heat-moisture-treated cassava starch and amaranth malt on the quality of sorghum-cassava-amaranth bread. Afr J Food Sci 7(5):80–86. https://doi.org/10.5897/AJFS2012.0612

Opara L (2003) Crop management and postharvest handling of horticultural products. In: Dris R, Niskanen R, Mohan Jain S (eds) Crop management and postharvest handling of horticultural products, vol II. Science Publishers Inc., Enfield, pp 381–406

Otálora González CM, Flores SK, Basanta MF, Gerschenson LN (2020) Effect of beetroot (*Beta vulgaris* L. *var conditiva*) fiber filler and corona treatment on cassava starch films properties. Food Packag Shelf Life 26:100605. https://doi.org/10.1016/j.fpsl.2020.100605

Othman Z, Hassan O, Hashim K (2015) Physicochemical and thermal properties of gamma-irradiated sago (*Metroxylon sagu*) starch. Radiat Phys Chem 109:48–53. https://doi.org/10.1016/J.RADPHYSCHEM.2014.12.003

Pasqualone A, Caponio F, Summo C, Paradiso VM, Bottega G, Pagani MA (2010) Gluten-free bread making trials from cassava (*Manihot Esculenta* Crantz) Flour and sensory evaluation of the final product. Int J Food Prop 13(3):562–573. https://doi.org/10.1080/10942910802713172

Perera A, Meda V, Tyler RT (2010) Resistant starch: a review of analytical protocols for determining resistant starch and of factors affecting the resistant starch content of foods. Food Res Int 43(8):1959–1974. https://doi.org/10.1016/j.foodres.2010.06.003

Pérez S, Bertoft E (2010) The molecular structures of starch components and their contribution to the architecture of starch granules: a comprehensive review. Starch/Stärke 62(8):389–420. https://doi.org/10.1002/star.201000013

Pinzon MI, Sanchez LT, Villa CC (2020) Chemical, structural, and thermal characterization of starches from four yellow Arracacha (*Arracacia xanthorriza*) roots produced in Colombia. Heliyon 6:e04763. https://doi.org/10.1016/j.heliyon.2020.e04763

Przetaczek-Rożnowska I, Dyrek K, Fortuna T, Wenda E, Bidzińska E, Jędrszczyk E (2018) Thermal properties and free radicals generation in starch isolated from pumpkin fruits. Int J Biol Macromol 108:1248–1254. https://doi.org/10.1016/j.ijbiomac.2017.11.037

Punia Bangar S, Kumar M, Whiteside WS (2021) Mango seed starch: a sustainable and eco-friendly alternative to increasing industrial requirements. Int J Biol Macromol. https://doi.org/10.1016/j.ijbiomac.2021.05.157

Punia Bangar S, Whiteside WS, Singh A, Ozogul F, Gupta A, Gahlawat SK (2022a) Properties, preparation methods, and application of sour starches in the food. Trends Food Sci Technol 121:44–58. https://doi.org/10.1016/j.tifs.2022.01.029

Punia Bangar S, Ashogbon AO, Singh A, Chaudhary V, Whiteside WS (2022b) Enzymatic modification of starch: a green approach for starch applications. Carbohydr Polym 119265. https://doi.org/10.1016/j.carbpol.2022.119265

Rahman MH, Zhang M, Sun HN, Mu TH (2022) Comparative study of thermo-mechanical, rheological, and structural properties of gluten-free model doughs from high hydrostatic pressure treated maize, potato, and sweet potato starches. Int J Biol Macromol 204:725–733. https://doi.org/10.1016/j.ijbiomac.2022.01.164

Rasper VF (1993) Dough rheology and physical testing of dough. Adv Baking Technol:107–133. https://doi.org/10.1007/978-1-4899-7256-9_5

Reddy CK, Luan F, Xu B (2017) Morphology, crystallinity, pasting, thermal and quality characteristics of starches from adzuki bean (*Vigna angularis* L.) and edible kudzu (*Pueraria thomsonii* Benth). Int J Biol Macromol 105:354–362. https://doi.org/10.1016/j.ijbiomac.2017.07.052

Ribeiro Oliveira A, Chaves Ribeiro AE, Gondim ÍC, dos Santos EA, de Oliveira ER, Mendes Coutinho GS, Soares Soares MJ, Caliari M (2021) Isolation and characterization of yam (Dioscorea alata L.) starch from Brazil. LWT 149:111843. https://doi.org/10.1016/j.lwt.2021.111843

Rodrigues Ferreira SM, de Mello AP, de Caldas Rosa dos Anjos M, Krüger CCH, Azoubel PM, de Oliveira Alves MA (2016) Utilization of sorghum, rice, corn flours with potato starch for the preparation of gluten-free pasta. Food Chem 191:147–151. https://doi.org/10.1016/j.foodchem.2015.04.085

Roman L, Sahagun M, Gomez M, Martinez MM (2019a) Nutritional and physical characterization of sugar-snap cookies: effect of banana starch in native and molten states. Food Funct 10(2):616–624. https://doi.org/10.1039/c8fo02266f

Roman L, Gomez M, Hamaker BR, Martinez MM (2019b) Banana starch and molecular shear fragmentation dramatically increase structurally driven slowly digestible starch in fully gelatinized bread crumb. Food Chem 274:664–671. https://doi.org/10.1016/j.foodchem.2018.09.023

Roman L, Reguilon MP, Martinez MM, Gomez M (2020) The effects of starch cross-linking, stabilization and pre-gelatinization at reducing gluten-free bread staling. LWT 2020:109908. https://doi.org/10.1016/j.lwt.2020.109908

Romano A, Gallo V, Ferranti P, Masi P (2021) Lentil flour: nutritional and technological properties, *in vitro* digestibility and perspectives for use in the food industry. Curr Opin Food Sci 40:157–167. https://doi.org/10.1016/J.COFS.2021.04.003

Ronda F, Gómez M, Caballero PA et al (2009) Improvement of quality of gluten-free layer cakes. Food Sci Technol Int 15:193–202. https://doi.org/10.1177/1082013208105170

Rożnowski J, Fortuna T, Przetaczek-Rożnowska I, Łabanowska M, Bączkowicz M, Kurdziel M, Nowak K (2014) Effect of enriching potato and corn starch with iron ions on selected functional properties. Starch-Stärke 66(11–12):1049–1059. https://doi.org/10.1002/star.201400070

Rübsam H, Krottenthaler M, Gastl M, Becker T (2012) An overview of separation methods in starch analysis: the importance of size exclusion chromatography and field flow fractionation. Starch– Stärke 64(9):683–695. https://doi.org/10.1002/star.201100188

Sajilata MG, Singhal R, Kulkarni P (2006) Resistant starch: a review. Compr Rev Food Sci F 5:1–17

Salazar D, Arancibia M, Ocaña I, Rodríguez-Maecker R, Bedón M, López-Caballero ME, Montero MP (2021) Characterization and technological potential of underutilized ancestral andean crop flours from Ecuador. Agronomy 11(9):1693. https://doi.org/10.3390/agronomy11091693

Saleh M, Ajo R, Al-Ismail K, Ondier G (2016) Effects of hydrocolloids on acorn starch physical properties. Starch/Staerke 68:1169–1179. https://doi.org/10.1002/star.201500304

Sancho RAS, Souza JDRP, de Lima FA, Pastore GM (2017) Evaluation of oligosaccharide profiles in selected cooked tubers and roots subjected to in vitro digestion. LWT 76:270–277. https://doi.org/10.1016/J.LWT.2016.07.046

Santacruz S, Koch K, Svensson E, Ruales J, Eliasson AC (2002) Three underutilised sources of starch from the Andean region in Ecuador Part I. Physico-chemical characterisation. Carbohydr Polym 49:63–70. https://doi.org/10.1016/S0144-8617(01)00305-8

Schamne C, Dutcosky SD, Demiate IM (2010) Obtention and characterization of gluten-free baked products. Cienc Tecnol Aliment 30(3):741–750

Schmiele M, Sampaio UM (2019) Chapter 1 – Basic principles: composition and properties of starch. In: Clerici MTPS, Schmiele M (eds) Starches for food application. Academic Press, Cambridge, MA, pp 1–22. https://doi.org/10.1016/B978-0-12-809440-2.00001-0

Sciarini LS, Rolland-Sabaté A, Guilois S, Decaen P, Leroy E, Le Bail P (2015) Understanding the destructuration of starch in water-ionic liquid mixtures. Green Chem 17(1):291–299. https://doi.org/10.1039/c4gc01248h

Semeijn C, Buwalda PL (2018) Chapter 9 – Potato starch. In: Sjöö M, Nilsson L (eds) Starch in food, 2nd edn. Woodhead Publishing, Sawston, pp 353–372. https://doi.org/10.1016/b978-0-08-100868-3.00009-3

Setiarto RHB, Kusumaningrum HD, Jenie BSL, Khusniati T, Widhyastuti N, Ramadhani I (2020) Microstructure and physicochemical characteristics of modified taro starch after annealing, autoclaving-cooling and heat moisture treatment. Food Res 4:1226–1233. https://doi.org/10.26656/FR.2017.4(4).079

Shen S, Hou H, Ding C, Bing DJ, Lu ZX (2016) Protein content correlates with starch morphology, composition and physicochemical properties in field peas. Can J Plant Sci 96:404–412. https://doi.org/10.1139/cjps-2015-0231

Shi X, Bemiller JN (2002) Effects of food gums on viscosities of starch suspensions during pasting. Carbohydr Polym 50:7–18. https://doi.org/10.1016/s0144-8617(01)00369-1

Shimelis EA, Meaza M, Rakshit SK (2006) Physico-chemical properties, pasting behaviorand functional characteristics of flours and starches from improved bean (*Phaseolusvulgaris* L.) varieties grown in East Africa. Agric Eng Int 8:1–19

Sigüenza-Andrés T, Gallego C, Gómez M (2021) Can cassava improve the quality of gluten free breads? LWT 149:111923. https://doi.org/10.1016/j.lwt.2021.111923

Silva Nykänen VP, Härkönen O, Nykänen A, Hiekkataipale P, Ruokolainen J, Ikkala O (2014) An efficient and stable star-shaped plasticizer for starch: cyclic phosphazene with hydrogen bonding aminoethoxy ethanol side chains. Green Chem 16(9):4339–4350. https://doi.org/10.1039/c4gc00794h

Silva E, Birkenhake M, Scholten E, Sagis LMC, Van der Linden E (2013) Controlling rheology and structure of sweet potato starch noodles with high broccoli powder content by hydrocolloids. Food Hydrocoll 30(1):42–52. https://doi.org/10.1016/j.foodhyd.2012.05.002

Singh J, Kaur L, McCarthy OJ (2007) Factors influencing the physico-chemical, morphological, thermal and rheological properties of some chemically modified starches for food applications – a review. Food Hydrocoll 21:1–22. https://doi.org/10.1016/j.foodhyd.2006.02.006

Singh J, Colussi R, McCarthy OJ, Kaur L (2016) Potato starch and its modification. In: Singh J, Kaur L (eds) Advances in potato chemistry and technology, 2nd edn. Academic Press, Amsterdam, pp 195–247. https://doi.org/10.1016/B978-0-12-800002-1.00008-X

Singh R, Kaur S, Aggarwal P (2021) Exploration of potato starches from non-commercial cultivars in ready to cook instant non cereal, non glutinous pudding mix. LWT 150:111966. https://doi.org/10.1016/j.lwt.2021.111966

Singla D, Singh A, Dhull SB, Kumar P, Malik T, Kumar P (2020) Taro starch: isolation, morphology, modification and novel applications concern – a review. Int J Biol Macromol 163:1283–1290. https://doi.org/10.1016/j.ijbiomac.2020.07.093

Šmídová Z, Rysová J (2022) Gluten-free bread and bakery products technology. Foods 11(3):480. https://doi.org/10.3390/foods11030480

Soison B, Jangchud K, Jangchud A, Harnsilawat T, Piyachomkwan K (2015) Characterization of starch in relation to flesh colors of sweet potato varieties. Int Food Res J 22(6):2302–2308

Soni PL, Sharma H, Dun D, Gharia MM (1993) Physicochemical properties of Quercus leucotnchophora (Oak) starch. Starch/Stärke 45:127–130. https://doi.org/10.1002/star.19930450403

Stevenson DG, Jane JL, Inglett GE (2007) Characterisation of jícama (Mexican potato) (*Pachyrhizus erosus* L. Urban) starch from Taproots grown in USA and Mexico. Starch/Staerke 59:132–140. https://doi.org/10.1002/star.200600596

Sun H, Fan J, Tian Z, Ma L, Meng Y, Yang Z, Zeng X, Liu X, Kang L, Nan X (2022) Effects of treatment methods on the formation of resistant starch in purple sweet potato. Food Chem 367:130580. https://doi.org/10.1016/j.foodchem.2021.130580

Swinkels JJM (1985) Composition and properties of commercial native starches. Starch/Stärke 37(1):1–5. https://doi.org/10.1002/star.19850370102

Tagliapietra BL, Felisberto MHF, Sanches EA, Campelo PH, Clerici MTPS (2021) Nonconventional starch sources. Curr Opin Food Sci 39:93–102. https://doi.org/10.1016/j.cofs.2020.11.011

Taib M, Bouyazza L (2021) Composition, physicochemical properties, and uses of acorn starch. J Chem 2021:9988570. https://doi.org/10.1155/2021/9988570

Tan X, Tan X, Li E, Bai Y, Nguyen TTL, Gilbert RG (2021) Starch molecular fine structure is associated with protein composition in chickpea seed. Carbohydr Polym 272:118489. https://doi.org/10.1016/J.CARBPOL.2021.118489

Tayade R, Kulkarni KP, Jo H, Song JT, Lee J-D (2019) Insight Into the prospects for the improvement of seed starch in legume – a review. Front Plant Sci 10:1213. https://doi.org/10.3389/fpls.2019.01213

Tester RF, Karkalas J, Qi X (2004) Starch – composition, fine structure and architecture. J Cereal Sci 39(2):151–165. https://doi.org/10.1016/j.jcs.2003.12.001

Tong C, Ru W, Wu L et al (2020) Fine structure and relationships with functional properties of pigmented sweet potato starches. Food Chem 311:126011. https://doi.org/10.1016/j.foodchem.2019.126011

Vamadevan V, Bertoft E (2015) Structure-function relationships of starch components. A review. Starch/Stärke 67:55–68. https://doi.org/10.1002/star.201400188

Vamadevan V, Blennow A, Buléon A, Goldstein A, Bertoft E (2018) Distinct properties and structures among B-crystalline starch granules. Starch/Staerke 70. https://doi.org/10.1002/star.201700240

van der Sman RGM, Broeze J (2013) Structuring of indirectly expanded snacks based on potato ingredients: a review. J Food Eng 114:413–425. https://doi.org/10.1016/j.jfoodeng.2012.09.001

Versino F, Lopez OV, Garcia MA, Zaritzky NE (2016) Starch-based films and food coatings: an overview. Starch-Stärke 68(11–12):1026–1037. https://doi.org/10.1002/star.201600095

Villanueva M, Pérez-Quirce S, Collar C, Ronda F (2018) Impact of acidification and protein fortification on rheological and thermal properties of wheat, corn, potato and tapioca starch-based gluten-free bread doughs. LWT 96:446–454. https://doi.org/10.1016/j.lwt.2018.05.069

Wang S, Guo P (2020) Botanical Sources of Starch. In: Wang S (eds) Starch Structure, Functionality and Application in Foods. Springer, Singapore. https://doi.org/10.1007/978-981-15-0622-2_2

Wang N, Maximiuk L, Toews R (2012) Pea starch noodles: effect of processing variables on characteristics and optimisation of twin-screw extrusion process. Food Chem 133(3):742–753. https://doi.org/10.1016/j.foodchem.2012.01.087

Wang N, Warkentin TD, Vandenberg B, Bing DJ (2014) Physicochemical properties of starches from various pea and lentil varieties, and characteristics of their noodles prepared by high temperature extrusion. Food Res Int 55:119–127. https://doi.org/10.1016/j.foodres.2013.10.043

Wang S, Li C, Copeland L, Niu Q, Wang S (2015) Starch retrogradation: a comprehensive review. C Compr Rev Food Sci Food Saf 14(5):568–585. https://doi.org/10.1111/1541-4337.12143

Wang M, Wu Y, Liu Y, Ouyang J (2020a) Effect of ultrasonic and microwave dual-treatment on the physicochemical properties of chestnut starch. Polymers 12:1718. https://doi.org/10.3390/POLYM12081718

Wang X, Hu A, Zheng J, Li L, Li L, Li Y (2020b) Physicochemical properties and structure of annealed sweet potato starch: effects of enzyme and ultrasound. Starch/Staerke 72:1900247. https://doi.org/10.1002/star.201900247

Wang Z, Mhaske P, Farahnaky A, Kasapis S, Majzoobi M (2022) Cassava starch: chemical modification and its impact on functional properties and digestibility, a review. Food Hydrocoll 129:107542. https://doi.org/10.1016/j.foodhyd.2022.107542

Wani IA, Sogi DS, Hamdani AM, Gani A, Bhat NA, Shah A (2016) Isolation, composition, and physicochemical properties of starch from legumes: a review. Starch/Staerke 68:834–845. https://doi.org/10.1002/star.201600007

Waterschoot J, Gomand SV, Fierens E, Delcour JA (2014) Production, structure, physicochemical and functional properties of maize, cassava, wheat, potato and rice starches. Starch/Stärke 67(1–2):14–29. https://doi.org/10.1002/star.201300238

Wieser H (2007) Chemistry of gluten proteins. Food Microbiol 24(2):115–119. https://doi.org/10.1016/j.fm.2006.07.004

Witczak M, Juszczak L, Ziobro R, Korus J (2012) Influence of modified starches on properties of gluten-free dough and bread. Part I: Rheological and thermal properties of gluten-free dough. Food Hydrocoll 28(2):353–360. https://doi.org/10.1016/j.foodhyd.2012.01.009

Witczak M, Ziobro R, Juszczak L, Korus J (2016) Starch and starch derivatives in gluten-free systems – a review. J Cereal Sci 67:46–57. https://doi.org/10.1016/j.jcs.2015.07.007

Witczak M, Korus J, Ziobro R, Juszczak L (2019) Waxy starch as dough component and anti-staling agent in gluten-free bread. LWT 99:476–482. https://doi.org/10.1016/j.lwt.2018.10.009

Woltjes JR, Meima HR, Buwalda PL (2004) Composition based on cross-linked starch and depolymerized starch suitable as gelatine replacement. US Patent 6749880.

Wongsagonsup R, Nateelerdpaisan T, Gross C, Suphantharika M, Belur PD, Agoo EMG, Janairo JIB (2021) Physicochemical properties and in vitro digestibility of flours and starches from taro cultivated in different regions of Thailand. Int J Food Sci Tech 56:2395–2406. https://doi.org/10.1111/ijfs.14865

Wu H, Lei Y, Lu J, Zhu R, Xiao D, Jiao C, Li S (2019) Effect of citric acid induced crosslinking on the structure and properties of potato starch/chitosan composite films. Food Hydrocoll 97:105208. https://doi.org/10.1016/j.foodhyd.2019.105208

Wu C, Sun R, Zhang Q, Zhong G (2020) Synthesis and characterization of citric acid esterified canna starch (RS4) by semi-dry method using vacuum-microwave-infrared assistance. Carbohydr Polym 250:116985. https://doi.org/10.1016/j.carbpol.2020.116985

Xu X, Huang XF, Visser RGF, Trindade LM (2017) Engineering potato starch with a higher phosphate content. PLOS ONE 12(1):e0169610. https://doi.org/10.1371/journal.pone.0169610

Yang B, Jiang G, Nagendra Prasad K, Gu C, Jiang Y (2010) Crystalline, thermal and textural characteristics of starches isolated from chestnut (*Castanea mollissima* Bl.) seeds at different degrees of hardness. Food Chem 119:995–999. https://doi.org/10.1016/j.foodchem.2009.08.002

Yang S, Dhital S, Zhang MN, Wang J, Chen ZG (2022) Structural, gelatinization, and rheological properties of heat-moisture treated potato starch with added salt and its application in potato starch noodles. Food Hydrocoll 131:107802. https://doi.org/10.1016/j.foodhyd.2022.107802

Yoo SH, Lee CS, Kim BS, Shin M (2012) The properties and molecular structures of gusiljatbam starch compared to those of acorn and chestnut starches. Starch/Staerke 64:339–347. https://doi.org/10.1002/star.201100104

Yu X, Chen L, Jin Z, Jiao A (2021a) Research progress of starch-based biodegradable materials: a review. J Mater Sci 56(19):11187–11208. https://doi.org/10.1007/s10853-021-06063-1

Yu B, Li J, Tao H, Zhao H, Liu P, Cui B (2021b) Physicochemical properties and in vitro digestibility of hydrothermal treated Chinese yam (*Dioscorea opposita* Thunb.) starch and flour. Int J Biol Macromol 176:177–185. https://doi.org/10.1016/j.ijbiomac.2021.02.064

Yulianto A, Kayati FN, Novariawan B, Supriyanti A (2020) The effect of extrusion temperature on changes of characteristics of partially pregelatinized cassava starch. Int J Chem Eng Appl 11(2):67–70. https://doi.org/10.18178/ijcea.2020.11.2.782

Zailani MA, Kamilah H, Husaini A et al (2022) Functional and digestibility properties of sago (Metroxylon sagu) starch modified by microwave heat treatment. Food Hydrocoll 122:107042. https://doi.org/10.1016/J.FOODHYD.2021.107042

Zandonadi RP, Botelho RBA, Gandolfi L, Ginani JS, Montenegro FM, Pratesi R (2012) Green banana pasta: an alternative for gluten-free diets. J Acad Nutr Diet 112(7):1068–1072. https://doi.org/10.1016/j.jand.2012.04.002

Zarroug Y, Boulares M, Mejri J, Slimi B, Hamdaoui G, Djebi S, Saidi F, Nasri H, Sfayhi DT, Kharrat M (2020) Extraction and characterization of tunisian quercus ilex starch and its effect on fermented dairy product quality. Int J Anal Chem 2020:868673. https://doi.org/10.1155/2020/8868673

Zhang M, Chen H, Zhang Y (2011) Physicochemical, thermal, and pasting properties of Chinese chestnut (*Castanea mollissima* Bl.) starches as affected by different drying methods. Starch/Staerke 63:260–267. https://doi.org/10.1002/star.201000146

Zhang D, Mu T, Sun H (2017) Comparative study of the effect of starches from five different sources on the rheological properties of gluten-free model doughs. Carbohydr Polym 176:345–355. https://doi.org/10.1016/j.carbpol.2017.08.025

Zhang Q, Zhang S, Deng L, Wu C, Zhong G (2018) Effect of vacuum treatment on the characteristics of oxidized starches prepared using a green method. Starch/Staerke:70. https://doi.org/10.1002/star.201700216

Zhao Y, Khalid N, Shu G, Neves MA, Kobayashi I, Nakajima M (2017) Formulation and characterization of oil-in-water emulsions stabilized by gelatinized kudzu starch. Int J Food Prop 20:1329–1341. https://doi.org/10.1080/10942912.2017.1347675

Zhao Y, Zhu X, Fang Y (2021) Structure, properties and applications of kudzu starch. Food Hydrocoll 119:106817. https://doi.org/10.1016/j.foodhyd.2021.106817

Zhu F (2015a) Composition, structure, physicochemical properties, and modifications of cassava starch. Carbohydr Polym 122:456–480. https://doi.org/10.1016/j.carbpol.2014.10.063

Zhu F (2015b) Isolation, composition, structure, properties, modifications, and uses of yam starch. Compr Rev Food Sci Food Saf 14:357–386. https://doi.org/10.1111/1541-4337.12134

Zhu, F (2017) Properties and Food Uses of Chestnut Flour and Starch. Food Bioproc Tech 10(7):1173–1191. https://doi.org/10.1007/s11947-017-1909-0

Zhu F (2019) Recent advances in modifications and applications of sago starch. Food Hydrocoll 96:412–423. https://doi.org/10.1016/J.FOODHYD.2019.05.035

Chapter 4
Use of Additives in Gluten-Free Formulations

Lorena Sciarini, Pablo Martín Palavecino, and Pablo Daniel Ribotta

Abbreviations

ADA	acetyl di-starch adipate
AMG	Amyloglucosidase
CGT	cyclodextrin glycosyltransferase
CMC	carboxymethyl cellulose
CSL	calcium stearoyl lactylate
DATEM	Diacetyl tartaric ester of monoglycerides
DM	distilled monoglycerides
G'	storage modulus
G"	loss modulus
GF	gluten-free
GMS	glycerol monostearate
GOX	glucose oxidase
GRAS	generally recognized as safe
HACS	high amylose starch
HLB	hydrophile-lipophile balance

L. Sciarini
Instituto de Ciencia y Tecnología de los Alimentos Córdoba (CONICET-UNC), Universidad Nacional de Córdoba (UNC), Córdoba, Argentina
e-mail: losciarin@agro.unc.edu.ar

P. M. Palavecino
Instituto de Ciencia y Tecnología de los Alimentos Córdoba (CONICET-UNC), Universidad Nacional de Córdoba (UNC), Córdoba, Argentina

Instituto de Ciencias Básicas y Aplicadas, Universidad Nacional de Villa María, Córdoba, Argentina
e-mail: pmpalavecino@agro.unc.edu.ar

P. D. Ribotta (✉)
Instituto de Ciencia y Tecnología de los Alimentos Córdoba (CONICET-UNC), Universidad Nacional de Córdoba (UNC), Córdoba, Argentina

Facultad de Ciencias Exactas, Físicas y Naturales, UNC, Córdoba, Argentina
e-mail: pribotta@agro.unc.edu.ar

M. F. de Escalada Pla, C. E. Genevois (eds.), *Designing Gluten Free Bakery and Pasta Products*, https://doi.org/10.1007/978-3-031-28344-4_4

HPMC	hydroxypropyl methyl cellulose
IR	infrared
LAB	lactic acid bacteria
LAC	Laccase
LE	lecithin
MC	methylcellulose
MW	microwave
O/W	oil-in-water
PGA	propylene glycol alginate
PSP	pomegranate seed powder
RS	resistant starch
SBV	specific bread volume
SSL	sodium stearoyl lactylate
tan δ	loss tangent
TG	transglutaminase
TYR	tyrosinase
UV	ultra violet
W/O	water-in-oil
WHC	water holding capacity
XYL	xylanase

4.1 Introduction

Many factors influence the quality of gluten-free (GF) products, such as bread, cakes, cookies and pasta; the most decisive factors being perhaps the characteristics of the different flour used and the processing conditions.

Gluten is the major structure-forming protein present in wheat and is responsible for the particular dough viscoelastic properties. The use of GF flour (e.g. rice, maize, sorghum, buckwheat, amaranth, quinoa, corn, chickpea, etc.) in bread making and pasta or noodles prevents the formation of a viscoelastic dough, which is necessary to hold the carbon dioxide produced during the fermentation process or to hold the pasta structure together during cooking. Another limitation associated with GF flours and their performance in bread making is the rapid onset of staling.

Also, variations in the quality of the flour and starch affect the quality of the finished products. For that reason, some ingredients have been incorporated, such as fat, milk, sugar and eggs, among the most used. These incorporate characteristics related to taste, colour, and texture. The rise in the research and production of GF products in recent decades has led to the systematic study of specific additives and ingredients in order to improve dough/batter handling, organoleptic properties, and product structure. From a GF bread industrial perspective, not only to get acceptable structure GF products is the problem, but it has also been shown that GF breads have shorter shelf-life and are less tasty when compared with gluten-containing bread (Nunes et al. 2009; Bender and Schönlechner 2020).

The simplest way to improve the structure of GF products is by adding functional ingredients and additives, such as gums, hydrocolloids, emulsifiers, starch, proteins; to the GF flour mixture.

The difficulty to elaborate GF products varies according to the role that gluten plays in the traditional product. Each product is prepared from a dough that should meet specific requirements. Bread dough has to be elastic and able to increase its volume as gasses are produced during fermentation, and expanded during baking (ovenspring). Without a continuous and elastic network, gasses would not be retained and the resulting loaf would be of an unacceptable low volume. A cookie dough, which is rich in fats and sugars, should laterally expand during baking producing a wide diameter and thin in-height, dry and crispy final product. For this to happen, dough should not be elastic but plastic, otherwise it would shrink during baking. This means that the gluten network should not be developed at all. Pasta is boiled before consumption. So in order to maintain the integrity of its structure, gluten network should be well-developed and coagulate during boiling thus avoiding pasta disintegration. Muffins and cakes are obtained from a batter formed by a complex fat-in-water emulsion as the continuous phase and gas bubbles as the discontinuous phase in which flour particles are dispersed. During baking, starch gelatinizes and proteins denature, which set the product structure. Gluten network in these products does not play a leading role. It is not surprising that the more critical the presence of a continuous network, the more difficult it is to develop its GF counterpart.

In GF systems, wheat flour is replaced by non-gluten flours from different origins, usually mixed with native starches. The most used raw materials are rice and maize flours most commonly combined with potato, corn or cassava starches. These ingredients are maybe the most abundant and the cheapest (Skendi et al. 2021); however, they are rich in carbohydrates and poor in proteins negatively affecting technological and nutritional quality of GF products. Commercial GF mixes scarcely contribute to the recommended daily protein intake, while they supply high amounts of dietary carbohydrates (Roman et al. 2019).

The present chapter is focused in the use of most common additives used either in the laboratory and industrial scale for the development of GF bread, cookies, cakes, muffins, and pasta. A technical and nutritional approach of non-starch polysaccharides, modified starches, proteins, enzymes, emulsifiers and antimicrobial agents is covered.

4.2 Gums and Non-starchy Polysaccharides

The term gums, or hydrocolloids, include a great diversity of compounds that share the ability to bind large amounts of water and interact with themselves. Therefore, they impart large rheological changes to aqueous systems at low concentrations and they are widely used as gelling agents, thickeners, stabilizers and emulsifiers. Gums are particularly valuable additives in GF products where they mainly contribute to the viscosity of mixtures and the texture of products. Most gums are polysaccharides, which are polymers of monosaccharides that can be structured as linear or branched chains. Gums are extracted from natural sources such as seeds, algae or animals and used as is, or chemically modified to obtain semi-synthetic compounds (Li and Nie 2016; Zoghi et al. 2021).

This section will focus on the non-starch hydrocolloids, among them guar gum, xanthan gum, pectin, agar and cellulose derivatives as carboxymethyl cellulose (CMC) and hydroxypropyl methyl cellulose (HPMC). In recent years, some experiments were carried out with less known gums like tragacanth (*Astragalus genus*), tara (*Caesalpinia spinosa*) and balangu (*Lallemantia royleana*), and several dietary fibers like arabinoxylans or inulin (Collar et al. 2015; Salehi 2020). In Fig. 4.1, the chemical composition of HPMC and xanthan gum is shown as an example of how diverse the hydrocolloids structure can be. More information about the chemical structure can be found in the literature (Phillips and Williams 2009).

In breadmaking applications, it is crucial the selection of structural ingredients that enhance dough physicochemical properties and at the same time prevent permanent disruption of the protein/starch networks and that would result in a weakening of the system matrix (Collar et al. 2015). In regular bakery products, the most used gums are κ-carrageenan, alginate and xanthan gum and they have the function of extending the shelf-life through two different mechanisms. First, the interactions with starch change pasting and gelatinization properties, interfering with the reassociation of amylose and promoting the formation of amylose-lipid complexes slowing down aging. Second, due to their great ability to bind water, they keep the product moist for long periods of time (Bender and Schönlechner 2020).

Particularly, in GF products the hydrocolloids are even a more important component, and play a key role in their basic formulation. The lack of gluten offers the advantage of avoiding the gluten development process but implies a whole new

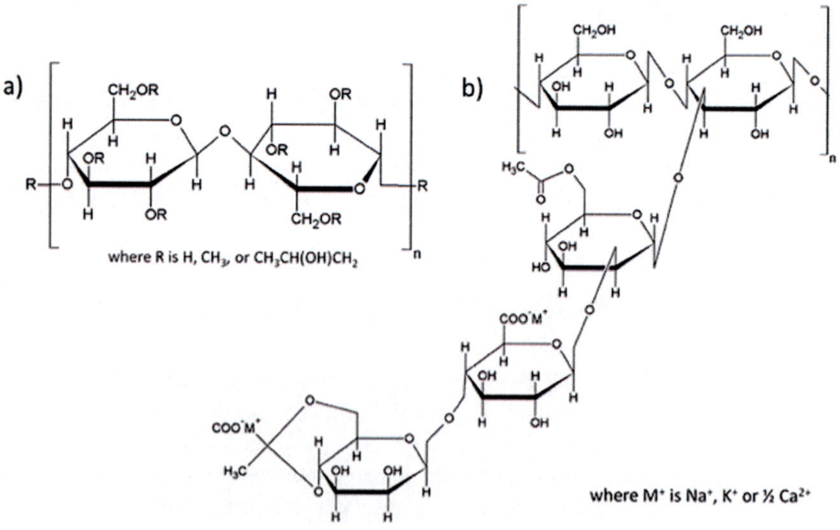

Fig. 4.1 Chemical structure of (**a**) hydroxypropyl methylcellulose (HPMC) and (**b**) xanthan gum

series of challenges to impart structure to the dough and to the final product. The production of GF breads differs greatly from its gluten-containing counterparts, mainly because there is no kneading, instead the mixture is battered like in muffins and cakes. In this sense, wheat bread preparation only needs hydration between 50% and 70% (flour basis), while GF breads requires hydration levels from 90% to 150%, making water binding components like gums so important (Sciarini et al. 2010a, b; Morreale et al. 2018).

No matter the type, from homemade flat bread to industrial pan bread, its high quality is synonym of high specific volume, tenderness, and uniform alveoli distribution (Salehi 2019). Gluten is unique and hardly replaceable, it is the main responsible of bread alveoli development during proofing and baking, and provides the structure to the final product and therefore its texture. Gums can interact with themselves and with several GF ingredients to allow the alveoli formation. What we know about gums behavior in GF bakery products is largely based upon empirical studies that investigate batter rheology, gas holding capacity in dough systems and final product texture (Zoghi et al. 2021).

The gums effect on the bread quality depends on its molecular composition (chain length, molecular mass, structure), the applied amount, the interaction with other ingredient components (starch, proteins, fiber, etc.) and process conditions (pH, temperature, stirring, shearing) (Sciarini et al. 2010a, b; Vidaurre-Ruiz et al. 2020; Zoghi et al. 2021).

In GF bakery goods, the most common approach to replace gluten functionality is to take advantage of hydrocolloids structuring properties to mimic the gluten viscoelastic properties, since rheological characteristics are key in product development. The gums goals are to reach dough consistency after mixing and to obtain desirable crumb textural values, so the correlation between dough viscosity and product texture is vital to understand the system and lead to its optimization. The dough and batters rheology can be measured through several devices that must be sensitive enough to assess its viscoelastic properties (Matos and Rosell 2015; Salehi 2020).

Usually, batter rheological characterization is carried out with a rheometer (fundamental viscoelasticity) through different methods. The results of both oscillatory shear tests and creep-recovery assay were successfully modeled and, in some cases, they were able to predict well the bread properties like specific volume (Mancebo et al. 2015; Zhao et al. 2021). Also, texturometer by compression-extrusion test, a farinograph, a Mixolab system or rotational viscometer can be used to assess batter empirical viscoelastic properties (Sciarini et al. 2010a, b; Morreale et al. 2018; Salehi et al. 2018). Beyond the selected method, there is a discrepancy about the effect of batter consistency on loaf volume. Some authors claimed that low consistency led to less resistant dough and greater expansion in proofing step (Renzetti and Arendt 2009a, b), while others suggested that higher consistency produce better dough development and gas retention in early stages (Gómez et al. 2007; Sciarini et al. 2010a, b). On the other hand, the relationship between textural parameters, dough consistency and starch gelling has been widely investigated presenting a strong correlation (Matos and Rosell 2015).

Generally, the texture of bread and cakes is assessed with the aid of a texturometer, and through the resultant parameters we can evaluate its tenderness and aging rate. These textural attributes are greatly affected by additives. The use of gums like CMC, HPMC or xanthan results in softer products with high specific volume, porosity and stable crumb texture during storage of both cakes and breads (Ferrero 2017; Herawati 2019). However, some gums can produce a negative effect on quality parameters like loaf volume, and present dissimilar behaviour when mixed with different flours (Hager and Arendt 2013; Mancebo et al. 2015).

Particularly, HPMC gelling properties and starch interactions allow gas cells development during proofing and baking, resulting in high specific volume loaf with soft texture (Ferrero 2017; Salehi 2019).

Psyllium fiber also has synergistic interactions with starch that result in a film-like structure with proper viscoelastic and thermal characteristics (Collar et al. 2015). In line with clean label requirements, arabinoxylans (hemicelluloses present in cereal cell walls) can be used as baking improvers. Particularly, GF formulations benefit from their functional properties that allow them to crosslink forming a stable network under oxidizing conditions. Despite the extraction method (water, alkaline, or enzymatic), rye arabinoxylans demonstrated to enhance GF buckwheat and millet batter rheology and sourdough-bread properties (Bender et al. 2018).

Gluten-free cakes produced with hydrocolloids addition resulted in softer products with high specific volume and increased the number of small porous (Turabi et al. 2010). Also, the staling process has been notably influenced by the type of gum involved where xanthan and xanthan–guar gum blend showed conservation of texture parameters during storage (Gómez et al. 2007; Sumnu et al. 2010). Also, methylcellulose (MC) is broadly employed in batter formulations due to its thickening and gelling agent abilities (Salehi 2019).

As mentioned above, the choice of an optimal gum for these kinds of products is not simple since their diverse chemical structure offers a world of different results, besides gums interact with other dough ingredients besides water. Thus, the ingredients characteristics (flour/starch origin, pretreatment, particle size, etc.) condition the hydrocolloid selection. Despite this, a few general rules can be suggested to choose the right additive to obtain a good quality GF bread. The literature suggests that the use of gum mixtures can lead to better products due to a synergistic effect (Morreale et al. 2018; Salehi 2019; Herawati 2019). This synergy can lead to improved rheological profiles and consequently lowers the total hydrocolloid content in the formulation and reduces cost of the product (Goff and Guo 2019).

The most successful combination of gums is HPMC and xanthan (Hager and Arendt 2013; Salehi 2019), so they are a must to test the appropriate additive in a new formulation; being a good control sample to compare the performance with other gums regarding the final product quality. Xanthan gum and HPMC can create a continuous network embedded with starch fragments resulting in a structure similar to gluten. Additionally, rice breads with this combination presented excellent mechanical properties and high sensory scores (Ahlborn et al. 2005).

Also, the combination of HPMC with CMC or propylene glycol alginate (PGA) is able to develop a cell structure that traps fermentation gasses resulting in good loaf volume and overcoming the texture defects (Cato et al. 2004; Zhao et al. 2021). The use of guar gum produces loaves with better volume, moisture content of crumb and baking efficiency than pectin, but the combination of both enhances the texture features (Gambuś et al. 2001).

In the case of low water content dough like the one used to prepare cookies, gums retain water and result in higher moisture content products. Also, they improve the emulsion activity which positively impacts cookies'shape and texture. Guar, acacia, xanthan and tragacanth gums were tested and in addition to the technological improvement they also increased sensory scores, particularly the formulation containing xanthan gum (Kaur et al. 2015). Guar gum was used as fat replacer in cookies to reduce the lipid content from 20 to 6% keeping the dough mobility and handling and improving product texture (Singh and Kumar 2018).

The short shelf life and the small market volume of GF products (compared to wheat-based bakery ones) generate a lack of fresh bread and cakes. Then, a solution to this obstacle is to use the frozen dough and partially baked frozen techniques. In the case of frozen dough process, it implies a freezing step during the product elaboration and the defrosting/cooking is performed later by the end-seller or the consumer. All three steps, freezing, storage and defrosting produce negative effects in the dough, but the use of hydrocolloids can help to prevent them. Gums are used to stabilize the frozen bread dough structure and as well to avoid ice-crystal formation and growth (Anton and Artfield 2008).

Storage of frozen dough changes rheological properties and results in longer proofing time and small loaf volume. In order to overcome these defects guar gum, locust bean gum, xanthan, and sodium alginate were employed in wheat bread (Sharadanant and Khan 2003; Ribotta et al. 2004a, b; Li et al. 2019). In GF breads guar gum, xanthan gum and locust bean gum were tested, where the mixture of guar and flaxseed exhibited the highest volume, softest texture (fresh and after the 3 days storage), and darkest colour (Ozkoc and Seyhun 2015). It would be interesting to undertake further research in this area to better understand the GF dough behavior and impulse the industrial implementation when it is possible.

Pasta is different from all other GF products because they have to be boiled before eating, so their structure needs to be capable of resisting this process and give the consumer a high firmness and low stickiness product. In GF pasta, the addition of gums improves dough handling because of their ability to provide high consistency, despite the low water content of the mixture (Sozer 2009; Palavecino et al. 2017). During pasta cooking gums help to create a tridimensional network that avoids material release to the medium but increases water absorption rate (Marti and Pagani 2013). Unfortunately, not everything is good; hydrocolloids affinity for water can impair the water intake of the other components and might thus reduce starch gelatinization. Regarding the texture of pasta, gums contribute to firmness, chewiness and mouthfeel, improving consumers' acceptance. Among hydrocolloids, HMPC, xanthan and guar gum are the most used to improve GF pasta formulations (Larrosa et al. 2013; Gao et al. 2018). Gum effectiveness is influenced by flour selected to produce GF pasta and can change the sensory and technological attributes leading to low cooking loss and high firmness (Palavecino et al. 2017; Culetu et al. 2021).

Another important topic that should be addressed is hydrocolloids amount to be used in the formulation. In this sense, in Table 4.1, the most relevant studies about hydrocolloids addition to GF at the present are summarised. In addition to the technological implications, it is central that updated legislation should be checked before using hydrocolloids in GF products. Most of the studies reported levels of gums between 0.1% and 5.0% on a flour basis, but authorities generally limit the use as a percentage of the final product. The maximum quantity permitted may vary considerably among countries, even though international organizations are looking to harmonize regulations (Anton and Artfield 2008).

4.3 Modified Starch and Starchy Polysaccharides

Starch is the major energy source in the human diet and it is incorporated in several forms, from boiled potatoes to noodles. Starch is a mixture of branched and linear glucose polymers (amylopectin and amylose, respectively) that build a granule from 1 to 200 μm depending on its botanical origin. Starch is widely used in food formulations because of its ability to thicken and gel all kinds of recipes, but to fulfil more exigent requirements (harder gels for example) and avoid some problems (like syneresis) starch is modified in several ways (Horstmann et al. 2017a, b). Starch gelatinization is critical in product baking and its extent depends on granule shape, size, crystallinity and composition, that in turn affect gelling and retrogradation during cooling (Witczak et al. 2016). Blends of starches from different botanical origins and the selection of starchy flours particle size are very common approaches to optimize bakery products and pasta (Matos and Rosell 2015). Nevertheless, the focus of this section is on starch derivatives that are added into formulations in small quantities, i.e., modified starches, dextrins and treated flours. The effect of physical and chemical starch modifications on the molecular structure are schematized in Fig. 4.2.

The physical modification of starch involves the use of energy (mainly heat and shear) to alter its semi-crystalline structure but not the chemical one, and as a result, products do not need to be labelled as modified starch (BeMiller and Huber 2015). From these, the most used is the pregelatinized starch that is produced by complete gelatinization and subsequent drying processes, among which we can mention drum drying, spray cooking and extrusion cooking (Horstmann et al. 2017a, b). Also, ultrasound, high pressure, hydrothermal treatments (annealing and high-moisture) are applied to starch in order to modify its structure (Park and Kim 2021). On the other hand, chemical and enzymatic modifications change the molecular structure of starch chains. Chemical modifications use reagents that provide a reactive substituent group like hydroxypropyl, long chain organic acids and carbonyl or cross-linking agents that replace starch hydroxyl (Calvin 2016). Enzymes are selected to produce starch modifications avoiding undesirable byproducts while decreasing

Table 4.1 Relevant studies on gluten-free (GF) cereal-based products containing hydrocolloids and their main results

Product	Hydrocolloid (amount)	Flour base	Results	References
Bread	Carrageenan, alginate, xanthan gum, CMC and gelatin (0.5%)	Rice, corn and soy flour	Hydrocolloids increased batter consistencies and bread specific volume, particularly xanthan	Sciarini et al. (2010a, b)
Bread	HPMC (1–3%)	Rice flour	Improved the batter consistency and textural features like crumb hardness and cohesiveness	Morreale et al. (2018)
Bread	HPMC (2–4%), psyllium (0–4%)	Rice flour	Both increased elastic modulus similarly, psyllium addition reduces bread specific volume and increase hardness	Mancebo et al. (2015)
Bread	HPMC, CMC, xanthan and propylene glycol alginate (0.5–3%)	Rice flour	HPMC significantly increased the specific volume and PGA promoted hardness, resilience and springiness	Zhao et al. (2021)
Bread	Pectin, guar gum (4%)	Corn starch	Guar gum increase the volume and retain moisture, but the combination with pectin enhances the texture	Gambuś et al. (2001)
Bread	HPMC and xanthan (1–3%)	Rice flour	Combination presented excellent mechanical and sensory properties exhibiting a continuous matrix	Ahlborn et al. (2005)
Bread	HPMC and xanthan (1–2%)	Rice, buckwheat, maize and teff	Dissimilar behavior with each flour in loaf volume and crumb hardness	Hager and Arendt (2013)
Bread	Guar gum, locust bean and psyllium fiber (1–2%)	Rice, amaranth and chickpea flours; corn and cassava starch	Psyllium fiber show synergistic interaction with starch with proper viscoelastic and thermal characteristics	Collar et al. (2015)
Bread	Arabinoxylans (3%)	Buckwheat and millet	Strengthen batter structure and improve the specific volume and firmness	Bender et al. (2018)
Bread (frozen)	Guar gum, xanthan gum, locust bean gum (1%)	Rice flour and potato starch	Gum and 5% flaxseed combination resulting in softer texture, lower staling rate and higher volume	Ozkoc and Seyhun (2015)

(continued)

Table 4.1 (continued)

Product	Hydrocolloid (amount)	Flour base	Results	References
Biscuits	Guar, acacia, xanthan, and tragacanth (1%)	Buckwheat flour	Increase moisture content, diameter, thickness, weight and decreased fracture strength and improved sensorial scores	Kaur et al. (2015)
Biscuits	Guar gum (1%)	Foxtail millet, amaranth and copra coconut by-product)	Keep dough mobility and handling and improving product texture despite fat and sugar reduction	Singh and Kumar (2018)
Cake	Balangu seed gum (0.5–1.5%)	Rice flour	Increased moisture content and volume of cakes with high consumer acceptability	Salehi et al. (2018)
Cake	Xanthan gum and guar gum (0.3–1% of a 1:1 blend)	Rice flour	Decreased the hardness, weight loss, retrogradation enthalpy and setback viscosity during storage	Sumnu et al. (2010)
Cake	Xanthan, guar, locust bean, κ-carrageenan and xanthan–guar blend (1%)	Rice flour	Increase pore area fraction and percent number of pores, especially with xanthan and xanthan–guar blend	Turabi et al. (2010)
Muffins	Bacterial nanocellulose (0.06–0.30%)	Rice flour, tapioca starch and corn-starch	Increase firmness, viscosity, and consistency indexes and retained more air during mixing	Marchetti et al. (2020)
Pasta	Guar gum (0.5%)	Rice flour	Act as a stabilizer and make the dough easy to handle and process	Sozer (2009)
Pasta	Xanthan gum (0–2.5%)	Sorghum flour	Reduce swelling index and significantly increase chewiness	Palavecino et al. (2017)
Pasta	Xanthan and locust bean (0.5–2.5%)	Corn-starch and corn flour	Increase dough storage and loss moduli and pasta break force	Larrosa et al. (2013)

production cost, and includes reactions like branching, hydrolysis and transfer (Park and Kim 2021). Table 4.2 summarises the use and effect of starch derivatives in GF formulations.

In GF bakery products and pasta starch is the major component because these foods are usually made from rice or corn flours. In turn, some starch-based additives can supplement GF flour to enhance the textural properties. As explained earlier, the addition of hydrocolloids brings positive technological and nutritional benefits, although consumers frequently perceive their presence as "artificial" possibly due to their chemical-sounding names and because they are classified as food additives (Šmídová and Rysová 2022). Then, starchy polysaccharides are adequate

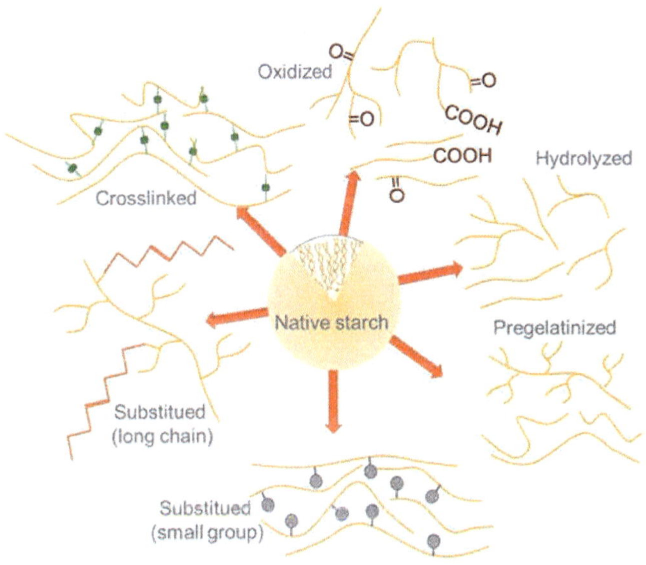

Fig. 4.2 Schematics of modified starches molecular structure

alternatives as they can impart similar characteristics to food products and, in some cases, allow the use of clean labels focused on health-conscious consumers (Marti and Pagani 2013; Park and Kim 2021).

Starch gelatinization plays a key role in the GF bread starchy matrix since it is the principal responsible of setting the structure through the viscosity rise during baking. Then, gelatinized starch added as an ingredient is very useful to dough consistency and has a positive effect in bread quality (Matos and Rosell 2015).

In breadmaking, the substitution of 3% of the raw flour with pregelatinized oat and barley flour resulted in firmer crumb, higher water retention during storage and lower amylopectin retrogradation (Purhagen et al. 2012). Pregelatinized rice flour by extrusion-cooking with lactic acid was added at 10% to GF rice bread resulting in products with similar crust and crumb colours and texture than those of wheat bread, but with lower specific volume (Pedrosa Silva Clerici et al. 2009).

The replacement of chemical substituent groups on starch hydroxyls reduces starch reassociation, and therefore bread staling rate (Calvin 2016). Chemically modified starch acetyl di-starch adipate (ADA) was incorporated at 10% and it reduced and delayed hardness and loss of cohesiveness in GF rice breads when comparing products with 1 and 7 days of storage; and presented similar specific volume to control (Roman et al. 2020). The use of ADA and another crosslinked starch, hydroxypropyl di-starch phosphate (HDP), changed system viscoelastic properties which resulted in bread loaves with high volume, elastic crumb and high number of small cells (Ziobro et al. 2012; Witczak et al. 2012). These authors also used high amylose starch (HACS), which significantly changed the thermograms,

Table 4.2 Effect of starch and starchy polysaccharides on gluten-free (GF) cereal-based products

Product	Starch amount	Flour base	Results	References
Bread	Pregelatinized flour (3%)	Commercial GF mix	Increase crumb firmness and water retention during storage while lower amylopectin retrogradation	Purhagen et al. (2012)
Bread	Acidic extruded flour (10%)	Rice flour	Similar crust and crumb colors and texture than those of wheat bread, but with lower specific volume	Pedrosa Silva Clerici et al. (2009)
Bread	Acetyl di-starch adipate (10%)	Rice flour	Exhibited reduced and delayed hardness and loss of cohesiveness in breads comparing day 1 product with day 7; and presenting specific volume similar to control	Roman et al. (2020)
Bread	High amylose corn starch, acetyl di-starch adipate and hydroxypropyl di-starch phosphate (5–15%)	Maize starch	Significant influence in dough viscoelastic, thermal and pasting properties. Increase volume of the loaves and decrease in hardness and chewiness of the crumb, particularly with HACS	Ziobro et al. (2012) and Witczak et al. (2012)
Bread	Pregelatinized cassava starch (0–15%)	Rice milling fractions	Significantly increase volume of the loaves	Genevois and de Escalada Pla (2021)
Bread	Pregelatinized cassava starch (17%)	Sorghum flour	Presented worst bread crumb textural properties compared to formulation containing native starch	Onyango et al. (2010)
Pasta	Pregelatinized cassava flour (10–40%)	Cassava starch and amaranth flour	Improve nutritional and technological properties to reach a product with adequate color and texture	Fiorda et al. (2013)
Pasta	Pregelatinized corn starch (15–30%)	Sorghum flour	Reduce material losses during cooking and increase luminosity	Palavecino et al. (2017)
Pasta	Precooked rice flour or pregelatinized rice starch (25%)	Buckwheat and rice flours	Improve the break strain and weight increase during cooking and enhance workability	Paiva et al. (2019)
Cookies	Debranched, annealed or acid and heat-moisture treated waxy rice starch (50%)	Rice flour	Increase significantly RS and a decrease of rapidly digestible starch	Giuberti et al. (2017)

(continued)

Table 4.2 (continued)

Product	Starch amount	Flour base	Results	References
Cookies	Maltodextrin (5–35%)	Copra, foxtail millet and amaranth	Improve mobility to allow the reduction of fat content and drastically reduce calories	Singh and Kumar (2018)
Cookies	Heat-moisture treated (0.3–0.9%)	Rice flour	Improved specific volume and contributed to maintaining the moisture	Mohammadi et al. (2022)
Cake	Ozone-treated sorghum flour	–	Increase number of cells per slice and specific volume while reducing crumb firmness	Marston et al. (2015)
Cake	Extruded rice flour	–	Changed batter rheological properties and improve cake textural properties and increase its sensory acceptance	Das and Bhattacharya (2019)
Cake	Commercial resistant starch (5–20%)	Rice flour and tapioca starch	Batters less elastic and thinner, increased cakes specific volume and average pore diameter, but decrease surface porosity and number of pores	Tsatsaragkou et al. (2015)

pasting profile and viscoelastic behaviour of the dough but weakened the crumb structure of bread resulting in poor mechanical properties.

Dextrins can be obtained from starch by enzymatical, chemical or physical treatments. Particularly, low molecular weight of dextrins retard the bread staling in both wheat and GF products (Witczak et al. 2016).

In GF pasta -which lacks the protein network- the structural role is most commonly assumed by (retrograded) starch. The retrogradation of amylose solubilized during gelatinization implies a double-helix formation stabilized through hydrogen bonding which gives rise to a continuous phase surrounding swollen and deformed starch granules. This retrograded amylose is thermally stable and can only be dissociated at temperatures higher than 100 °C. Thus, gelatinized starch is often selected as the main structuring agent of GF pasta, where it can be added as an ingredient or generated in the making process by extrusion-cooking (Palavecino et al. 2020). The addition of heat-treated starch into the formulation produces pasta with lower water absorption, higher firmness and a smoother starchy matrix than pasta prepared by extrusion cooking (Marti and Pagani 2013).

The use of pregelatinized corn, potato and cassava starches, or heat-treated maize flour reduces cooking loss and increases water absorption yet improving the pasta structure and consequently its texture parameters (Fiorda et al. 2013; Ferreira et al. 2016; Palavecino et al. 2017; Paiva et al. 2019). The hydration level and the time-temperature conditions of the pregelatinisation process significantly affect the pasta-making procedure and the cooking quality of pasta. There is a thin equilibrium between pasta with low amounts of gelatinized starch where it is enough to create an ultrastructure and excessive quantity that absorbs large amounts of water and results in a soft texture pasta (Marti and Pagani 2013).

Asian rice noodles are starch-based products that after the forming step (sheeting and cutting or extrusion) are subjected to cooking-cooling cycles where starch is gelatinized and retrograded (Gao et al. 2018). Also, GF pasta and noodles might be produced by the extrusion-cooking method where forming and heat-treatment happen simultaneously (Marti et al. 2011). These popular heat-treated products usually do not include a pregelatinized starch or any other kind of starchy additive because the process creates the continuous starchy matrix.

Generally, the use of pregelatinized flour is a cheap approach to produce noodles and pasta because it can be carried out in a conventional press and its industrial adoption is relatively easy with good results (Alamprese et al. 2007; Palavecino et al. 2017). Also, the traditional noodle making process is hard to apply at an industrial scale due to the enormous amounts of energy and water to perform the cooking and cooling cycles (Marti and Pagani 2013).

Starch modified by annealing (humidity higher than 40% and temperature between 40 and 60 °C) and heat-moisture treatment (humidity lower than 40% and temperature between 90 and 110 °C) were successfully used to produce fresh and dried rice noodles, respectively (Cham and Suwannaporn 2010).

Different modified waxy rice starch (hydrolysis by pullulanase debranching enzyme, annealing and a combination of acid and heat-moisture treatments) were added to rice cookies resulting in a significative increase in resistant starch (RS) and a diminution of rapidly digestible starch (Giuberti et al. 2017). Also, the use of maltodextrin as a texture modifier allows the reduction of fat content in GF biscuits achieving up to 33% calorie reduction (Singh and Kumar 2018). The use of heat-moisture treated wheat starch is also a valid but controversial approach, with positive effect in moisture retention, specific volume and sensory acceptance of rice-based cookies (Mohammadi et al. 2022).

The quality of sweet products obtained from batters, such as cakes and muffins, is highly dependent on uniform air incorporation, air retention, and bubble stability during mixing. Air incorporation into batter can be determined by batter specific gravity or viscosity. Viscous batter is necessary to trap gas bubbles during mixing and retain the shape during baking (Wilderjans et al. 2008). Of utmost importance is the gas bubble stability during baking but prior to the formation of cake structure. The efficacy of air retention in batter has a proportional relationship with batter viscosity (Sahi and Alava, 2003). Product volume is greatly dependent on the starch gelatinization temperature. Higher gelatinization temperature leads to better batter expansion (Gularte et al. 2012).

In products like muffins and sponge cakes, the structure is formed mainly of egg proteins and starch, therefore, the processes of denaturation and gelatinization are responsible for preventing them from collapsing during baking and cooling (Hesso et al. 2014, 2015). Therefore, the use of oxidized starches that have a low gelatinization temperature and develop high viscosity can be positive in this type of product. Ozone-treated sorghum flour has been reported to produce GF cake with higher number of cells per slice and specific volume while reducing crumb firmness (Marston et al. 2015). The addition of extrusion-cooked rice flour changed the batter rheological properties, the textural attributes of the cake and increased its sensory acceptance (Das and Bhattacharya 2019). Cakes from rice flour and tapioca starch with high amounts of RS were also successfully obtained with good technological (porosity, number of pores, staling rate), nutritional (up to 20% RS) and sensory (consumer acceptance) properties (Tsatsaragkou et al. 2015).

4.4 Proteins

As mentioned before, the most common approach for the development of GF products consists in trying to replace gluten functionality for another network with similar viscoelastic properties. Thus, it is generally proposed to add a source of proteins alone or together with an enzyme to produce a viscoelastic dough. In other words, the focus is to extrapolate wheat breadmaking technology to GF systems. However, contrary to wheat-systems, GF-systems are very heterogeneous, and the effect of different protein sources on the technological properties of GF products is very dependent on the flours/starches used, other ingredients and additives, and the water amount. Thus, the effect of various protein ingredients on dough/batter properties and the quality of the end-products cannot be fully predicted. However, the intrinsic properties of each type of protein will partially determine its behaviour.

The properties of proteins vary according to their origin. These properties are related to protein structure, which is considered on four levels: the primary structure, i.e., the specific sequence of amino acids linked by peptide bonds; the secondary structure, based on how amino acids interact, promoting protein folding; the tertiary structure, which defines the three-dimensional shape of the protein; and the quaternary structure, where single proteins, or subunits, combine to make up a multisubunit protein (Table 4.3). The structure of proteins from animal and plant sources is inherently different because they have different polypeptide sequences and are within different native environments (Day 2016). This means that they differ in the amount of each of the secondary structures and thus have different tertiary structures. Ultimately, the conformation of a protein determines its functional properties such as solubility, water holding capacity, gelation, emulsification, and foaming properties (Zayas 1997). It also influences the nutritional function of the protein in a food, *e.g.* the accessibility to digestive enzyme attack, fragmentation into peptides, and availability of essential amino acids (Day et al. 2022).

A fundamental difference between animal and plant proteins is that the plant proteins are mostly storage proteins with large and compact structures. According to Osborne (1907), plant proteins can be divided into four major classes based on their solubility in various solvents: albumins, globulins, prolamins and glutelins. The major storage proteins in cereals are prolamins and glutelins, which are generally insoluble in aqueous solvents. On the other hand, while salt-soluble globulins are the major protein fraction of legumes, water-soluble albumins are more

Table 4.3 Levels of proteins structure

Level of structure	Primary	Amino acid sequence	
	Secondary	α-helix	Regular right-hand turns of amino acids 3.6 residues long.
		β-sheet	Formed by the interactions between parallel regions of a protein chain. These either run in the same direction (parallel) or in the opposite direction (antiparallel).
		β-turn	Connect two other elements of secondary structure. The change of direction occurs in the space of four residues.
	Tertiary	α-domain	Given by α-helices at the protein's core.
		β-domain	Mainly antiparallel β-sheets at the protein's core.
		α/β-domain	β-sheets surrounded by α-helices in a βαβ conformation.
	Quaternary	Protein subunits (tertiary structures) linked to produce a multisubunit protein. Two or several identical or different subunits.	

prevalent in oilseeds and legumes (Day et al. 2022). It has to be considered that solubility is a key factor determining a protein's functionality. Another important protein property is its water holding capacity (WHC): plant proteins (less soluble) usually have higher WHC than animal proteins (more soluble) (Zayas, 1997).

Another factor to consider when analysing a protein source is their concentration and related processing history. According to the *Codex Alimentarius* Commission (1989) a protein product is defined as a protein concentrate if it has 65–90% protein content, and as a protein isolate when it contains 90% of proteins and above. Soy, whey and casein are maybe the most common sources of proteins processed as concentrates and isolates in the bakery industry.

The presence of proteins modifies the sensory properties of foods, mainly through the Maillard reaction. This group of reactions is responsible for the development of desirable aroma and colour in baked goods, although it is also associated with some undesirable effects, such as nutritional damage because of loss in lysine availability, and the formation of potentially toxic compounds (e.g. acrylamide) (Ames 1992).

Many different proteins have been used in GF breadmaking. They generally affect bread final quality because they modify dough/batter rheology; while proteins with high WHC increase batter consistency, proteins with low WHC decrease it. It has been well established that batter consistency plays a key role in determining bread quality. When the batter is too stiff, a decrease in consistency may improve batter development owing to a reduced resistance to expansion during proofing, whereas when batter is too liquid, an increase in consistency leads to higher specific bread volumes (SBV), because it improves gas retention, thereby increasing loaf volume (Sciarini et al. 2010a, b; Ziobro et al. 2016; Mancebo et al. 2017; Miś et al. 2018; Sahagún and Gómez 2018a). A "limiting consistency" (or consistency "threshold") has been defined as the consistency at which the batter is no longer capable of retaining air bubbles during baking, and therefore a drop in volume occurs (Sciarini et al. 2010a, b; Bravo-Núñez et al. 2019). This consistency value is different for each batter and depends on the formulation used. It is therefore difficult to predict the exact influence of the rheological properties of the batter on bread characteristics; the optimum formulation should combine relatively low viscosity with the ability to form sufficiently strong and rigid structure, which would hold enough gas during proofing and provide crumb with appropriate structure and texture (Ziobro et al. 2016). Sahagún and Gómez (2018a) assayed both animal (egg white and whey protein) and plant (rice, pea) proteins with different hydration levels and found that the optimum moisture level (to achieve highest specific volume) was lower for animal proteins, even lower than the control, without protein addition. They also found that the maximum SBV was achieved with plant proteins compared to animal ones (always lower than the control with no exogenous protein added). The lower amount of water needed for animal proteins was also confirmed by Bravo-Núñez et al. (2019).

As mentioned earlier, protein intrinsic properties, such as WHC, foaming or emulsifying capacity also play a role on bread properties. WHC and foaming ability greatly influence both consistency and air entrapment during mixing and proofing. These properties have a stabilizing effect on bread crumb. Proteins of animal origin are highly soluble, have high emulsifying and foaming capacity and high stability; thus, they generally impart good quality properties to breads. The use of egg white results in a high SBV due to its foaming capacity as well as its low denaturation temperature, which would stabilize crumb structure in early stages of baking (Ziobro et al. 2013a, b). The spatial arrangement of proteins may also influence their behaviour. For example, Ziobro et al. (2013a, b) found that collagen application resulted in a strong decrease in tan δ (meaning an increase in viscoelasticity) with values typical from a strong gel, and proposed that this was due to collagen structure, with regularly occurring amino acid triplets, which ultimately results in the formation of tight triple helix. Despite this higher viscoelasticity, breads supplemented with collagen presented worse overall properties than control bread (with no protein added) maybe due to its stiff structure. In other work, Ribotta et al. (2004a, b) found that soy flour with its proteins in a native state exerted a positive effect on bread quality whereas soy flour with denatured proteins had a detrimental effect on bread quality. More recently, Genevois and de Escalada Pla (2021) reported higher specific bread volume, softer crumb, and faster recuperation of resilience and springiness with the addition of 6% of soybean extruded-expelled meal to GF bread based on pregelatinised starch.

It is accepted that legume proteins in GF formulations have a potential role to play in terms of technofunctional properties and the improvement of the nutritional profile of these products (Foschia et al. 2017). Horstmann et al. (2017a, b) assayed different plant proteins in GF breads, and found that both potato and soy proteins resulted in breads with lower specific volume and a denser crumb; but carob, lupin and pea proteins, resulted in a high volume with greater cell pores and a softer bread crumb. These authors found that foaming properties and solubility of the proteins correlated with dough properties: high foaming ability was related to higher dough viscosity which reduced specific volume of the bread.

Pasting behaviour of the GF dough, related to starch properties, is also affected by protein addition. In general, the addition of proteins results in a decrease in peak and final viscosities, and setback of dough. This decrease is usually related to starch dilution (Sciarini et al. 2010a, b). In addition, protein-starch interactions established in the presence of proteins stabilize starch structure, and hence delay swelling and overall gelatinization process (Crockett et al. 2011). High breakdown viscosities are usually associated with low specific volume (Matos and Rosell 2013; Horstmann et al. 2017a, b). A higher breakdown viscosity indicates a lower stability as granules are less resistant to shear during heating; on the other hand, a high dough peak viscosity restrains the cell expansion, leading to smaller, finer cells, which further leads to a smaller bread volume. Finally, higher gelling temperatures were associated with increased specific volume (Horstmann et al. 2017a, b), since air bubbles are able to expand longer, until the structure is set due to a sudden increase in viscosity.

Several proteins have been assayed in GF pasta-making in order to reduce cooking losses and improve pasta texture. Among commonly used proteins, egg white (Marti et al. 2014; Larrosa et al. 2016; Phongthai et al. 2017), whey protein (Susanna and Prabhasankar 2013; Marti et al. 2014), and soy protein (Rachman et al. 2020) are the most frequent. Phongthai et al. (2017) reported that the addition of egg proteins had a positive effect on the cooking quality, resulting in firm and elastic pasta with low cooking loss. Egg albumen in pasta made from parboiled rice flour improved more than whey proteins, the cooking quality (firm and elastic pasta with low cooking loss), and this result was attributed to the formation of a compact network that did not allow the material release during cooking (Marti et al. 2014). Schoenlechner et al. (2010) found similar results when adding egg white powder to GF noodles based on quinoa, amaranth and buckwheat flour blends.

Muneer et al. (2018) studied the behaviour of a mixture of pea protein isolate and pea fibre in a pasta-sheet like product and found that protein polymerisation via disulphide bonds resulted in pasta of enhanced cooking properties. Shukla et al. (2021) evaluated pasta with pea and faba protein isolates and found that both provided desirable extrudability, water uptake and cooking loss characteristics similar to those presented by to semolina pasta to extruded pasta.

Positive results were obtained when substituting rice flour by rice proteins for the production of rice-based noodles, especially when treated with transglutaminase (Kim et al. 2014). In a technological study, Detchewa et al. (2022) confirmed that rice protein had a positive impact on rice-based pasta, with lower cooking times, water absorption and cooking loss when increasing protein content from 0% to 10%, with 2.5 and 5% presenting higher liking scores in a hedonic scale.

Rice flour is still the most popular flour for GF cookies, and it is commonly blended with other flours, starches, and/or proteins for better functionality and product quality (Xu et al. 2020). As it happens in GF breadmaking, the incorporation of a protein source in cookie formulation increases the water absorption of the dough which in turn reduces cookie hardness and spread ratio, related to changes in dough rheology. Sarabhai and Prabhasankar (2015) studied the effect of substituting 5%,

7.5% and 10% of chestnut flour by whey protein concentrate on cookie quality and dough rheological properties and microstructure. An increase in whey protein concentrate resulted in more elastic doughs, with increased tenacity and resistance to deformation. At higher protein substitution, starch granules were covered by a protein matrix which was responsible for good handling of GF dough and cookies with proper technological quality.

Sarabhai et al. (2015) incorporated soy protein isolate or whey protein concentrate and evaluated sensory and textural characteristics of rice-cookies. They found that both proteins improved cookie quality compared to control, and contributed to obtaining cookies more similar to wheat-based cookies. The effect of different protein sources at two substitution levels (15% and 30%) on the characteristics of corn flour cookies were evaluated by Sahagún and Gómez (2018b). They found that animal (egg white and whey) proteins led to a more pronounced decrease in dough consistency (given by a reduction in the rheological parameters G' and G"), while increasing tan δ (decreased viscoelasticity) compared to vegetable (pea and potato) proteins. Samples with lower G' and G" moduli values also presented lower water binding capacity. Regarding cookie quality, cookie width was negatively associated with G' and G"; so that a low consistency provided a higher dough expansion during baking. Good quality cookies were obtained using whey proteins, while egg white and potato protein had a detrimental effect on cookie quality compared to the control, without protein addition.

Matos et al. (2014) studied the effect of a variety of proteins (soy and pea protein isolates, egg white protein, and casein) on rice-based muffins. They found that casein and soy and pea protein isolates significantly increased the elastic modulus (G') of the batter, while both casein and egg white protein increased specific volume of the muffins. Soy protein isolate did not influence the texture profile of muffins; however, pea protein isolate resulted in softer and springier muffins. Shevkani and Singh (2014) studied the incorporation of protein isolates from kidney bean, field pea, and amaranth on muffins based on corn starch. Specific volume, springiness and cohesiveness of the muffins were improved due to the incorporation of all protein isolates, and this finding was explained as a result of increased batter viscoelasticity after protein addition. Sahagún et al. (2018) substituted 15% and 30% of rice flour by plant (pea and rice protein) and animal (egg white and whey protein) proteins for GF cake production. These authors found that proteins in general increased batter viscosity, whereas their effect on cake texture varied from one protein to another: while animal proteins increased hardness, cohesiveness and springiness, vegetable proteins reduced the hardness and cohesiveness. Animal protein reduced the bubble size due to its intrinsic foaming properties, resulting in a general stabilizing effect. However, all protein-enriched cakes presented significantly lower sensory acceptability relative to the non-protein-enriched cake, and this effect was even more pronounced when rice protein or egg white were added. In Table 4.4, representative works about GF formulation with protein addition were summarised.

Table 4.4 Relevant studies on gluten-free (GF) cereal-based products containing proteins and their main results

Product	Protein[a]	% flour basis	Flour base	Results	References
Bread	*Chlorella sorokiniana* flour	2.5–5%	Rice flour, corn starch and pea flour	SBV and crumb firmness were not modified. Global acceptance decreased	Diprat et al. (2020)
Bread	Sunflower protein concentrate (85%)	5–20%	Rice flour, corn starch and pea flour	SBV decreased, firmness increased. No difference in global acceptance between 5–10–20% Sunflower protein concentrate	Zorzi et al. (2020)
Bread	Rapeseed protein isolate (96%)	6–15%	Corn and potato starches	SBV and firmness increased. increased sensory acceptability	Korus et al. (2021)
Bread	Pea protein powder (78%)	5–25%	Buckwheat and flaxseed flours	SBV decreased and increased firmness. More than 10% reduced sensory score	Wójcik et al. (2021)
Bread	Rice protein (79%), pea protein (78%), EWP (82%), WPC (92%)	5–10%	Rice flour and corn starch	5% protein slightly decreased SBV. 10% decreased SBV. Increased volatile compounds production. Decreased crust crispiness	Pico et al. (2019)
Bread	Zein (93%)	2.5–10%	Corn and potato starches	Increased crumb firmness, decreased crust firmness	Berta et al. (2019)
Bread	EWP (82%)	5–15%	Commercial mix (chickpea flour, potato starch, tapioca flour, wholegrain sorghum flour, faba bean flour)	SBV increased, no significant effect on firmness	Han et al. (2019)
Bread	Spray dried EWP (88%), Dry heated EWP (91%), SPI (84%)	EWP 6% SPI 4%	Rice flour	EW increased SBV, increased crumb homogeneity. Decreased batter viscosity SPI did not modify SBV, crumb was inhomogeneous. Increased batter viscosity	Masure et al. (2019)

(continued)

Table 4.4 (continued)

Product	Protein[a]	% flour basis	Flour base	Results	References
Bread	Rice protein (79%), pea protein (78%), EWP (82%), WPC (92%)	30%	Corn starch	All proteins decreased SBV. Animal proteins increased crumb firmness	Sahagún and Gómez (2018a)
Bread	Potato protein (85%), SPI (92%), pea protein (76%), lupin protein (39%), carob germ protein (55%)	2%	Corn starch	Best bread properties (highest SBV and lowest firmness) with carob germ protein; worst results were obtained with pea protein	Horstmann et al. (2017)
Pasta	EWP (75%), WPC (75%), SPI (81%), rice bran protein concentrate (68%)	6–9%	Rice flour	EWP and SPC has low cooking loss. SPI presented good color Pasta with animal protein higher water absorption EWP and WPC improved texture; rice protein and SPI decreased firmness. EWP and SPI had the highest potential	Phongthai et al. (2017)
Pasta	EWP (80%), SPI (91%)	5–15%	Banana and cassava flours	Proteins increased water absorption and decreased cooking loss. Proteins increased firmness (EWP more than SPI). EWP increased cooking time	Rachman et al. (2020)
Pasta	Potato protein isolate (>90%), pea protein isolate (84–88%), rice protein isolate (79%)	6–12%	Quinoa flour, potato starch and lupine flour	Pea protein was superior to potato and rice protein (increased firmness and acceptable cooking loss)	Linares-García et al. (2019)
Pasta	Sodium caseinate, WPC	10–20%	Millet flour	The mixture of both proteins decreased cooking loss and maintained pasta firmness	Kumar et al. (2019)

(continued)

Table 4.4 (continued)

Product	Protein[a]	% flour basis	Flour base	Results	References
Pasta	Liquid egg albumen, WPC (80%)	Egg 15% WPC 3%	Parboiled rice flour	Egg albumen lowered cooking loss and increased firmness	Marti et al. (2014)
Cookies	Pea protein (78%), potato protein (90%), EWP (85%), WPC (89%)	15–45%	Corn flour	EWP and WPC produced harder and wider cookies. Potato protein produced darker cookies, Pea protein did not change any cookie parameters	Sahagún and Gómez (2018b)
Cookies	Pea protein (80%)	10–20%	Rice flour and corn starch	Reduced the size of cookies (thickness and width), produced softer and darker cookies	Mancebo et al. (2016)
Cookies	SPI (89%), WPC (69%)	5–10%	Rice flour	SPI increased spread ratio; WPC reduced spread ratio and cookies were too firm	Sarabhai et al. (2015)
Cookies	WPC	5–15%	Sweet potato, rice, sorghum and corn flour	WPC decreased spread ratio and increased sensory score	Giri and Sakhale (2019)
Cakes	Rice protein (79%), pea protein (78%), EWP (82%), WPC (92%)	15–45%	Rice flour	WPC increased specific volume and hardness. Pea and rice proteins were similar to control. All proteins decreased sensory acceptability	Sahagún et al. (2018)
Cakes	WPC (25%)	0–15%	Corn and rice flours	WPC had positive effects on specific volume and baking loss of cakes and increased hardness	Ammar et al. (2021)
Muffins	Chickpea protein isolate	7–14%	Millet flour	Protein slightly decreased specific volume and increased hardness	Shaabani et al. (2018)

[a]Protein concentration is included in parenthesis when provided
EWP egg white powder, *WPC* whey protein concentrate, *SPI* soy protein concentrate, *SBV* specific bread volume

4.5 Enzymes

Enzymes are widely used as technological aids in numerous processes of food technology, as they are considered clean label compounds. They are considered as the best and safest alternative to chemical compounds because enzymes are proteins which have the ability to catalyse chemical reactions, they can be labelled as generally recognized as safe (GRAS), and do not remain active after breadmaking due to their protein structure being denatured during baking (Rosell 2009).

The enzymes used in GF breadmaking differ from those used in wheat breadmaking since the whole system behaves differently. For practical reasons, the enzymes will be grouped in two different categories according to the dough/batter component they mainly affect, *i.e.* enzymes that modify polysaccharide, and enzymes that modify proteins (Table 4.5). In the first category, the following enzymes are included: (i) the broad group of *starch converting enzymes* (endoamylases, exoamylases, debranching enzymes, and transferases). Representative elements of this group are α-amylases (endoamylase), undoubtedly the most popular starch converting enzyme used in bakery; amyloglucosidase and α-glucosidase (exoamylases), and cyclodextrin glycosyltransferases (transferase). (ii) *Xylanases* that act on arabinoxylans and cleave the xylan backbone of arabinoxylan which increases water solubility and thus have a direct impact on dough/batter properties. (iii) *Glucose oxidase* that catalyses, in the presence of oxygen, the oxidation of glucose to gluconolactone and hydrogen peroxide (H_2O_2). This H_2O_2 oxidizes free sulfhydryl groups present in proteins producing S-S bonds, and also leads to the gelation of soluble arabinoxylans, which modifies the rheological behaviour of the systems in which it is present (Vemulapalli and Hoseney 1998). Although the substrate of glucose oxidase is glucose, and thus a polysaccharide modifying enzyme, it indirectly produces protein cross-linking thus it could also be grouped with protein modifying enzymes.

The enzymes acting on the protein fraction can be roughly classified as polymerizing and depolymerizing enzymes. In the first group we include transglutaminase and, with an indirect effect on proteins, laccase and tyrosinase. In the latter, we include proteases. Transglutaminase is an acyltransferase that catalyses three type of reactions, but the most important reaction for the bakery industry is the formation of intra- or inter-chain isopeptide bonds between glutamine and lysine residues (Seguro et al. 1996). Laccase catalyses the oxidation of a variety of organic substrates such as phenols and aromatic amines and thiols, producing reactive radicals. Further reactions of these radicals may result in crosslinking of monomers, degradation of polymers and cleavage of aromatic rings (Flander et al. 2011). Tyrosinase catalyses the hydroxylation of monophenols (but not ferulic acid) to diphenols and the subsequent oxidation of these to quinones. Tyrosine side chains in proteins can be oxidized by this enzyme, and lysyl, tyrosyl, cysteinyl, and histidine moieties may react further with oxidized tyrosine residues producing protein crosslinking. *Proteolytic enzymes*, or proteases, catalyse the hydrolysis of peptide bonds. Two main protease groups are described: endoproteases, which randomly break peptide bonds producing peptides of lower molecular mass; and exoproteases, which split single amino acids either from amino-terminal extreme (aminopeptidase) or from carboxy-terminal extreme (carboxypeptidase).

The activity of amylases has several consequences on dough/batter and bread properties. During batter mixing and proofing, amylases degrade the damaged starch fraction which increases fermentable sugars and thus favour yeast

Table 4.5 Most representative enzymes used in bakery

Enzyme type		Substrate	Reaction	Product
Enzymes that modify polysaccharides				
Starch converting enzymes	Endoamylases *(e.g. α-amylases)*	Starch	Random hydrolysis of α,1–4 glycosidic bonds in the inner part of amylose and amylopectin	Glucose, maltose, dextrins, limit dextrin
	Exoamylases *(e.g. β-amylases, amyloglucosidase, α-glucosidase)*	Starch	Hydrolysis of external α,1–4 glycosidic bonds of amylose and amylopectin	Glucose (amyloglucosidase and α-glucosidase) or maltose (β-amylase), limit dextrin
	Debranching enzymes *(e.g. Isoamylases, pullanases)*	Starch	Hydrolysis of α,1–6 glycosidic bonds	Linear dextrins
	Transferases *(e.g. cyclodextrin glycosyltransferases, amylomaltase)*	Starch	Hydrolysis of α,1–4 glycosidic bond and transfer part of the donor to a glycosidic acceptor	Oligosacharides, ciclic oligosacharides, highly branched high-molecular-weight dextrins
Xylanases		(Arabino) xylans	Random hydrolysis of β,1–4 xylosidic bonds	Lower molecular weight (arabino) xylans
Glucose oxidase		Glucose	Oxidation of α-glucose	α-gluconolactone and hydrogen peroxide (H_2O_2). H_2O_2 further oxidise proteins

(continued)

Table 4.5 (continued)

Enzyme type		Substrate	Reaction	Product
Enzymes that modify proteins (directly or indirectly)				
Polymerizing enzymes	Transglutaminase	Glutamine-lysine	Isopeptide bond formation	Cross-linked protein and ammonia (NH_3)
		Glutamine-primary amine	Acyl transfer reaction	Polyamine and ammonia (NH_3)
		Glutamine-water	Glutamine deamination	Glutamate and ammonia (NH_3)
	Laccase	Organic compounds and molecular oxygen	Oxidation of organic substrates and reduction of oxygen to water	Reactive radicals and water
	Tyrosinase	Monophenols (*e.g.* tirosine)	Oxidation	Quinones that may further react with lysyl, tyrosyl, and cysteinyl residues, resulting in the inter- and intra-molecular cross-linking of proteins
Proteolytic enzymes	Endoproteases	Proteins	Cleave inner peptide bonds	Peptides
	Exoproteases	Proteins	Cleave peptide bond proximal to the amino or carboxy termini of the substrate	Peptides and amino acids

metabolism increasing bread volume. Damaged starch has a large hydration capacity and its disappearance leads to a decrease in batter/dough consistency (Barrera et al. 2007), and the impact of this decrease depends on the amount of damaged starch present. As mentioned before, the reduction in batter consistency might have both a positive or negative effect on bread properties depending on the "limiting consistency" of the working system. It has to be considered that most amylases are stable at temperatures below 50 °C, however, some amylases maybe active at higher temperatures (Leman et al. 2005), thus can exert their hydrolysing activities not only during proofing but also during the first stage of baking, *i.e.* when starch gelatinisation has already begun. Of especial interest is the effect of α-amylase when a pregelatinised starch is used in GF formulation, since this starch is already available for hydrolysis. This gelatinised starch is now available for hydrolysis and this may affect gas-holding/expansion during baking. Finally, the products of the reaction also increase the substrates for the Maillard reaction which improves bread flavour and crust colour (Goesaert et al. 2009).

Another effect of amylases activity, especially endo-amylases, is the liberation of dextrins and oligosaccharides that affect starch retrogradation during storage which is of especial interest for GF breads since they are prone to a rapid staling. This reduced starch retrogradation has an implication in bread firming during storage. It has been reported that increasing α-amylase concentration decreases crumb firmness of rice bread up to 30% (Rosell 2009). However, the use of α-amylases has some drawbacks because even a slight overdose results in sticky bread associated with the production of branched maltodextrins of DP20-100. It was suggested that this problem could be solved using an exoamylase, since these do not produce these branched maltooligosaccharides. Such enzymes, like maltogenic amylases, produce linear oligosaccharides of 2–6 glucose residues, and are active during baking, modifying starch at a temperature when most of the starch starts to gelatinize (van der Maarel et al. 2002). Microencapsulation has been proposed as another alternative to minimize the negative effect of a possible overdose of α-amylase (Haghighat-Kharazi et al. 2018).

Amyloglucosidase (AMG) also proved to increase bread quality, as reported by Elgeti et al. (2014). These authors found that refined quinoa flour increased bread volume, and ascribed this result to the high α-glucosidase activity of this flour. To verify this result they added AMG or α-amylase to a control bread made with rice and corn flours, and corn starch and found an increase in bread volume, when both enzymes were used, especially AMG.

Gujral et al. (2003) evaluated the incorporation of cyclodextrin glycosyltransferase (CGT) to rice doughs. This enzyme catalyses different reactions by cleaving α-1,4 glycosidic bonds present in the inner part of a polysaccharide chain. The production of cyclodextrins is the specific reaction of CGT; cyclodextrins have a polar surface, responsible for the aqueous solubility, and a hydrophobic inner core (Gujral et al. 2003). These authors found that CGT reduced the viscoelasticity of the rice doughs, and this was explained as a result of the hydrolysis of damaged starch during mixing and proofing. They also found that bread specific volume increased by 73% when CGT was used, and attributed this result to higher concentration of fermentable sugars. An increase was also observed when α-amylase was used, but the increase was lower than for CGT, thus the effect of this enzyme cannot only be explained in terms of the presence of fermentable sugars. Crumb firmness was lowered by both enzymes, but α-amylase produced sticky crumbs, suggesting that CGT did decrease bread firmness by a hydrolytic mechanism but also by the cyclization of the hydrolysis products (resulting in the formation of cyclodextrins) and latter complexation with proteins and lipids, which has a significant role in decreasing crumb firmness and increased specific volume.

Xylanases (XYL) modify batter/dough properties by converting water-unextractable arabinoxylans to water-extractable. Since water-extractable arabinoxylans have lower WHC, a decrease in firmness, an increase in bread volume, and a uniform and finer crumb is obtained after XYL treatment. It showed varied effects on baking quality of GF bread. This enzyme has not been extensively applied in GF systems. Sarabhai et al. (2021) evaluated the effect of XYL on batter rheology and bread quality using foxtail millet flour as main ingredient. Treated batters presented a decreased resistance to deformation, and increased bread overall quality, *i.e.*, higher specific volume, lower crumb firmness and increased air fraction in the crumb.

Gujral and Rosell (2004a) first pointed out that the formation of a protein network in GF systems was necessary to hold the gas produced during fermentation. These authors found that transglutaminase (TG) produced a crosslinked network in rice-based batters, and that this crosslinking resulted in a dough with improved viscoelastic behaviour. Moore et al. (2006) carried out a study on the effect of TG on batters added with different protein sources (soy flour, skim milk powder and egg powder) and found that a network was actually formed after TG addition, and that the TG effect was protein source and dose dependent. Later, Renzetti et al. (2008) studied the effect of this enzyme on the properties of dough and breads made of different flours (buckwheat, brown rice, oat, sorghum, teff and corn). They found that the enzyme modified differently dough rheology and that the effect on bread quality was also flour dependent. For some flours, TG increased dough resistance to deformation and elasticity, obtaining breads with better technological parameters (*i.e.*, higher specific volume and lower crumb firmness). For other flours, TG did not affect dough rheology while bread quality was neither improved nor worsen, and finally, for other flours, TG decreased dough resistance to deformation, and this improved bread properties. Marco and Rosell (2008) evaluated the effect of TG and HPMC on the rheological properties of soybean-enriched rice batters and bread quality. HPMC and soy protein isolate (SPI) increased batter consistency, but while HPMC increased rice bread volumes, TG showed no significant effect; after adding SPI, the trend was the same: while HPMC counteracted the detrimental effect of soy protein, the enzyme had no significant effect. More recently, Tomić et al. (2020) evaluated the effect of TG addition on GF breads formulated with millet flour enriched with different protein sources (pea, rice and whey concentrates). They reported improved viscoelastic properties (higher G' and G") in batters enriched with rice and whey proteins when TG was added, although this did not result in better technological quality of breads; moreover, a detrimental effect of TG was found on bread quality when pea and rice were used, while no effect was reported on whey-enriched bread. These authors suggested that this negative effect was probably due to an extensive crosslinking that resulted in a compact dough structure unable to expand during the fermentation. From these overall results, it can be concluded that the protein source is a key element determining the impact of the enzyme, and that no generalisation about TG effect on batter and bread is plausible.

Protein crosslinking was also reported after glucose oxidase (GOX) addition by Gujral and Rosell (2004b), Renzetti and Arendt (2009a) and Sciarini et al. (2012). In the first study, a rice-based bread was evaluated; in the second, corn, sorghum, buckwheat or teff flours were used individually, and in the third, a formulation made of rice, soy and cassava was evaluated. In all cases, protein crosslinking increased the elastic properties of dough/batter, but the effect on bread quality was not consistent. While Gujral and Rosell (2004b) obtained breads of higher overall quality, no significant effect was reported by Sciarini et al. (2012), whereas Renzetti and Arendt (2009a) concluded that the result largely depended on the type of flour used.

As previously addressed, tyrosinase and laccase are enzymes capable of catalysing biopolymers cross-linking via their phenolic moieties. Laccase (LAC) is able to stabilize the dough/batter structure by crosslinking proteins and proteins with arabinoxylans, resulting in a strong arabinoxylan network. However, the application of this enzyme to GF systems has been poorly explored. Renzetti et al. (2010) reported an increase in bread specific volume and a softening of the crumb when this enzyme was added to oat-based breads, and explained that these findings were partly a result of β-glucan depolymerisation. Flander et al. (2011) also found an increase in specific volume of oat bread combining laccase and xylanase, although crumb softness was not increased. These authors also explored the use of tyrosinase (TYR) and reported that it effectively induced the formation of higher molecular weight proteins and assumed this to be the result of the cross-linking of oat globulins. TYR alone or combined with xylanase increased specific volume and the softness of the bread. Ayala-Soto et al. (2017) evaluated the effect of LAC in GF batter made of rice flour, corn starch and brown rice, and added with corn fibre arabinoxylans. They found no effect on batter consistency nor bread specific volume when the enzyme was used, and they ascertained this result to insufficient time for LAC action.

Renzetti and Arendt (2009b) proposed that mild protein hydrolysis could improve the foaming properties of the batter and consequently its breadmaking performance. They assayed a protease treatment in batters made of brown rice, and found a decrease in batter resistance to deformation, and suggested that this decreasing improved batter development due to a reduced resistance to expansion during proofing. Sarabhai et al. (2021) also found better bread quality when including proteases in bread formulation. Hatta et al. (2015) assayed proteases with different catalytic activities (metalloenzymes, serine, cysteine and aspartyl-proteases) and found an improvement in rice bread quality with metalloenzymes, serine, and cysteine, but not aspartyl, proteases. These authors reported the formation of fine networks of small protein in rice batters treated with metalloenzymes, serine or cysteine proteases, and that this network was effective for retaining CO_2 during the fermentation process, resulting in an increase in the specific volume and a decrease in the crumb hardness of rice bread. Kawamura-Konishi et al. (2013) described, on the other hand, that the protease Thermoase PC10F exhibited limited hydrolysis of rice prolamins and glutelins, but readily hydrolysed globulins and albumins, and that this hydrolysis was probable the responsible of the increased bread volume and overall technological quality.

It has been reported that the pasting properties of flours are also modified after protease treatment, decreasing peak and final viscosities (Renzetti and Arendt 2009b) and these changes are most probably due to the modification of protein-starch interactions (Ragaee and Abdel-Aal 2006).

As reported for the other enzymes, the effect of proteases proved to be dependent on the source of flour used. Thus, in those systems where proteins play a structural role (*e.g.* corn, sorghum and buckwheat), protease activity could be detrimental to bread quality. In such cases, TG treatment, instead, may improve crumb texture after reinforcing such protein structure (Renzetti et al. 2008), while proteolytic activity disrupts its continuity leading to breads of inferior overall quality.

The use of enzymes is less widespread for GF pasta production than for GF bread production. Due to the specific structure required for pasta-making, enzymes acting on the protein fraction have been more explored. Pyranose-2-oxidase has a catalytic activity similar to that of GOX, although its use in food products is still rare. Linares-García et al. (2019) reported that adding this enzyme to quinoa-based pasta improved the quality of the product due to the formation of chemical intermolecular cross-links. Also, noodles containing lupine flour, pea protein, and pyranose-2-oxidase exhibited acceptable quality and had high protein and dietary fibre contents.

Takács et al. (2007) demonstrated that TG produced the polymerisation of pea proteins, and that this polymerisation would be responsible for the increased pasta quality (improved sensory properties, high water uptake and low cooking loss). Yalcin and Basman (2008) reported that adding TG to rice-based noodles improved the machinability of the dough, and that this led to a smooth noodle surface and improved noodle quality, based on cooking loss reduction. The beneficial effects of TG on pasta quality were also confirmed by Kim et al. (2014), on rice-based pasta with rice protein isolate; Kumar et al. (2019) on pearl millet-pasta added with whey and cascinate proteins concentrates; and by Shokri et al. (2016) on rice flour/corn starch-pasta.

The use of enzymes in GF cookies is not a common practice. On the one hand, polysaccharides modifying enzymes tend to increase water absorption/retention and dough stickiness, which are negative for cookie production; and on the other, dough with plastic (extensible) behaviour is preferred for cookie development since it is more easily handled, thus cross-linking enzymes tend to produce viscoelastic doughs that may result in shrinkage during sheeting.

Altindağ et al. (2015) evaluated the addition of transglutaminase in GF cookies made of buckwheat, corn and rice flours, and their mixtures. The addition of TG resulted in increased moisture content and fracturability and decreased hardness values.

Saeidi et al. (2018) evaluated the use of TG and pomegranate seed powder (PSP) in rice-based cakes. The presence of PSP and TG reduced the overall quality of cake which was related to the high fibre content in PSP and to the formation of a protein network after enzyme addition. Both factors could prevent the expansion of gas cells, consequently decreasing specific volume. Shaabani et al. (2018) included TG in millet-cakes fortified with chickpea protein isolate, and found that the protein and transglutaminase together helped in the development of muffin sponge-like structure and argued that this was the result of a cross-linked network formed within muffins that was able to entrap and retain more air. With a technological standpoint, transglutaminase was also evaluated in revani, a cake-like Turkish dessert, made from corn, rice and potato flours, and corn and tapioca starches, and added with two different protein sources (soy and pea proteins). The combined effect of TG and proteins resulted in revani with ideal hardness properties, while they did not affect the sensory quality of the end-products (Yildirim et al. 2018). In Table 4.6, representative works about the effect of enzymes addition in GF formulation are presented.

Table 4.6 Relevant studies on gluten-free (GF) cereal-based products containing enzymes and their main results

Product	Enzyme	Flour base	Results	References
Bread	Pr and Lip	Rice and quinoa flours and corn starch	Protease and lipase improved bread quality by increasing SBV	Azizi et al. (2020)
Bread	CGT and TG	Chickpea flour and cassava starch	CGT reduced crumb firming rate. TG had no effect	Santos et al. (2020)
Bread	GOX, XYL, Pr	Millet flour	Enzymes increased SBV and decreased crumb hardness and cohesiveness. Pr had better taste, aroma and overall quality	Sarabhai et al. (2021)
Bread	GOX, Pr (endo-protease and alcalase)	*Colocasia* spp. (taro) flour	GOX did not modify SBV but reduced firmness. Endo-protease increased SBV and firmness, and alcalase decreased both SBV and firmness	Calle et al. (2020)
Bread	TG, Pr	Quinoa flour	Pr improved dough characteristics, but produced bitter peptides. TG improved bread appearance and taste	Romano et al. (2018)
Bread	Acidic-thermostable α-Am	Rice, quinoa and buckwheat flours, and potato starch	Enzyme increased SBV, porosity and moisture content of crumb. Decreased crumb firmness and decreased crust luminosity (L*)	Motahar et al. (2021)
Bread	maltogenic Am encapsulated in beeswax	Rice and chickpea flours	Encapsulated enzyme produced darker crust, whiter and softer crumb, and more aerated structure. Also increased sensorial acceptability during storage	Haghighat-Kharazi et al. (2020)
Bread	POX (in presence of AX)	Buckwheat or millet flours (both refined and wholemeal)	In the presence of AX the enzyme produced softer crumbs, and increased water binding (related to the shelf-life of the products)	Farkas et al. (2021)
Pasta	TG	Millet flour	TG increased cooking loss but improved pasta texture by increasing firmness	Kumar et al. (2019)
Pasta	TG	*Colocasia esculenta* (taro flour)	In the presence of egg white, TG produced pasta with good colour, cooking properties, and texture	Campos and Almeida (2021)

(continued)

Table 4.6 (continued)

Product	Enzyme	Flour base	Results	References
Cookies	TG	Corn and rice flours	TG increased moisture content, spread ratio, and fracturability, but decreased hardness values	Altındağ et al. (2015)
Cakes	TG	Rice flour	Optimized breads showed decreased specific volume and L* values (crust and crumb), and increased overall acceptability	Saeidi et al. (2018)
Cakes	TG	Brown, red or black rice flours	TG only affected the technological properties of brown rice cake (decreased crumb firmness and increase in the specific volume)	Lang et al. (2020)
Muffins	TG	Millet flour	TG increased specific volume and firmness in the presence of a protein source	Shaabani et al. (2018)

Pr protease, *Lip* lipase, *CGT* cyclodextrin glycosyltransferase, *TG* transglutaminase, *GOX* glucose oxidase, *XYL* xylanase, *Am* amylase, *POX* pyranose-2-oxidase, *SBV* specific bread volume, *AX* arabinoxylans

4.6 Emulsifiers

Food emulsifiers do more than simply stabilize emulsions; they are more accurately termed surfactants (Hasenhuettl 2008). However, the term emulsifier has been used so extensively in the food industry, particularly in baking, it will be used in this section.

Most foods are complex mixtures of different ingredients. In some cases, these components have such different chemical compositions that they are immiscible, but they also form systems where one phase is dispersed in another. An emulsion is a heterogeneous system, consisting of two or more immiscible phases intimately dispersed in one to another, forming small droplets. These systems are characterised by their low stability, since the droplets tend to merge and form larger droplets, and the matrix tends to separate in phases. So, emulsifiers are necessary to form this type of immiscible system and keep it stable.

Surface-active compounds have a lipophilic and a hydrophilic region in the same molecule. The hydrophilic head group is attracted to the aqueous phase, and the often-larger lipophilic tail prefers to be in the oil phase. The surfactant therefore positions itself to some extent, at the air/water or oil/water interface where it can act to lower surface or interfacial tension (Hasenhuettl 2008).

The hydrophilic region can be non-ionic (contains no charge, they are dipoles), anionic (contains a negative charge), cationic (positively charged), or amphoteric (contains both positive and negative charges on the same molecule). On the other hand, the lipophilic functional groups are derived from fatty acids with a number of carbon atoms between 16 and 22 and their source can be vegetable (sunflower, palm and soybean oil) or animal (pork or beef fat).

One of the two regions of the same molecule exerts a more marked effect than the other in the system, which determines its hydrophile-lipophile balance (HLB). The number and relative polarity of functional groups in a surface-active molecule determine whether the molecule will be water or oil "soluble" (or dispersible). Since conventional practice is to disperse the surfactant into the continuous phase, an arbitrary scale was created to classify these compounds, where lipophilic compounds assume low values (from 1 to 9) and hydrophilic compounds high values (10–18) of HLB. Oil-in-water (O/W) emulsifiers have high HLB values and water-in-oil (W/O) emulsifiers have low HLB values. Extreme high or low values are not functional as emulsifiers since almost all of the molecule will be solubilised in the continuous phase (Hasenhuettl 2008).

When emulsifiers are used in breadmaking, they contribute to increase the stability of a thermodynamically unstable system. In addition to the function of producing and stabilising emulsions, food emulsifiers in baking contribute to other functional roles, as blending and emulsification of ingredients, foam aeration and stabilisation, dough strengthening and lubricating, and starch complexation (anti-staling) (Gómez et al. 2004; Nunes et al. 2009).

As mentioned before, in the elaboration of conventional bread, the development of gluten is essential. The non-covalent interactions between gliadins, glutenins and the components that surround them are of vital importance for the properties of gluten. Lipophilic region of the emulsifiers can interact with hydrophobic amino acids, which are mainly present in glutenins. These bonds are stronger than those generated by the lipids that are normally found in flour. On the other hand, emulsifiers neutralise electrostatic positive charges that are normally found in gliadins. In consequence, the complex emulsifier-protein strengthens the dough allowing a better CO_2 retention during ovenspring, resulting in breads with greater volume and better structure (Kamel and Ponte 1993; Atwell and Finnie 2016; Palavecino and Sciarini 2019).

It is known that the formation of amylose-lipid complexes retards the process of recrystallization of starch, and consequently, delay bread staling. Similarly, the lipid region of the emulsifiers interacts with amylose and interferes with starch retrogradation in GF breads. Also, emulsifiers interact with the starch granule surface retarding the ingress of water as the temperature increases. As a consequence, a softer breadcrumb is obtained and a reduction in the rate of hardening (Orthoefer 2008).

Diacetyltartaric ester of monoglycerides (DATEM), lecithin (LE), distilled monoglycerides (DM), sodium stearoyl lactylate (SSL), calcium stearoyl lactylate (CSL), sodium stearoyl fumarate, sodium lauryl sulfate, glycerol monostearate (GMS), dioctyl sodium sulfosuccinate, polyglycerol esters and sucrose esters are some of the commonly used emulsifiers in wheat-based bakery products (Gómez et al. 2004; Orthoefer 2008; Nunes et al. 2009).

Emulsifiers are also used in GF bakery products to assist blending and emulsification of ingredients, to enhance the properties of the shortening, and to interact with the components of the flour and other ingredients in the mix for softer crumb (Palav et al. 2009). Emulsifiers proved to be beneficial in improving texture and softness of wheat bread crumb and crust and enhancing loaf volume, however, controversial results about their function in GF bread can be found in the literature (Rao et al. 2017).

Onyango et al. (2009) made GF bread based on pregelatinised cassava starch and found that emulsifier addition (GMS, SSL, CSL, and DATEM) reinforced dough structure and decreased crumb firmness as well, except for DATEM. Nunes et al. (2009) analysed the effects of the LE, DATEM, DM, and SSL on GF batter and bread quality at three different levels. The effect depended on the type and level of emulsifier used. Emulsifiers affected the rheological properties of the batters and showed great ability to modify the characteristics of the bread quality; they had very little effect on the melting of the starch components. Main results showed that lecithin reduced the elasticity of the batter and increased the batter consistency during gelatinisation. Distilled monoglycerides improved bread volume. However, DATEM decreased it. These authors concluded that GF bread quality can be greatly enhanced with the correct emulsifier and optimal addition level.

However, some authors found negative results when emulsifiers were used in GF breads. López-Tenorio et al., (2015) analysed the effects of DATEM and SSL on dough rheology and GF bread quality. They found that emulsifiers had no significant effect on dough rheology. However, they affected the physical and textural characteristics of GF cheese bread. The height, diameter and specific volume of the samples decreased with higher concentrations of emulsifiers in the formula, while the yield and crumb hardness increased. Crust fracture and crumb hardness of samples increased during storage; thus the emulsifiers did not affect product behaviour during aging. Purhagen et al. (2012), analysed the effect of a monoglyceride diacetyltartaric acid ester in a commercial GF mix to produce bread. The addition of the emulsifier improved the water retention and decreased the amount of retrograded amylopectin as compared to both the gluten-free and the gluten-containing controls, and the crumb was softer than for the gluten-containing control; however, the structure of these loaves containing the emulsifier was impaired and not acceptable. Sciarini et al. (2012) concluded that the addition of DATEM and SSL affected batter rheology but they did not improve specific loaf volume. The authors concluded that these additives are not essential for GF bread production.

The described controversial results about the use of emulsifiers on GF bread quality could be related to the different formulations used, different quality of ingredients (flours, starches, and proteins), different water content of dough/batter, and different bread-making procedure (Yano 2019). Some general conclusions arise from literature review, emulsifiers used to strengthen gluten doughs, such as DATEM or SSL, do not seem to have the same effect on GF systems since they do not produce important changes on bread quality and in some cases, they have a negative effect. On the other hand, emulsifiers with better air-stabilizing properties, such as monoglycerides or lecithins, lead to better GF bread quality.

During pasta cooking, starch granules swell and partly solubilize, while the protein becomes insoluble and coagulates, so it influences the texture of cooked pasta. For continuous pasta extrusion, a satisfactory GF pasta product is usually smooth, mechanically strong and of uniform colour. It should maintain its shape when cooked, and cooked pasta should have a firm consistency without a sticky surface. It should also be resistant to disintegration due to overcooking (Lai 2002). Although many additives have been used to improve the quality of GF pasta (Palavecino et al. 2017; Gao et al. 2018), emulsifiers are one of the most used compounds.

According to Lai (2002), the fatty nature of emulsifiers enables them to act as a lubricant in the extrusion process, resulting in less nozzle wear and tear and thus making production easier. Some emulsifiers also provide a firmer consistency, a less sticky surface and better starch retention properties during cooking. Emulsifiers possess the ability to form complexes with starch, which could be important for the structure of the noodles (Schoenlechner et al. 2010). Kovacs et al. (2001) described that emulsifiers have effects in gluten-free pasta; they found protein-emulsifier and emulsifier-carbohydrate interactions with a high complexing rate of 50–90%.

According to De Arcangelis et al. (2020), in GF doughs, the functions of gluten are partially performed by the starch and their gelatinization process. So, substances whose action can occur at the starch level, for example, inhibiting swelling during cooking or accelerating the phenomenon of gelatinization, can facilitate proteins crosslinking. At an industrial level, emulsifier such as mono and di-glycerides of fatty acids are added to the GF flours with the aim to form complexes with amylose and limiting its passage in the cooking water with consequent improvement of the quality characteristics of the pasta itself (Kovacs et al. 2001; Schoenlechner et al. 2010).

Schoenlechner et al. (2010) tested DATEM and DM on GF pasta produced from amaranth, quinoa and buckwheat; and they found the best results with 1.2% of distilled monoglycerides. Pasta firmness was increased and cooking loss decreased. Additionally cooking weight showed increased values after addition of DM. However, addition of DATEM showed negative effects on firmness.

Most recently, the gelatinization of mixed flours (buckwheat, maize, and rice) with the combined use of 0.1% of propylene glycol alginate and 0.5% of monoglycerides of fatty acids was found to be the best combination to obtain gluten-free pasta with good cooking quality (De Arcangelis et al. 2020).

Mono- and di-glycerides are the surfactants commonly used to soften cake crumbs. Dough strengtheners include SSL, DATEM, sorbitan monostearate, and ethoxylated mono-and diglycerides. Propylene glycol esters are indicated as foam aeration and stabilisation for cakes and whipped toppings. DATEM, DM, monoglycerides of fatty acids, LE and propylene glycol alginate were tested in conventional and GF pasta or noodles.

4.7 Antimicrobial Agents

Chemical preservatives are used in order to guarantee consumer safety, prolonging the shelf life of the product. These must inhibit the growth of pathogenic microorganisms and limit the production of toxins, preventing the deterioration of the food without significantly modifying its organoleptic characteristics.

During the baking, a large part of the microbial load present in the bread is destroyed. The intermediate-low water activity of bread limits the growth of microorganisms to almost exclusively moulds, mainly *Penicillium* species, *Aspergillus* species and *Clodosporium*, *Mucorales* and *Neurospora*. However, the most common bread spoilage moulds are *Penicillium* spp. The development of microorganisms not only alters the organoleptic characteristics making it inedible, but some of these microorganisms can produce toxins that are harmful to health. Another type of microorganism can develop in bread if its spores survive cooking and then find favourable conditions to germinate: *Bacillus subtilis*. This contaminant degrades the internal structure of the crumb, producing unpleasant flavours and a greasy texture (Legan 1993; Pateras 2007, Melini and Melini 2018). On rye bread, *P. roqueforti* was the major contaminant (Lund et al. 1996).

Although all bread has a low bacterial load immediately after baking, airborne mould spores can contaminate bread after it has been baked. Special attention must be paid to the end stages (cooling, slicing and packaging) of the production process of sliced bread, where a low amount of free water and microbial load must be ensured. Hence preservatives are often added to reduce the development of mould on the surface of bread products.

The principal mould inhibitors used in bread world-wide are propionic, sorbic and acetic acids and certain of their salts, which are more soluble in aqueous solution. The most commonly employed preservative is calcium propionate. Potassium sorbate is used sometimes in spray operations to reduce mould growth, but some consumers perceive an undesirable off-flavour. The effectiveness of the preservatives is dependent on the pH of the product, as the antimicrobial effect of the undissociated acid is much stronger than the dissociated acid. Maximum pH for activity is around 6.0–6.5 for sorbate, 5.0–5.5 for propionate and 4.0–4.5 for benzoate (Suhr and Nielsen 2004; Pateras 2007). However, the status and use of these materials is controlled in many countries by legislation which limits the type and concentration of preservatives that may be used. Legislation varies considerably among countries, so it is not possible to generalise about maximum doses. The European Regulation establishes 0.2% (w/w) and 0.3% (w/w) limits for sorbate and propionate addition, respectively, in both prepacked sliced bread and rye bread; and a maximum of 0.1% propionate in case of prepacked unsliced bread (European Parliament and the Council 2004).

Weak-acids, such as acetic, lactic, citric, and malic, can help inhibiting the growth of microorganisms, this effect is linked both to specific properties of these compounds and to the reduction of the pH of the medium, which in turn enhances the activity of other antimicrobials (Gurtler and Mai 2014).

Addition of ethanol concentrations ranging between 0.2% and 12% are reported to increase bread shelf-life. Also, ethanol addition on bread surface contributes to improving sorbate and propionate effect, as reviewed by Melini and Melini (2018).

The use of proper packaging is needed to extend the shelf life of bakery products.

Other methodologies can be used to extend the product shelf-life. Physical procedures, such as the modified atmospheres and active packaging, ultra violet (UV) light, infrared (IR), and microwave (MW) heating; the application of gamma/UV irradiation, the processes including biopreservation, and the action of antimicrobial compounds extracted from plants have been analysed in the literature (Smith et al. 2004; Melini and Melini 2018). Therefore, according to Garcia and Copetti (2019) the large-scale use of these methods still depend on further studies for their validation, and on factors related to economic viability and consumers' acceptance.

Gluten-free bread, sliced or not, is a product with high added value and short shelf-life. Baked good shelf-life is limited by different deterioration processes including fungal growth, the loss of moisture, and the staling. According to Melini and Melini (2018), GF bread shelf-life deserves a separate analysis and discussion, because of their different formulation. They have higher levels of water (and higher water activity) and, in some cases, the addition of fat ingredients. Staling represents the major issues in GF bread, as it is often mainly based on starchy ingredients (Schiraldi and Fessas 2001). However, GF bread should be protected from spoilage.

Traditional methods to improve GF bread shelf-life are similar to those used by many decades in wheat bread: physical treatments (UV light, IR radiation are some examples), and chemical preservatives (weak organic acids such as propionic and sorbic acid and combined with other weak-acids).

The sourdough, an ancient technology, is being increasingly revalued because of its impact on bread texture, flavour and its nutritional effects. Sourdough has also been reconsidered as a form of food bio-preservation and a possible way to replace chemical preservatives and thus guarantee a clean label, due to the role played by lactic acid bacteria (LAB) as bio-agents and inhibitors to bread spoilage. Important scientific work has been made to probe the ability of sourdough to retard staling, protect bread from spoilage, and subsequently contribute to extending bread shelf-life (Axel et al. 2016; Melini and Melini 2018).

Fresh pasta and noodles show a short shelf-life because of the high water activity. They deteriorate quickly if not stored under refrigeration, being bacteria the most common spoilage organisms in fresh noodles, followed by yeast and moulds (Ray 2001). For example, fresh rice noodles are more susceptible to contamination by amylolytic bacteria such as *Bacillus* sp., *Clostridium* sp., and molds such *as Aspergillus flavus*, *Penicillium citrinum*, *Monascus ruber*, and *Fusarium graminearum* (Tantala et al. 2022).

Hence, extending the shelf-life of traditional or GF fresh pasta and noodles is a crucial problem to be solved. Physical treatments, such as refrigeration, steam, irradiation, microwave, modified atmosphere packaging and active packaging and ozone, are employed to extend the shelf life of these fresh type foods (Bai et al. 2017; Li et al. 2011; Tuersuntuoheti et al. 2019: Li et al. 2021). Also, chemical preservatives, such as calcium propionate, potassium sorbate, sodium benzoate, and sodium dehydroacetate, are used (Li et al. 2011; CODEX 2017).

Moreover, weak-acid can be added to exert a pH regulation and a bactericidal effect and thus enhance the storage stability (Kobayashi 2012). Combination effects of chemical preservatives with different concentrations and physical treatments on shelf-life extension have been proposed (Tuersuntuoheti et al. 2019; Yang et al. 2021; Tantala et al. 2022).

However, it must be noted that consumers demand products free of chemical preservatives or with reduced levels of them. Among alternatives of chemical preservatives, natural antibacterial compounds (Li et al. 2014; Tuersuntuoheti et al. 2019; Tantala et al. 2022; Lucera et al. 2012) or modified packing conditions, as antifungal packaging of sorbate and benzoate incorporated biodegradable films have been assayed (Wangprasertkul et al. 2021).

4.8 Nutritional Considerations

Gluten-free baked goods in general have unsatisfactory nutritional value, which is why the number of studies on its fortification with proteins, fibre and/or bioactive compounds, mineral salts have increased in recent years. From a nutritional point of view, hydrocolloids are soluble dietary fibers generally associated with health promoting claims (Collar et al. 2015). Also, hydrocolloids can be used to reduce the lipid and sugar content in cookies formulations producing low-calorie products (Singh and Kumar 2018). In turn, additives like inulin can be added to GF formulations. Inulin is a linear fructan that acts as prebiotics because it cannot be digested by humans but it is fermented by colonic microbiota. Besides the nutritional enhancement, inulin incorporation into GF bread may also result in higher loaf volume (though less uniform) and with slower crumb hardening rate (Sciarini et al. 2017), and better results can be obtained using inulin of low degree of polymerization (Ziobro et al. 2013a, b).

The starch that cannot be hydrolysed in the human digestive tract is considered as dietary fibre and known as Resistant Starch (RS) (Englyst and Hudson 1996). The starch retrograded as a consequence of processing and storage is considered RS type III, the chemically modified that cannot be hydrolysed by enzymes is RS type IV, and the amylose–lipid complexes have been recently considered as RS type V (Lockyer and Nugent 2017). Despite RS IV is classified as a food additive and labelled as such, health allegations can be attached to these modified starches as well (Witczak et al. 2016). Then, GF formulations have to be designed to allow the use and/or formation of these RS to enhance its nutritional profile.

It is clear that modified starch and non-starchy polysaccharides are useful to improve the technological properties of GF cereal-based products while generally enhance its soluble dietary fibre content. Therefore, the application of these materials to GF should be more deeply researched. The nutritional value of proteins differs substantially depending upon their amino acid composition and digestibility. Protein nutritional quality is a measure of bioavailability, and its evaluation is a means of determining the capacity of food proteins and diets to satisfy metabolic demands for amino acids and nitrogen (Gilani 2012). In general, plant proteins are less digestible than animal proteins, as a result of a number of factors. One is the structural differences between animal and plant proteins. Carbonaro et al. (2012) and Nguyen et al. (2015) found that plant proteins have more β-sheet structures and relatively low α-helixes compared to animal proteins, which makes them resistant to digestion.

Then, the fact that more fibers are associated with plant proteins (Duodu et al. 2003) and the presence of antinutritive factors are additional factors for the lower proteolytic digestibility of plant-based proteins in the human gastrointestinal tract compared to animal proteins. Understanding protein nutritive factors is essential in product development formulation strategies for alternative protein products to meet the human body's protein needs (Ismail et al. 2020).

The presence of proteins, on the other hand, usually decreases the starch digestibility of baked goods, decreasing their glycaemic index. Enzymes such as transglutaminase reduces the *in vitro* starch hydrolysis index of GF pasta probably as a result of the cross-linkings in the protein network (Rosa-Sibakov et al. 2016).

This chapter summarises the most relevant advances in gluten free product's additives, some of them being incorporated into current legislation, and in some cases, they are yet to be regulated.

References

Ahlborn GJ, Pike OA, Hendrix SB et al (2005) Sensory, mechanical, and microscopic evaluation of staling in low-protein and gluten-free breads. Cereal Chem 82:328–335

Alamprese C, Casiraghi E, Pagani MA (2007) Development of gluten-free fresh egg pasta analogues containing buckwheat. Eur Food Res Technol 225:205–213

Altındağ G, Certel M, Erem F et al (2015) Quality characteristics of gluten-free cookies made of buckwheat, corn, and rice flour with/without transglutaminase. Food Sci Technol Int 21:213–220

Ames JM (1992) The Maillard reaction. In: Hudson BJF (ed) Biochemistry of food proteins. Springer, Boston, pp 99–153

Ammar I, Gharsallah H, Brahim AB et al (2021) Optimization of gluten-free sponge cake fortified with whey protein concentrate using mixture design methodology. Food Chem 343:128457

Anton AA, Artfield SD (2008) Hydrocolloids in gluten-free breads: a review. Int J Food Sci Nutr 59:11–23

Atwell W, Finnie S (2016) Wheat flour, 2nd edn. American Association of Cereal Chemists International, St. Paul

Axel C, Brosnan B, Zannini E et al (2016) Antifungal sourdough lactic acid bacteria as biopreservation tool in quinoa and rice bread. Int J Food Microbiol 239:86–94

Ayala-Soto FE, Serna-Saldívar SO, Welti-Chanes J (2017) Effect of arabinoxylans and laccase on batter rheology and quality of yeast-leavened gluten-free breads. J Cereal Sci 73:10–17

Azizi S, Azizi MH, Moogouei R et al (2020) The effect of quinoa flour and enzymes on the quality of gluten-free bread. Food Sci Nutr 8:2373–2382

Bai Y, Guo X, Zhu K et al (2017) Shelf-life extension of semidried buckwheat noodles by the combination of aqueous ozone treatment and modified atmosphere packaging. Food Chem 237:553–560

Barrera GN, Pérez GT, Ribotta PD et al (2007) Influence of damaged starch on cookie and bread-making quality. Eur Food Res Technol 225:1–7

BeMiller JN, Huber KC (2015) Physical modification of food starch functionalities. Annu Rev Food Sci Technol 6:19–69

Bender D, Schönlechner R (2020) Innovative approaches towards improved gluten-free bread properties. J Cereal Sci 91:102904. https://doi.org/10.1016/j.jcs.2019.102904

Bender D, Regner M, D'Amico S et al (2018) Effect of differently extracted arabinoxylan on gluten-free sourdough-bread properties. J Food Qual. https://doi.org/10.1155/2018/5719681

Berta M, Koelewijn I, Öhgren C et al (2019) Effect of zein protein and hydroxypropyl methylcellulose on the texture of model gluten-free bread. J Texture Stud 50:341–349

Bravo-Núñez Á, Sahagún M, Gómez M (2019) Assessing the importance of protein interactions and hydration level on protein-enriched gluten-free breads: a novel approach. Food Bioprocess Technol 12:820–828

Calle J, Benavent-Gil Y, Rosell CM (2020) Development of gluten free breads from Colocasia esculenta flour blended with hydrocolloids and enzymes. Food Hydrocoll 98:105243

Calvin O (2016) Starch and modified starch in bread making: a review. Afr J Food Sci 10:344–351

Campos BVP, Almeida EL (2021) Gluten-free pasta elaborated with taro flour (Colocasia esculenta): a study of the employ of egg white and transglutaminase on the technological properties. Res Society Dev 10:e52710111454

Carbonaro M, Maselli P, Nucara A (2012) Relationship between digestibility and secondary structure of raw and thermally treated legume proteins: a Fourier transform infrared (FT-IR) spectroscopic study. Amino Acids 43:911–921

Cato L, Gan JJ, Rafael LGB, Small DM (2004) Gluten free breads using rice flour and hydrocolloid gums. Food Aust 56:75–78

Cham S, Suwannaporn P (2010) Effect of hydrothermal treatment of rice flour on various rice noodles quality. J Cereal Sci 51:284–291

Codex (2017) Codex general standard for food additives (GSFA) online database. http://www.fao.org/fao who codexalimentarius/codex-texts/dbs/gsfa/en/. Accessed 12 Jan 2022

Codex Alimentarius Commission (1989) Codex standards for vegetable proteins and general guidelines for the utilization of vegetable protein products, 1st edn. FAO-WHO, Rome, supplement 1 to Codex Alimentarius. CODEX STAN 175

Collar C, Conte P, Fadda C, Piga A (2015) Gluten-free dough-making of specialty breads: significance of blended starches, flours and additives on dough behaviour. Food Sci Technol Int 21:523–536

Crockett R, Ie P, Vodovotz Y (2011) Effects of soy protein isolate and egg white solids on the physicochemical properties of gluten-free bread. Food Chem 129:84–91

Culetu A, Duta DE, Papageorgiou M, Varzakas T (2021) The role of hydrocolloids in gluten-free bread and pasta; rheology, characteristics, staling and glycemic index. Foods 10:1–19

Das AB, Bhattacharya S (2019) Characterization of the batter and gluten-free cake from extruded red rice flour. LWT Food Sci Technol 102:197–204

Day L (2016) Protein: food sources. In: Caballero B, Finglas PM, Toldrá F (eds) Encyclopedia of food and health. Academic, London, pp 530–537

Day L, Cakebread JA, Loveday SM (2022) Food proteins from animals and plants: differences in the nutritional and functional properties. Trends Food Sci Technol 119:428–442

De Arcangelis E, Cuomo F, Trivisonno MC et al (2020) Gelatinization and pasta making conditions for buckwheat gluten-free pasta. J Cereal Sci 95:103073. https://doi.org/10.1016/j.jcs.2020.103073

Detchewa P, Prasajak P, Phungamngoen C et al (2022) Substitution of rice flour with rice protein improved quality of gluten-free rice spaghetti processed using single screw extrusion. LWT Food Sci Technol 153:112512

Diprat AB, Thys RCS, Rodrigues E et al (2020) Chlorella sorokiniana: a new alternative source of carotenoids and proteins for gluten-free bread. LWT Food Sci Technol 134:109974

Duodu KG, Taylor JRN, Belton PS, and Hamaker BR (2003) Factors affecting sorghum protein digestibility. J Cereal Sci 38:117–131

Elgeti D, Nordlohne SD, Föste M et al (2014) Volume and texture improvement of gluten-free bread using quinoa white flour. J Cereal Sci 59:41–47

Englyst HN, Hudson GJ (1996) The classification and measurement of dietary carbohydrates. Food Chem 57:15–21

European Parliament and the Council. Regulation (EC) No 1935/2004 of the European Parliament and of the Council of 27 October 2004 on materials and articles intended to come into contact with food and repealing Directives 80/590/EEC and 89/109/EEC. Off J Eur Union 2004, L 338, 4-17.004

Farkas A, Szepesvari P, Németh R et al (2021) Comparative study on the rheological and baking behaviour of enzyme-treated and arabinoxylan-enriched gluten-free straight dough and sourdough small-scale systems. J Cereal Sci 101:103292

Ferreira SMR, de Mello AP, de Caldas Rosa dos Anjos M et al (2016) Utilization of sorghum, rice, corn flours with potato starch for the preparation of gluten-free pasta. Food Chem 191:147–151

Ferrero C (2017) Hydrocolloids in wheat breadmaking: a concise review. Food Hydrocoll 68:15–22. https://doi.org/10.1016/j.foodhyd.2016.11.044

Fiorda FA, Soares MS, da Silva FA et al (2013) Microestructure, texture and colour of gluten-free pasta made with amaranth flour, cassava starch and cassava bagasse. LWT Food Sci Technol 54:132–138

Flander L, Holopainen U, Kruus K et al (2011) Effects of tyrosinase and laccase on oat proteins and quality parameters of gluten-free oat breads. J Agric Food Chem 59:8385–8390

Foschia M, Horstmann SW, Arendt EK et al (2017) Legumes as functional ingredients in gluten-free bakery and pasta products. Annu Rev Food Sci Technol 8:75–96

Gambuś H, Nowotna A, Ziobro R et al (2001) The effect of use of guar gum with pectin mixture in gluten-free bread. Electron J Polish Agric Univ 4:1–11

Gao Y, Janes ME, Chaiya B et al (2018) Gluten-free bakery and pasta products: prevalence and quality improvement. Int J Food Sci Technol 53:19–32

Garcia MV, Copetti MV (2019) Alternative methods for mould spoilage control in bread and bakery products. Int Food Res J 26:737–749

Genevois CE, de Escalada Pla MF (2021) Soybean by-products and modified cassava starch for improving alveolar structure and quality characteristics of gluten-free bread. Eur Food Res Technol 247:1477–1488

Gilani GS (2012) Background on international activities on protein quality assessment of foods. Br J Nutr 108:S168–S182

Giri NA, Sakhale BK (2019) Development of sweet potato flour based high protein and low calorie gluten free cookies. Curr Res Nutr Food Sci 7:427–435

Giuberti G, Marti A, Fortunati P, Gallo A (2017) Gluten free rice cookies with resistant starch ingredients from modified waxy rice starches: nutritional aspects and textural characteristics. J Cereal Sci 76:157–164

Goesaert H, Slade L, Levine H et al (2009) Amylases and bread firming–an integrated view. J Cereal Sci 50:345–352

Goff HD, Guo Q (2019) Chapter 1. The role of hydrocolloids in the development of food structure. In: Part a food structure development: the interplay between processing routes and formulation elements, pp 1–28

Gómez M, Del Real S, Rosell CM, Ronda F et al (2004) Functionality of different emulsifiers on the performance of breadmaking and wheat bread quality. Eur Food Res Technol 219:145–150

Gómez M, Ronda F, Caballero PA et al (2007) Functionality of different hydrocolloids on the quality and shelf-life of yellow layer cakes. Food Hydrocoll 21:167–173

Gujral HS, Rosell CM (2004a) Functionality of rice flour modified with a microbial transglutaminase. J Cereal Sci 39:225–230

Gujral HS, Rosell CM (2004b) Improvement of the breadmaking quality of rice flour by glucose oxidase. Int Food Res 37:75–81

Gujral HS, Guardiola I, Carbonell JV et al (2003) Effect of cyclodextrin glycosyl transferase on dough rheology and bread quality from rice flour. J Agric Food Chem 51:3814–3818

Gularte MA, de la Hera E, Gómez M et al (2012) Effect of different fibers on batter and gluten-free layer cake properties. LWT Food Sci Technol 48:209–214

Gurtler J, Mai TL (2014) Traditional preservatives – organic acids. In: Batt C, Tortorello M (eds) Encyclopedia of food microbiology, 2nd edn. Academic, New York, pp 119–130

Hager AS, Arendt EK (2013) Influence of hydroxypropylmethylcellulose (HPMC), xanthan gum and their combination on loaf specific volume, crumb hardness and crumb grain characteristics of gluten-free breads based on rice, maize, teff and buckwheat. Food Hydrocoll 32:195–203

Haghighat-Kharazi S, Milani JM, Kasaai MR et al (2018) Microencapsulation of α-amylase in beeswax and its application in gluten-free bread as an anti-staling agent. LWT Food Sci Technol 92:73–79

Haghighat-Kharazi S, Reza Kasaai M, Milani JM et al (2020) Antistaling properties of encapsulated maltogenic amylase in gluten-free bread. Food Sci Nutr 8:5888–5897

Han A, Romero HM, Nishijima N et al (2019) Effect of egg white solids on the rheological properties and bread making performance of gluten-free batter. Food Hydrocoll 87:287–296

Hasenhuettl GL (2008) Overview of food emulsifiers. In: Hasenhuettl GL, Hartel RW (eds) Food emulsifiers and their applications, 2nd edn. Springer Science, New York

Hatta E, Matsumotov K, Honda Y (2015) Bacillolysin, papain, and subtilisin improve the quality of gluten-free rice bread. J Cereal Sci 61:41–47

Herawati H (2019) Hydrocolloids to the effects of gluten free bakery products. J Phys Conf Ser 1295:012052. https://doi.org/10.1088/1742-6596/1295/1/012052

Hesso N, Loisel C, Chevallier S, Le-Bail A (2014) Impact of pregelatinized starches on the texture and staling of conventional and degassed pound cake. Food Bioprocess Technol 7:2923–2930

Hesso N, Garnier C, Loisel C et al (2015) Formulation effect study on batter and cake microstructure: correlation with rheology and texture. Food Struct 5:31–41. https://doi.org/10.1016/j.foostr.2015.03.002

Horstmann SW, Foschla M, Arendt EK (2017a) Correlation analysis of protein quality characteristics with gluten-free bread properties. Food Funct 8:2465–2474

Horstmann SW, Lynch KM, Arendt EK (2017b) Starch characteristics linked to gluten-free products. Foods 6:1–21

Ismail BP, Senaratne-Lenagala L, Stube A, Brackenridge A (2020) Protein demand: Review of plant and animal proteins used in alternative protein product development and production. Anim Front 10(4):53–63

Kamel BS, Ponte JG (1993) Emulsifiers in baking. In: Kamel BS, Stauffer CE (eds) Advances in baking technology. Springer, Boston

Kaur M, Sandhu KS, Arora AP, Sharma A (2015) Gluten free biscuits prepared from buckwheat flour by incorporation of various gums: physicochemical and sensory properties. LWT Food Sci Technol 62:628–632

Kawamura-Konishi Y, Shoda K, Koga H et al (2013) Improvement in gluten-free rice bread quality by protease treatment. J Cereal Sci 58:45–50

Kim Y, Kee JI, Lee S et al (2014) Quality improvement of rice noodle restructured with rice protein isolate and transglutaminase. Food Chem 145:409–416

Kobayashi T (2012) Manufacturing method of gluten-free noodle. JP2019092526A

Korus J, Chmielewska A, Witczak M et al (2021) Rapeseed protein as a novel ingredient of gluten-free bread. Eur Food Res Technol 247:2015–2025

Kovacs ET, Maraz-Szabo L, Varga J (2001) Examination of the protein-emulsifier-carbohydrate interactions in amaranth based pasta products. Acta Aliment Hung 30:173–187

Kumar CM, Sabikhi L, Singh AK et al (2019) Effect of incorporation of sodium caseinate, whey protein concentrate and transglutaminase on the properties of depigmented pearl millet based gluten free pasta. LWT Food Sci Technol 103:19–26

Lai H-M (2002) Effects of rice properties and emulsifiers on the quality of rice pasta. J Sci Food Agric 82:203–216

Lang GH, Kringel DH, dos Santos Acunha T et al (2020) Cake of brown, black and red rice: influence of transglutaminase on technological properties, in vitro starch digestibility and phenolic compounds. Food Chem 318:126480

Larrosa V, Lorenzo G, Zaritzky N, Califano A (2013) Optimization of rheological properties of gluten-free pasta dough using mixture design. J Cereal Sci 57:520–526

Larrosa V, Lorenzo G, Zaritzky N et al (2016) Improvement of the texture and quality of cooked gluten-free pasta. LWT Food Sci Technol 70:96–103

Legan JD (1993) Mould spoilage of bread: the problem and some solutions. Int Biodeter Biodegr 32:33–53

Leman P, Goesaert H, Vandeputte GE et al (2005) Maltogenic amylase has a non-typical impact on the molecular and rheological properties of starch. Carbohydr Polym 62:205–213
Li JM, Nie SP (2016) The functional and nutritional aspects of hydrocolloids in foods. Food Hydrocoll 53:46–61. https://doi.org/10.1016/j.foodhyd.2015.01.035
Li M, Zhu K, Guo X et al (2011) Effect of water activity (aw) and irradiation on the shelf life of fresh noodles. Innov Food Sci Emerg Technol 12:526–530
Li M, Zhu K-X, Guo X-N et al (2014) Natural additives in wheat-based pasta and noodle products: opportunities for enhanced nutritional and functional properties. Comprehens Rev Food Sci Food Saf 13:347–357
Li J, Zhu Y, Yadav MP, Li J (2019) Effect of various hydrocolloids on the physical and fermentation properties of dough. Food Chem 271:165–173
Li C, You Y, Chen D et al (2021) A systematic review of rice noodles: raw material, processing method and quality improvement. Trends Food Sci Technol 107:389–400
Linares-García L, Repo-Carrasco-Valencia R, Glorio Paulet P et al (2019) Development of gluten-free and egg-free pasta based on quinoa (Chenopdium quinoa Willd) with addition of lupine flour, vegetable proteins and the oxidizing enzyme POx. Eur Food Res Technol 245:2147–2156
Lockyer S, Nugent AP (2017) Health effects of resistant starch. Nutr Bull 42:10–41
López-Tenorio J, Rodriguez-Sandoval E, Sepúlveda-Valencia J (2015) The influence of different emulsifiers on the physical and textural characteristics of gluten-free cheese bread: emulsifiers on gluten-free cheese bread. J Texture Stud 46:227–239
Lucera A, Costa C, Conte A, Del Nobile MA (2012) Food applications of natural antimicrobial compounds. Front Microbiol 3:1–13. https://doi.org/10.3389/fmicb.2012.00287
Lund F, Filtenborg O, Westall S et al (1996) Associated mycoflora of rye bread. Lett Appl Microbiol 23:213–217
Mancebo CM, San Miguel MÁ, Martínez MM, Gómez M (2015) Optimisation of rheological properties of gluten-free doughs with HPMC, psyllium and different levels of water. J Cereal Sci 61:8–15
Mancebo CM, Rodriguez P, Gómez M (2016) Assessing rice flour-starch-protein mixtures to produce gluten free sugar-snap cookies. LWT Food Sci Technol 67:127–132
Mancebo CM, Martínez MM, Merino C et al (2017) Effect of oil and shortening in rice bread quality: relationship between dough rheology and quality characteristics. J Texture Stud 48:597–606
Marchetti L, Andrés SC, Cerruti P, Califano AN (2020) Effect of bacterial nanocellulose addition on the rheological properties of gluten-free muffin batters. Food Hydrocoll 98:105315
Marco C, Rosell CM (2008) Breadmaking performance of protein enriched, gluten-free breads. Eur Food Res Technol 227:1205–1213
Marston K, Khouryieh H, Aramouni F (2015) Evaluation of sorghum flour functionality and quality characteristics of gluten-free bread and cake as influenced by ozone treatment. Food Sci Technol Int 21:631–640
Marti A, Pagani MA (2013) What can play the role of gluten in gluten free pasta? Trends Food Sci Technol 31:63–71. https://doi.org/10.1016/j.tifs.2013.03.001
Marti A, Pagani MA, Seetharaman K (2011) Understanding starch organisation in gluten-free pasta from rice flour. Carbohydr Polym 84:1069–1074
Marti A, Barbiroli A, Marengo M et al (2014) Structuring and texturing gluten-free pasta: egg albumen or whey proteins? Eur Food Res Technol 238:217–224
Masure HG, Wouters AG, Fierens E et al (2019) Impact of egg white and soy proteins on structure formation and crumb firming in gluten-free breads. Food Hydrocoll 95:406–417
Matos ME, Rosell CM (2013) Quality indicators of rice-based gluten-free bread-like products: relationships between dough rheology and quality characteristics. Food Bioprocess Technol 6:2331–2341
Matos ME, Rosell CM (2015) Understanding gluten-free dough for reaching breads with physical quality and nutritional balance. J Sci Food Agric 95:653–661
Matos ME, Sanz T, Rosell CM (2014) Establishing the function of proteins on the rheological and quality properties of rice based gluten free muffins. Food Hydrocoll 35:150–158

Melini V, Melini F (2018) Strategies to extend bread and GF bread shelf-life: from sourdough to antimicrobial active packaging and nanotechnology. Fermentation 4:1–18

Miś A, Nawrocka A, Lamorski K et al (2018) Dynamics of gas cell coalescence during baking expansion of leavened dough. Food Res Int 103:30–39

Mohammadi M, Khorshidian N, Yousefi M, Khaneghah AM (2022) Physicochemical, rheological, and sensory properties of gluten-free cookie produced by flour of chestnut, date seed, and modified starch. J Food Qual. https://doi.org/10.1155/2022/5159084

Moore MM, Heinbockel M, Dockery P et al (2006) Network formation in gluten-free bread with application of transglutaminase. Cereal Chem 83:28–36

Morreale F, Garzón R, Rosell CM (2018) Understanding the role of hydrocolloids viscosity and hydration in developing gluten-free bread. A study with hydroxypropylmethylcellulose. Food Hydrocoll 77:629–635

Motahar SFS, Ariaeenejad S, Salami M et al (2021) Improving the quality of gluten-free bread by a novel acidic thermostable α-amylase from metagenomics data. Food Chem 352:129307

Muneer F, Johansson E, Hedenqvist MS et al (2018) The impact of newly produced protein and dietary fiber rich fractions of yellow pea (Pisum sativum L.) on the structure and mechanical properties of pasta-like sheets. Food Res Int 106:607–618

Nguyen TTP, Bhandari B, Cichero J, Prakash S (2015) Gastrointestinal digestion of dairy and soy proteins in infant formulas: an in vitro study. Food Res Int 76(Pt 3):348–358

Nunes M, Moore M, Ryan L et al (2009) Impact of emulsifiers on the quality and rheological properties of gluten-free breads and batters. Eur Food Res Technol 228:633–642

Onyango C, Unbehend G, Lindhauer M (2009) Effect of cellulose-derivatives and emulsifiers on creep-recovery and crumb properties of gluten-free bread prepared from sorghum and gelatinised cassava starch. Food Res Int 42:949–955

Onyango C, Mutungi C, Unbehend G, Lindhauer MG (2010) Batter rheology and bread texture of sorghum-based gluten-free formulations modified with native or pregelatinised cassava starch and α-amylase. Int J Food Sci Technol 45:1228–1235

Orthoefer F (2008) Applications of emulsifiers in baked foods. In: Gerard LH, Hartel RW (eds) Food emulsifiers and their applications, 2nd edn. Springer, New York

Osborne TB (1907) Proteins of the wheat kernel. Publ Carnegie Inst Washington 84:1–119

Ozkoc SO, Seyhun N (2015) Effect of gum type and flaxseed concentration on quality of gluten-free breads made from frozen dough baked in infrared-microwave combination oven. Food Bioprocess Technol 8:2500–2506

Paiva CL, Queiroz VAV, Garcia MAVT (2019) Características tecnológicas, sensoriais e químicas de massas secas sem glúten à base de farinhas de sorgo e milho. Braz J Food Technol 22. https://doi.org/10.1590/1981-6723.09518

Palav T, Bhatia S, Perks C (2009) Formula and process for producing gluten-free bakery products. CA2740382A. Canadian Intellectual Property Office

Palavecino PM, Sciarini LS (2019) Aditivos para panificacion. In: León AE, Ribotta PD, Pérez GT (eds) Trigo: un cereal único. EDUVIN, Villa MAría, pp 381–386

Palavecino PM, Bustos MC, Heinzmann Alabí MB et al (2017) Effect of ingredients on the quality of gluten-free sorghum pasta. J Food Sci 82:2085–2093

Palavecino PM, Curti MI, Bustos MC et al (2020) Sorghum pasta and noodles: technological and nutritional aspects. Plant Foods Hum Nutr 75:326–336

Park S, Kim YR (2021) Clean label starch: production, physicochemical characteristics, and industrial applications. Food Sci Biotechnol 30:1–17

Pateras IM (2007) Bread spoilage and staling. In: Technology of breadmaking. Springer, Boston. ISSN: 978-0-387-38565-5

Pedrosa Silva Clerici MT, Airoldi C, El-Dash AA (2009) Production of acidic extruded rice flour and its influence on the qualities of gluten-free bread. LWT Food Sci Technol 42:618–623

Phillips GO, Williams PA (2009) Handbook of hydrocolloids, 2nd edn. Woodhead Publishing Limited, Duxford

Phongthai S, D'Amico S, Schoenlechner R et al (2017) Effects of protein enrichment on the properties of rice flour based gluten-free pasta. LWT Food Sci Technol 80:378–385

Pico J, Reguilón MP, Bernal J et al (2019) Effect of rice, pea, egg white and whey proteins on crust quality of rice flour-corn starch based gluten-free breads. J Cereal Sci 86:92–101
Purhagen JK, Sjöö ME, Eliasson AC (2012) The anti-staling effect of pre-gelatinized flour and emulsifier in gluten-free bread. Eur Food Res Technol 235:265–276
Rachman A, Brennan MA, Morton J et al (2020) Gluten-free pasta production from banana and cassava flours with egg white protein and soy protein addition. Int J Food Sci Technol 55:3053–3060
Ragaee S, Abdel-Aal EM (2006) Pasting properties of starch and protein in selected cereals and quality of their food products. Food Chem 95:9–18
Rao K, Ketola V, Lapic S et al (2017) Gluten-free compositions and methods for producing shelf-stable breads and other bakery products. US11102986B2. United State Patent
Ray B (2001) Fundamental food microbiology, 2nd edn. CRC Press, London, pp 228–233
Renzetti S, Arendt EK (2009a) Effects of oxidase and protease treatments on the breadmaking functionality of a range of gluten-free flours. Eur Food Res Technol 229:307–317
Renzetti S, Arendt EK (2009b) Effect of protease treatment on the baking quality of brown rice bread: from textural and rheological properties to biochemistry and microstructure. J Cereal Sci 50:22–28
Renzetti S, Dal Bello F, Arendt EK (2008) Microstructure, fundamental rheology and baking characteristics of batters and breads from different gluten-free flours treated with a microbial transglutaminase. J Cereal Sci 48:33–45
Renzetti S, Courtin CM, Delcour JA et al (2010) Oxidative and proteolytic enzyme preparations as promising improvers for oat bread formulations: rheological, biochemical and microstructural background. Food Chem 119:1465–1473
Ribotta PD, Ausar SF, Morcillo MH et al (2004a) Production of gluten-free bread using soybean flour. J Sci Food Agric 84:1969–1974
Ribotta PD, Pérez GT, León AE, Añón MC (2004b) Effect of emulsifier and guar gum on micro structural, rheological and baking performance of frozen bread dough. Food Hydrocoll 18:305–313
Roman L, Belorio M, Gomez M (2019) Gluten-free breads: the gap between research and commercial reality. Compr Rev Food Sci Food Saf 18:690–702
Roman L, Reguilon MP, Martinez MM, Gomez M (2020) The effects of starch cross-linking, stabilization and pre-gelatinization at reducing gluten-free bread staling. LWT Food Sci Technol 132:109908. https://doi.org/10.1016/j.lwt.2020.109908
Romano A, Masi P, Bracciale A et al (2018) Effect of added enzymes and quinoa flour on dough characteristics and sensory quality of a gluten-free bakery product. Eur Food Res Technol 244:1595–1604
Rosell CM (2009) Enzymatic manipulation of gluten-free breads. In: Gallagher E (ed) Gluten-free food science and technology. Blackwell Publishing Ltd, Oxford, pp 83–98
Rosa-Sibakov N, Heiniö RL, Cassan D, Holopainen-Mantila U, Micard V, Lantto R, Sozer N (2016) Effect of bioprocessing and fractionation on the structural, textural and sensory properties of gluten-free faba bean pasta. LWT – Food Sci Technol 67:27–36
Saeidi Z, Nasehi B, Jooyandeh H (2018) Optimization of gluten-free cake formulation enriched with pomegranate seed powder and transglutaminase enzyme. J Food Sci Technol 55:3110–3118
Sahagún M, Gómez M (2018a) Assessing influence of protein source on characteristics of gluten-free breads optimising their hydration level. Food Bioprocess Technol 11:1686–1694
Sahagún M, Gómez M (2018b) Influence of protein source on characteristics and quality of gluten-free cookies. J Food Sci Technol 55:4131–4138
Sahagún M, Bravo-Núñez Á, Báscones G et al (2018) Influence of protein source on the characteristics of gluten-free layer cakes. LWT Food Sci Technol 94:50–56
Sahi SS, Alava JM (2003) Functionality of emulsifiers in sponge cake production. J Sci Food Agric 83:1419–1429
Salehi F (2019) Improvement of gluten-free bread and cake properties using natural hydrocolloids: a review. Food Sci Nutr 7:3391–3402

Salehi F (2020) Effect of common and new gums on the quality, physical, and textural properties of bakery products: a review. J Texture Stud 51:361–370

Salehi F, Amin Ekhlas S, Pavee S, Zandi F (2018) Effect of balangu seed gum on rheological, physical and sensory properties of gluten free rice cake. J Food Technol Nutr 15:61–68

Santos FG, Aguiar EV, Centeno ACL et al (2020) Effect of added psyllium and food enzymes on quality attributes and shelf life of chickpea-based gluten-free bread. LWT Food Sci Technol 134:110025

Sarabhai S, Prabhasankar P (2015) Influence of whey protein concentrate and potato starch on rheological properties and baking performance of Indian water chestnut flour based gluten free cookie dough. LWT Food Sci Technol 63:1301–1308

Sarabhai S, Indrani D, Vijaykrishnaraj M et al (2015) Effect of protein concentrates, emulsifiers on textural and sensory characteristics of gluten free cookies and its immunochemical validation. J Food Sci Technol 52:3763–3772

Sarabhai S, Tamilselvan T, Prabhasankar P (2021) Role of enzymes for improvement in gluten-free foxtail millet bread: it's effect on quality, textural, rheological and pasting properties. LWT Food Sci Technol 137:110365

Schiraldi A, Fessas D (2001) Mechanism of staling: an overview. In: Chinachoti P, Vodovotz Y (eds) Bread staling. CRC Press, London

Schoenlechner R, Drausinger J, Ottenschlaeger V et al (2010) Functional properties of gluten-free pasta produced from amaranth, quinoa and buckwheat. Plant Foods Hum Nutr 65:339–349

Sciarini LS, Ribotta PD, León AE et al (2010a) Influence of gluten-free flours and their mixtures on batter properties and bread quality. Food Bioprocess Technol 3:577–585

Sciarini LS, Ribotta PD, León AE, Pérez GT (2010b) Effect of hydrocolloids on gluten-free batter properties and bread quality. Int J Food Sci Technol 45:2306–2312

Sciarini LS, Ribotta PD, León AE et al (2012) Incorporation of several additives into gluten free breads: effect on dough properties and bread quality. J Food Eng 111:590–597

Sciarini LS, Bustos MC, Vignola MB et al (2017) A study on fibre addition to gluten free bread: its effects on bread quality and in vitro digestibility. J Food Sci Technol 54:244–252

Seguro K, Kumazawa Y, Kuraishi C et al (1996) The epsilon-(gamma-glutamyl) lysine moiety in cross-linked casein is an available source of lysine for rats. J Nutr 126:2557–2562

Shaabani S, Yarmand MS, Kiani H et al (2018) The effect of chickpea protein isolate in combination with transglutaminase and xanthan on the physical and rheological characteristics of gluten free muffins and batter based on millet flour. LWT Food Sci Technol 90:362–372

Sharadanant R, Khan K (2003) Effect of hydrophilic gums on the quality of frozen dough: II. Bread characteristics. Cereal Chem 80:773–780

Shevkani K, Singh N (2014) Influence of kidney bean, field pea and amaranth protein isolates on the characteristics of starch-based gluten-free muffins. Int J Food Sci Technol 49:2237–2244

Shokri F, Salehi Far M, Azizi MH (2016) Effect of hydroxy propyl methyl cellulose and microbial transglutaminase enzyme on farinograph and quality characteristics of gluten-free pasta. J Food Sci Technol (Iran) 13:123–132

Shukla V, Carlos-Martínez A, Li YO et al (2021) Optimization of gluten-free pasta formulation enriched with pulse protein isolates. J Culin Sci Technol:1–19

Singh A, Kumar P (2018) Gluten free approach in fat and sugar amended biscuits: a healthy concern for obese and diabetic individuals. J Food Process Preserv 42. https://doi.org/10.1111/jfpp.13546

Skendi A, Papageorgiou M, Varzakas T (2021) High protein substitutes for gluten in gluten-free bread. Foods 10:1997

Šmídová Z, Rysová J (2022) Gluten-free bread and bakery products technology. Foods 11:480. https://doi.org/10.3390/foods11030480

Smith JP, Daifas DP, El-Khoury W et al (2004) Shelf life and safety concerns of bakery products – a review. Crit Rev Food Sci Nutr 44:19–55

Sozer N (2009) Rheological properties of rice pasta dough supplemented with proteins and gums. Food Hydrocoll 23:849–855

Suhr KI, Nielsen PV (2004) Effect of weak acid preservatives on growth of bakery product spoilage fungi at different water activities and ph values. Int J Food Microbiol 95:67–78

Sumnu G, Koksel F, Sahin S et al (2010) The effects of xanthan and guar gums on staling of gluten-free rice cakes baked in different ovens. Int J Food Sci Technol 45:87–93

Susanna S, Prabhasankar P (2013) A study on development of gluten free pasta and its biochemical and immunological validation. LWT Food Sci Technol 50:613–621

Takács K, Nemedi E, Marta D et al (2007) Use of the enzyme transglutaminase for developing glutenfree noodle products from pea flour. J Acta Alimentaria 36:195–205

Tantala J, Meethongchai S, Suethong W et al (2022) Mold-free shelf-life extension of fresh rice noodles by synergistic effects of chitosan and common food preservatives. Food Control 133:108597

Tomić J, Torbica A, Belović M (2020) Effect of non-gluten proteins and transglutaminase on dough rheological properties and quality of bread based on millet (Panicum miliaceum) flour. LWT Food Sci Technol 118:108852

Tsatsaragkou K, Papantoniou M, Mandala I (2015) Rheological, physical, and sensory attributes of gluten-free rice cakes containing resistant starch. J Food Sci 80:341–348

Tuersuntuoheti T, Wang Z, Zheng Y et al (2019) Study on the shelf life and quality characteristics of highland barley fresh noodles as affected by microwave treatment and food preservatives. Food Sci Nutr 7:2958–2967

Turabi E, Sumnu G, Sahin S (2010) Quantitative analysis of macro and micro-structure of gluten-free rice cakes containing different types of gums baked in different ovens. Food Hydrocoll 24:755–762. https://doi.org/10.1016/j.foodhyd.2010.04.001

Van Der Maarel MJ, Van der Veen B, Uitdehaag JC et al (2002) Properties and applications of starch-converting enzymes of the α-amylase family. J Biotechnol 94:137–155

Vemulapalli V, Hoseney RC (1998) Glucose oxidase effects on gluten and water soluble. Cereal Chem 75:859–862

Vidaurre-Ruiz J, Salas-Valerio F, Schoenlechner R, Repo-Carrasco-Valencia R (2020) Rheological and textural properties of gluten-free doughs made from Andean grains. Int J Food Sci Technol 56:468. https://doi.org/10.1111/ijfs.14662

Wangprasertkul J, Siriwattanapong R, Harnkarnsujarit N (2021) Antifungal packaging of sorbate and benzoate incorporated biodegradable films for fresh noodles. Food Control 123:107763

Wilderjans E, Pareyt B, Goesaert et al (2008) The role of gluten in a pound cake system: a model approach based on gluten–starch blends. Food Chem 110:909–915

Witczak M, Juszczak L, Ziobro R, Korus J (2012) Influence of modified starches on properties of gluten-free dough and bread. Part I: rheological and thermal properties of gluten-free dough. Food Hydrocoll 28:353–360

Witczak M, Ziobro R, Juszczak L, Korus J (2016) Starch and starch derivatives in gluten-free systems – a review. J Cereal Sci 67:46–57

Wójcik M, Różyło R, Schönlechner R et al (2021) Physico-chemical properties of an innovative gluten-free, low-carbohydrate and high protein-bread enriched with pea protein powder. Sci Rep 11:1–10

Xu J, Zhang Y, Wang W et al (2020) Advanced properties of gluten-free cookies, cakes, and crackers: a review. Trends Food Sci Technol 103:200–213

Yalcin S, Basman A (2008) Effects of gelatinisation level, gum and transglutaminase on the quality characteristics of rice noodle. Int J Food Sci Technol 43:1637–1644

Yang S, Shan C-S, Xu Y-Q et al (2021) Dissimilarity in sensory attributes, shelf life and spoilage bacterial and fungal microbiota of industrial-scale wet starch noodles induced by different preservatives and temperature. Food Res Int 140:109980

Yano H (2019) Recent practical researches in the development of gluten-free breads. npj Sci Food 3:7–15

Yildirim RM, Gumus T, Arici M (2018) Optimization of a gluten free formulation of the Turkish dessert revani using different types of flours, protein sources and transglutaminase. LWT Food Sci Technol 95:72–77

Zayas JF (1997) Functionality of proteins in food. Springer Science & Business Media, Berlin
Zhao F, Li Y, Li C et al (2021) Co-supported hydrocolloids improve the structure and texture quality of gluten-free bread. LWT Food Sci Technol 152:112248. https://doi.org/10.1016/j.lwt.2021.112248
Ziobro R, Korus J, Witczak M, Juszczak L (2012) Influence of modified starches on properties of gluten-free dough and bread. Part II: quality and staling of gluten-free bread. Food Hydrocoll 29:68–74
Ziobro R, Korus J, Juszczak L, Witczak T (2013a) Influence of inulin on physical characteristics and staling rate of gluten-free bread. J Food Eng 116:21–27. https://doi.org/10.1016/j.jfoodeng.2012.10.049
Ziobro R, Witczak T, Juszczak L et al (2013b) Supplementation of gluten-free bread with non-gluten proteins. Effect on dough rheological properties and bread characteristic. Food Hydrocoll 32:213–220
Ziobro R, Juszczak L, Witczak M et al (2016) Non-gluten proteins as structure forming agents in gluten free bread. J Food Sci Technol 53:571–580
Zoghi A, Mirmahdi RS, Mohammadi M (2021) The role of hydrocolloids in the development of gluten-free cereal-based products for coeliac patients: a review. Int J Food Sci Technol 56:3138–3147
Zorzi CZ, Garske RP, Flôres SH et al (2020) Sunflower protein concentrate: a possible and beneficial ingredient for gluten-free bread. Innov Food Sci Emerg Technol 66:102539

Chapter 5
Fermented Gluten-Free Baked Goods

Karen F. Irigoytia, Nancy N. Espósito, Verónica M. Busch, Marina F. de Escalada Pla, and Carolina E. Genevois

Abbreviations

ABTS	$ABTS^{\bullet+}$ radical cation scavenging activity
DPPH	2,2-diphenyl-1-picrylhidrazyl free radical
EPs	exopolysaccharides
FRAP	ferric ion reducing antioxidant power
GF	gluten-free
GI	glycaemic index
GRD	gluten-related disorders
HR	relative humidity
LAB	lactic acid bacteria
LSV	loaf specific volume
Mw	molecular weigh
NA	not applicable
NR	not reported
PD	protected designation of origin
PGI	protected by geographical indication
r	Pearson's product-moment correlations
RDS	rapidly digested starch
RS	resistant starch
SDS	slowly digestible starch
TPC	total phenolic content

K. F. Irigoytia · N. N. Espósito · V. M. Busch · C. E. Genevois (✉)
Instituto de Ciencia y Tecnología de los Alimentos de Entre Ríos (ICTAER, CONICET-UNER), Gualeguaychú, Entre Ríos, Argentina

Universidad Nacional de Entre Ríos (UNER), Facultad de Bromatología, Gualeguaychú, Entre Ríos, Argentina
e-mail: carolina.genevois@uner.edu.ar

M. F. de Escalada Pla
Departamento de Industrias, Universidad de Buenos Aires (UBA), Facultad de Ciencias Exactas y Naturales (FCEN), Ciudad Autónoma de Buenos Aires, Argentina

Instituto de Tecnología de Alimentos y Procesos Químicos (ITAPROQ, CONICET-UBA), Ciudad Autónoma de Buenos Aires, Argentina
e-mail: marina@di.fcen.uba.ar

M. F. de Escalada Pla, C. E. Genevois (eds.), *Designing Gluten Free Bakery and Pasta Products*, https://doi.org/10.1007/978-3-031-28344-4_5

5.1 Introduction of Fermented Gluten-Free Bread Making

Bread is a staple food in Western countries that provides essential macronutrients to the organism, especially those related to energy supply and, simple and complex, carbohydrates. The increasing demand for gluten-free (GF) products, including bakery goods, can be explained, in part, by the greater prevalence of the diseases related to gluten intake such as celiac disease, non-celiac gluten sensitivity and wheat allergy, around the world (Ortiz et al. 2017; Cabanillas 2019; Taraghikhah et al. 2020).

From a technological perspective, the replacement of gluten in baked goods still represents a challenge for the food industry and science. In wheat products, the gluten is crucial for building the protein network that gives the unique dough viscoelastic properties capable of retaining the carbon dioxide (CO_2). This latter is produced by yeasts during fermentation, particularly, in high-quality leavened bakery products. The GF flours are not able to mimic the viscoelastic doughs of wheat flour when kneaded with water, and no single ingredient or raw material can completely replace the wheat gluten so far. This is the main reason why formulations of bakery products involve several ingredients, e.g. different flours and starches, milk powder, isolate proteins, additives, etc. as is detailed in Table 5.1. The process of obtaining high-quality GF bread comprises the development and optimisation of raw materials and/or traditional or novel ingredients, and the inclusion of hydrocolloids, native or modified starches, enzymes, emulsifiers, and/or alternative sources of protein.

In order to achieve the bakery industry requirements and fulfil the consumer acceptance, GF doughs should be extensible and also present the appropriate tenacity to allow gas cell expansion over the fermentation process and, to increase the loaf volume during proofing and baking. Additionally, loaf bread might have a crispy crust, and a soft and resilient crumb. Over the last years, unconventional ingredients such as certain cereals or pseudocereals have been investigated in the development of GF breads in an effort to reach a product with desired characteristics.

In the previous Chaps. 2, 3, and 4, a complete revision of available GF raw material as well as additives, is approached. Therefore, this chapter is centred in the breadmaking processes reviewing different technological strategies and focusing on sourdough fermentation.

5.2 Challenges and Alternatives

Usually, in fermented bakery such as bread, pizza, or breadsticks, *Saccharomyces cerevisiae* yeast is responsible for providing CO_2 to the crumb structure. In general, time and fermentation conditions are fitted for reaching the maximum loaf volume avoiding the collapse of the pieces before baking is completed (Sahagún and Gómez 2018). It is important to consider that *S. cerevisiae* performance can be affected by

Table 5.1 List of gluten-free (GF) sourdough breads and sourdough baking mixtures commercially available around the world

Sourdough GF breads			Sourdough baking mixes		
Company	Country	Ingredients	Company	Country	Ingredients
Cook's GF Sourdough	USA	Fermented sourdough starter (filtered water, organic brown rice flour, organic sorghum flour), organic brown rice flour, organic tapioca flour, organic potato starch, organic evaporated cane sugar, sea salt, xanthan gum, organic guar gum, ascorbic acid	Alnavit	Germany	Wholemeal oat flour GF, corn starch, wholemeal rice flour, potato starch, buckwheat flour, buckwheat sourdough powder (buckwheat flour, quinoa flour*, starter cultures), chestnut flour, sea salt, xanthan gum and psyllium husks ground
Simple Kneads	USA	Water, organic millet flour, organic sorghum flour, organic teff flour, organic buckwheat flour, organic quinoa flour, *Psyllium* seed husk powder, sunflower oil, raisin juice concentrate, flax meal, salt, sunflower seeds	The GF Bakery	UK	Brown rice, potato starch, sorghum flour, teff flour, tapioca flour, buckwheat flour, sourdough starter (3%), xanthan gum, caraway seeds, salt, fennel seed, coconut sugar
The Whole Kitchen	Singapur	Sorghum flour, oat flour, chickpea flour, organic buckwheat flour, sourdough starter (buckwheat flour, water), arrowroot starch, tapioca starch, golden flaxseed, *psyllium* husk, olive oil, yeast, sea salt	The GF Bakery	UK	Potato starch, tapioca flour, brown rice flour, sorghum flour, millet flour, GF oat flour, stabiliser: xanthan gum, salt, sourdough starter (1%), coconut sugar, gluten free oats, garlic
Zukkee	USA	Organic sourdough starter, organic sorghum flour, arrowroot flour, millet flour, organic brown rice flour, xanthan gum, salt	The GF Bakery	UK	Brown rice flour, potato starch, tapioca flour, sorghum flour, Sourdough starter (9%), millet flour, salt, Stabiliser: Xanthan gum
New Grain	USA	White rice flour, water, eggs, tapioca flour, sugar, potato flour, palm fruit oil, yeast, *Psyllium* husk powder, vinegar, sea salt, xanthan gum, powdered sugar, enzyme	The GF Bakery	UK	Potato starch, brown rice flour, tapioca flour, sorghum flour, GF oats, GF oat flour, sourdough starter (3%), stabiliser: xanthan gum, salt, coconut sugar

(continued)

Table 5.1 (continued)

Sourdough GF breads			Sourdough baking mixes		
Company	Country	Ingredients	Company	Country	Ingredients
Young Kobras	USA	Sourdough starter (organic brown rice, water), organic sorghum flour, organic millet flour, organic tapioca flour, *psyllium* husk, organic apple cider vinegar, sea salt	Hunorganic Kft	Hungary	Tapioca starch, bamboo fibre, millet flour, dried rice sourdough (5%), brown rice flour, psyllium husk fibre, chicory inulin 4%, salt, sodium carbonates, ascorbic acid, citric acid
SRLY Bread	USA	Wild fermented sourdough (water, organic white rice flour, organic millet flour, organic sorghum flour, arrowroot, xanthan gum, sea salt)	Bauckhof	Germany	Rice whole grain flour, corn starch, rice whole grain flakes, Teffvollkornmehl, buckwheat sourdough powder (buckwheat flour, quinoa flour, starter cultures), buckwheat wholemeal flour, carob seed flour, coriander, cumin, fennel, baking powder, sodium bicarbonate, monopotassium tartrate, corn starch, sea salt, xanthan gum
Zealia bio	Spain	Flours (corn starch, chickpea), sourdough (20%, whole buckwheat, whole teff, quinoa), water, virgin olive oil, xanthan gum, yeast, prebiotic vegetable fibre (2%), apple cider vinegar, *psyllium*, apple concentrate, salt, sesame			
Schär	Italy	Corn starch, water, sourdough (11%; rice flour, water), buckwheat flour, rice flour, rice syrup, ground *psyllium* fibre, rice starch, sunflower oil, soy protein, sorghum flour, hydroxypropyl-methylcellulose (HPMC), yeast, salt, sugar			

(continued)

Table 5.1 (continued)

Sourdough GF breads			Sourdough baking mixes		
Company	Country	Ingredients	Company	Country	Ingredients
Leon Bakers	USA	Water, rice sourdough (20%), flour mix (tapioca starch, whole buckwheat flour, whole rice flour), extra virgin olive oil, *psyllium*, salt			
El horno de leña	Spain	Water, corn starch, high oleic sunflower oil, vegetable fibre (*psyllium* and bamboo), whole rice flour, dextrose, (HPMC and xanthan gum), powdered egg albumin, yeast, devitalized sourdough, salt, preservatives (cropionate calcium and potassium sorbate), raising agent (sodium hydrogen carbonate), emulsifiers (mono and diglycerides of fatty acids), antioxidant (ascorbic acid)			
Airos	Spain	Water, corn starch, tapioca starch, sourdough (rice flour, water), rice syrup, buckwheat flour, high oleic sunflower oil 3.8%, vegetable fiber (psyllium), potato protein, yeast, thickeners (HPMC, xanthan gum), sugar, salt, emulsifiers (mono- and diglycerides of fatty acids, sodium stearoyl-2-lactylate), aroma, preservatives (sorbic acid, calcium propionate)			

(continued)

Table 5.1 (continued)

Sourdough GF breads			Sourdough baking mixes		
Company	Country	Ingredients	Company	Country	Ingredients
Semper	Sweden	Water, 24% sourdough (water, rice flour, sourdough culture), GF whole grain oat flour, corn starch, modified tapioca starch, rice flour, yeast, potato flour, broad bean protein, rapeseed oil, GF oat fibre (3%), psyllium husk, xanthan gum, HPMC, salt			
Ener G	USA	Filtered water, Rice flour (White & sweet rice), sourdough starter (Rice flour, tapioca syrup, yeast, salt), high oleic safflower oil, tapioca starch, sugar, yeast, pear juice concentrate, microcrystalline cellulose, egg white powder, modified cellulose, baking powder (Glucono Delta Lactone, calcium carbonate, magnesium carbonate), salt, orange citrus fiber, vegetable glycerin, dough conditioner (calcium sulfate, enzyme). Enriched with thiamin (vitamin B1), riboflavin (vitamin B2), niacin, iron, folic acid			

the different processes used to bread production. Nowadays, the application of frozen technology, for instance, frozen dough and pre-baked frozen bread, as well as the use of active packaging are alternatives commonly found in the bread market (Luo et al. 2018; Qian et al. 2021).

When bread is frozen before proofing, the loaf volume is significantly lower, being an advantage from the logistic point of view since lower refrigerated space is required for the transport. Nevertheless, yeast cells can die because of ice crystals formation on their surface during freezing. In pre-baked frozen breads, the fermentation as well as a partial baking occur before freezing. In this case, the quality of the product is more controlled since almost all the process is carried out before the product distribution. In addition, active packaging leads to increase the shelf life of the baked products.

On the other hand, biotechnology offers alternative tools for improving the quality of baked goods. For instance, enzymes catalysed reactions such as starch or protein hydrolysis that provoke viscoelastic changes in dough. Phytases can hydrolyse phytic acid and consequently improve the mineral bio-accessibility. In this sense, the use of flour obtained from germinated grains or legumes has been widely studied in recent years (Aparicio-García et al. 2020; Rodríguez-España et al. 2022; Heberle et al. 2022). Germination is the process that occurs when seeds begin to become plants. In this process, some enzymes like amylases, proteases, phytases, lipases, and fibre-degrading are activated leading to the breakdown of macromolecules into simple molecules. The conditions of this germination, like moisture, temperature, and time, can be controlled to achieve a desirable composition in the flour (Rodríguez-España et al. 2022).

The other biotechnological tool is the fermentation by addition of sourdough to the bread formulation as natural leavening agent. This chapter will focus on this last technology, since this process involves the widest range of biological reactions and biochemical changes in bread dough.

Fermentation is the oldest biological technology to produce bread. Meanwhile the concept of sourdough refers to a mixture containing flour and water which is spontaneously fermented by native lactic acid bacteria (LAB) and yeast, being the most ancient technological process to obtain leavened breads. However, other microorganisms (e.g., acetic acid bacteria) can be present, but in general, only at the beginning of fermentation (De Vuyst et al. 2017; Bender and Schönlechner 2020).

The use of sourdough in the leavening of bread has data in ancient Egypt in approximately 3000 BC. After the Middle Ages, the barm obtained from beer brewing was identified as a substitute agent for sourdough in the bread leavening process. Since the nineteenth century, the sourdough was almost completely replaced by baker's yeast, mainly due to the faster and simple leavening process, and the greater suitability for the requirements of modern industrial baking processes. The rapid fermentation using only commercial yeast, is currently the most common technique in artisanal or industrial bread production.

In the last years, the use of sourdough as a leavening agent for bread fermentation has gained popularity in consumers who demand breads with pronounced flavour and taste, healthy properties, without addition of additives and an extended shelf life. In addition, the traditional aspect of sourdough bread represents another attractive concept.

The sourdough process has been traditionally used in rye- and wheat-based bread production giving as result a larger specific volume, a softer and more elastic structure, a wide range of flavour notes, and longer shelf life in baked goods.

There are some commercial breads produced by sourdough, which are protected by geographical indication (PGI) or protected designation of origin (PDO) in the European Community and North America not only to protect the traditional breadmaking process, but also because they are products that have a particular loaf form, size and sensory characteristics. These identified products are produced in a specific world area using the recognized *"know-how"* of local producers and ingredients from the concerned region with a particular microbiome. For instance, *Pane Toscana*, *Coppia Ferrarese*, *Pane di Altamura*, *Pane di Genzano*, *Pagnotta del Dittaino* and *Pane di Matera* from Italy; *San Francisco* from United States; a homemade bread of *Daujėnai* from Lithuania; and *Pan de Cruz de Ciudad Real*, *Pan de Alfacar*, *Pan de Cea* and *Pan de Payés* from Spain.

Although the use of sourdough has been extensively studied in the traditional wheat counterpart bread (Lattanzi et al. 2014; Van Kerrebroeck et al. 2016; Cizeikiene et al. 2020; Debonne et al. 2020), over the last years similar approaches have been made in GF bread-making as well (Axel et al. 2015; Różyło et al. 2016; Rinaldi et al. 2017; Bender et al. 2018; Nami et al. 2019; Olojede et al. 2020; Carbó et al. 2020; Lancetti et al. 2022). GF breads are produced by the traditional fermentation process using fresh compressed or dried yeast as leavening agent. It is important to highlight that PGI or PDO sourdough GF breads haven't been found in bibliography so far.

Nevertheless, currently there are several companies that produce GF sourdough bread and baking mixtures around the world, giving different alternative to consumers with gluten-related disorders (GRD). In Table 5.1 are listed the GF sourdough breads and sourdough baking mixtures that are commercially available per country with their list of ingredients.

Furthermore, there are commercial starter cultures in powder, ready to use by professional bakers or consumers in order to prepare homemade sourdough bread [Freshly Fermented (UK); Lallemand Ink. (Canada); Böcker (Germany)]. The advantage of these powder leavening agents is that they reduce the time consuming of daily dough propagation and minimise the mutation, variation of microorganism, and, therefore, the microbial risk. In general, they are based on species of lactobacilli and/or yeast.

5.3 Microorganisms Association in GF Sourdough

The use of sourdough is, in general, associated with loaf bread with higher specific volume, softer crumb, higher size of alveoli, wide range of notes and intense flavour, acidic taste and improved nutritional value. These effects have been related to the metabolic activities associated to lactic acid and acetic acid fermentation, the enzymatic proteolytic activity, the bacterial production of exopolysaccharides, the synthesis of volatile compounds, and the antimicrobial metabolites of microorganisms present in sourdough (De Vuyst and Vancanneyt 2007; Suo et al. 2021; Gobbetti et al. 2014).

The propagation of sourdough using the back sloping technique in the same area over a long period gives as result a stable adapted microbial association (Cizeikiene et al. 2020; Ma et al. 2021). The sourdough microbiome can be developed spontaneously from the native microorganism present in GF flours or can be added as live or dried commercial starter culture at laboratory scale or home based (Table 5.2). In the latter scenario, the sourdough could be inoculated with a pure single culture (e.g. *L. sanfranciscensis*) or with a mixed culture (e.g. *L. sanfranciscensis* and *L. plantarum*) as starter culture (Bender et al. 2018; Nami et al. 2019).

It is important to highlight that sourdough ecosystem is a very specific, stressful, microbial ecosystem, characterised by specific adaptations of the microbiota to the carbohydrate and nutrient contents, low pH (<4.5), oxygen and redox potential. Processing conditions factors such as fermentation temperature and time, nutrients and water availability, and number of dough propagation give as result a different microbial association in sourdough. Furthermore, the composition of flours could have a strong influence on the microorganisms adapted, which finally will dominate the sourdough ecosystem (Van Kerrebroeck et al. 2016; Vogelmann and Hertel 2011).

Therefore, the stability of sourdough relies on either specific technological parameters or parameters not fully controllable (Ramos et al. 2021; De Vuyst et al. 2017). The most significant technological parameters are detailed below:

- Flour composition: e.g., the ash content in the bran fraction of flours can promote the growth of LAB in the sourdough.
- Nutrient availability: e.g., fermentable carbohydrate could enhance the cell count of specific LAB strains.
- Addition of other ingredients such as mono- and disaccharides or different amino acid sources could affect the microbial growth and the final microbial composition.
- Water level. The flour and water ratio determines the sourdough viscosity and is expressed as dough yield (DY) according to Eq. 5.1:

$$\mathrm{DY} = (\text{amount of flour} + \text{amount of water}) \times 100 / (\text{amount of flour}) \quad (5.1)$$

DY values around 250–300 are represented by liquid dough, 150–250 are paste-like dough, <150 are firm dough. For instance, high DY results in higher rate of acidification due to a greater diffusion of acids in the hydrated dough.

- pH: the synthesis of organic acids by endogenous microorganism reduces the pH of dough excluding the growth of microorganisms which are not acid-tolerant, having a positive effect on the product shelf-life.
- Oxygen and redox potential: the consistency and the refreshment of sourdough have an impact in oxygen availability favouring the growth of certain LAB and yeast strains. For instance, some yeast and LAB species such as, *P. kudriavzevii* and *L. amylovorus* DCE 471, only grow with enough oxygen availability (De Vuyst et al. 2017; Calvert et al. 2021).
- Leavening temperature: e.g. high temperature of fermentation favour the growth of microorganisms that are resistant to heat stress.
- Number of dough propagation cycles: the use of several back slopping over long periods gives as result a mature sourdough with stablished microbial association between LAB and yeast (De Vuyst et al. 2017; Calvert et al. 2021; Comasio et al. 2020).

Table 5.2 Main characteristics of sourdough development and, effect of its addition on the technological and sensorial parameters of GF bread

Main flour in sourdough	Starter culture of sourdough and initial inoculum size	Fermentation conditions, dough yield and proportion of sourdough addition in a bread recipe	Dominate microorganism at the end of the fermentation	Effect of sourdough addition on:						Author
				Dough rheology	Crumb texture	Specific loaf volume (LSV)	Alveolar structure	Sensorial characteristics	Shelf life	
Germinated sorghum flour (*Sorghum bicolour*) (0.2–0.6 μm)	*P. pentosaceus* (2×10^{10} CFU/mL) or *S. cerevisiae* (3×10^{9} cfu/mL), and a mixture culture of both	Fermentation at 28 °C for 48 h. Control system with 2.5% baker's yeast DY = 200	36 LAB and 30 yeast isolates were identified from the spontaneously fermenting sorghum meal, being *P. pentosaceus* and *S. cerevisiae* the dominant species	NA	NA	Bread with *P. pentosaceus* ↑ LSV	NA	Bread with *P. pentosaceus*, *S. cerevisae* and, a mixture culture received a punctuation >5-point in a 9-point hedonic scale (n = 12) in appearance, taste, texture, aroma, crumb, and overall acceptability	Shelf life (visible moulds) was prolonged up to 6 days in bread sourdough with *P. pentosaceus* respect to *S. cerevisae* and mixture culture	Ogunsakin et al. (2015)
Legumes flours (*Phaseolus vulgaris, Cicer arietinum, Lathyrus sativus, Lens culinaris* and *Pisum sativum*)	*L. plantarum* C48 and *L. brevis* AM7 (initial cell density of 7.0 log CFU/g dough for each strain)	Fermentation at 30 °C for 24 h DY = 160	NA	NA	NA	NA	NA	NA	NA	Curiel et al. (2015)
Commercial quinoa flour	*L. amylovorus* DSM19280 (initial inoculum size of 7 log CFU/g dough)	Fermentation at 30 °C for 48 h Quinoa sourdough added at 20% DY = 200	NA	NA	Softer crumb for fresh breads (day 0) and stored breads (day 2–5)	↑ LSV (6%)	NA	NA	Bread with *L. amylovorus* prolonged the shelf life up to 4 days	Axel et al. (2015)
Rice and chesnut flour	*L. plantarum* (GF commercial starter, 0.6 g)	Fermentation at 30 °C – 85% RH for 72 h Sourdough addition added at 20, 40 and 60% DY = 200	NA	↓ complex modulus G*, promoting the softening of dough	↓ crumb firmness; however, higher levels of sourdough (60%) had a detriment in texture	↑ LSV at lower level of sourdough addition (20%)	Homogenous structure and higher number of smaller pores with 20% of sourdough addition. Higher values of sourdough showed a denser crumb structure	NA	NA	Demirkesen et al. (2016)

White and whole rice flours	Commercial starter culture of LAB and yeast (1%; LV1-SAF Levain-Lessafre)	Initial fermentation at 30 °C and 75–88% HR until pH was stabilized (pH 3.63) by dough propagation Fresh and freeze-dried whole rice sourdough was added at 10, 20, 30 and 40% of DY = 100	NA	NA	↑ cohesiveness and springiness	↑ LSV at lower level of sourdough addition (10%)	↑ size and area of pores. Addition of fresh sourdough increase the pore area (26%) compared to freeze-dried sourdough (21–22%)	Addition of 10% rice sourdough had the highest score in taste Breads with 10 and 20% of rice sourdough had the best overall sensory score (n = 52)	Breads produced with 10% of fresh and freeze-dried sourdough presented the lowest degree of crumb staling (lower firmness) after 3 days of storage	Różyło et al. (2016)
Bread recipe (corn starch, rice flour)	Fresh commercial yeast and/or *L. sanfranciscensis* (9.1 log CFU/g) and *C. humilis* (7.7 log CFU/g) species	Fermentation at 25 °C until pH 4.0 was reached. Sourdough was added at 20%	Type I sourdough composed with *L. sanfranciscensis* and *C. humilis* species	Sourdough positively affects the proofing curves – dough height (13.3 mm/h). The sourdough leavening time increased compared to fresh yeast	Softer crumb with both, sourdough and fresh yeast	↓ LSV (~26%) respect to fresh yeast	Denser crumb with higher percentage of size pores >3 mm^2	NA	Bread with sourdough increased the hardening kinetics compared to the breads with fresh compressed yeast or both	Cappa et al. (2016)
Commercial quinoa flour	Spontaneous fermentation	Fermentation at 30 °C for 24 h, and then propagated for 10 days (LAB count 8.1–8.4 CFU/g) DY = 200	*L. plantarum*, *L. brevis* and *Leuconostoc mesenteroides* were predominant in stable sourdough	NA	NA	NA	NA	NA	NA	
Bread recipe (corn starch, rice flour)	*L. sanfranciscensis* UMB26 and *C. humilis* CHV	Fermentation at 25 °C till a pH value of 4.0 was reached Dough consistency 230 BU	Cell concentrations of yeasts (7.74 log CFU/g) and lactobacilli (9.08 log CFU/g)	NA	NA	NA	NA	NA	NA	Picozzi et al. (2016)

(continued)

Table 5.2 (continued)

Main flour in sourdough	Starter culture of sourdough and initial inoculum size	Fermentation conditions, dough yield and proportion of sourdough addition in a bread recipe	Dominate microorganism at the end of the fermentation	Effect of sourdough addition on:						Author
				Dough rheology	Crumb texture	Specific loaf volume (LSV)	Alveolar structure	Sensorial characteristics	Shelf life	
Germinated white sorghum flour	Spontaneous fermentation	Fermentation at 27 °C for 48 h DY = 200	Main LAB and yeast identified were: *Pediococcus pentosaceus* SA8 and LD7, *Weissella confusa* SD8, and *S. cerevisae*	NA	NA	NA	NA	NA	NA	Ogunsakin et al. (2017)
Bread recipe (corn starch, rice flour)	Spontaneous fermentation (*L. sanfranciscensis* UMB26 and *C. humilis* CHV)	Fermentation at 25 °C till a pH value of 4.0 was reached. Sourdough was added at 20% Dough consistency 230 BU	Cell concentrations of yeasts (7.74 log CFU/g) and lactobacilli (9.08 log CFU/g)	Sourdough bread showed the lowest height during proofing phase, and required a longer time in proofing phase time (4 h)	Sourdough bread had the lowest softness values at low deformation (Young's modulus), and during storage	↓ LSV (~36%) respect to compressed yeast	Homogenous, and compact structure crumb	NA	Sourdough bread was less prone to fracture during storage compared with fresh compressed yeast	Mariotti et al. (2017)
Organic buckwheat flour	*Gluconobacter (G.) albidus* TMW 2.1191 isolated from water kefir, *Kozakia (K.) baliensis* NBRC 16680 from Indonesian ragi starter and *Neoasaia (N.) chiangmaiensis* NBRC 101099 from a Thai red ginger flower	Fermentation at 30 °C for 24 and 48 h DY = 250 and 350	*G. albidus* was the most competitive strain to grow in buckwheat dough. *Pediococcus pentosaceus* was the main LAB observed at the end of fermentation process	NA	NA	NA	NA	NA	NA	Ua-Arak et al. (2016)

Organic buckwheat flour	*G. albidus* TMW 2.1191 or *Kozakia* (K.) *baliensis* NBRC 16680	Fermentation at 30 °C for 24, 30 and 48 h Sourdough was added at 40% DY = 200	The LAB cell count increased from 3×10^7 to $\sim 2 \times 10^8$ CFU/g dough after 24 h and, slightly reduced to 10^6–10^7 after 72 h. The LAB increased from 10^2 to 10^7–10^8 after 24 h (*P. pentosaceus* 70.4%, *Weissella cibaria* 28.7%) and remained in higher concentration	NA	↓ crumb hardness	↑ LSV	Sourdough breads from 24 h had slightly larger pore size than control; while sourdough breads from 48 h had finer pore size and denser crumb in both strains	Sourdough breads with *G. albidus* and *K. baliensis* at 24 and 30 h obtained higher punctuation (>6 in a 9-point hedonic scale, n = 18) in colour, taste and overall acceptance compared to the control and 48 h sourdough breads. Sourdough breads with 48 h were described as "too sour"	NA	Ua-Arak et al. (2017)
Rice flour; chesnut flour addition (40%)	NR	Fermentation at 22–24 °C with dough propagation at least three times. Sourdough was added at 20%	NR	NR	↑ crumb hardness with sourdough and/or chestnut flour addition	↓ LSV (1.6 ml/g) the chestnut flour and/or sourdough addition (~32%) compared to yeast	Highest class of pores (>10 mm²) were reduced by sourdough addition. Meanwhile, simultaneous addition of chestnut flour and sourdough increased the number of alveoli with highest size (>1 mm²)	NA	Sourdough delayed the amylopectin retrogradation enthalpies	Rinaldi et al. (2017)

(continued)

Table 5.2 (continued)

Main flour in sourdough	Starter culture of sourdough and initial inoculum size	Fermentation conditions, dough yield and proportion of sourdough addition in a bread recipe	Dominate microorganism at the end of the fermentation	Effect of sourdough addition on:						Author
				Dough rheology	Crumb texture	Specific loaf volume (LSV)	Alveolar structure	Sensorial characteristics	Shelf life	
Teff flour (size <0.5 mm)	Inoculum obtained from wheat sourdough provided by an artisan bakery of North Italy	Fermentation at 20 °C for 24 h with daily dough propagation for 8 days Sourdough teff was added at 25%	Cell count of LAB was 2.4×10^6 CFU/g and yeast was 1×10^3 CFU/g	The pasting profile of fermented dough presented a higher onset gelatinization temperature (76.1 °C) and loss of viscosity at high temperatures (70 °C, breakdown). The tendency to retrogradation (setback) was not affected by fermentation of teff flour	Sourdough teff bread showed a softer crumb compared to bread enriched with teff flour	↑ LSV (1.3 mL/g) in bread with fermented teff; however no changes ($p > 0.05$) were observed with control system	Sourdough teff bread showed a more open crumb structure with a lower number of cells	NA	Sourdough teff breads and breads enriched with teff flour showed a higher firmness crumb during storage (3 days)	Marti et al. (2017)
Refined buckwheat flour (size <250 µm)	Commercial GF rice-based sourdough starter culture	Fermentation at 30 °C – 85% RH for 20 h Sourdough was added at 18, 36 and 54%	NR	NA	↓ crumb firmness and relative elasticity	LSV was not affected (1.7–1.8 cm^3/g)	A non-homogenous pore structure was observed in breads with sourdough (18, 36 and 54%)	NA	NA	Zand et al. (2018)

Rice flour and soy protein isolate/soy flour (2:1)	*L. paracasei*/*L. casei*, *L. paracasei* E3, *L. plantarum* E4, *L. plantarum* E5, *L. plantarum* E36, *L. parabuchneri* E7, *L. fermentum* E28, and *L. brevis* E38	Fermentation at 30 °C for 18–20 h Sourdough was added at 40–50%	NR	NA	↑ crumb compressibility (1.8–2.0 times)	↑ LSV (~19% respect to control)	↑ crumb porosity by 9.8–11.5% compared to the control bread	Sourdough bread received a punctuation >4 in a 5-point scale in colour, taste, smell, texture and porosity	NA	Dubrovskaya et al. (2018)
Buckwheat and millet flour	Commercial GF sourdough starter culture and *Lactobacillus* spp. (*L. fermentum* LMG 6902, *L. hammesii* DSM 16381, *L. paralimentarius* LMG 19152, *L. pentosus* LMG 10755, *L. pentosus* LMG 10755, *L. plantarum* subsp. *plantarum*, *L. sanfranciscensis* LMG 16002 and DSM 20663)	Fermentation at 25–27 °C and 85% RH for 16–18 h DY = 200	NR	NA	↓ crumb firmness by specific *Lactobacillus spp.* strains in millet and buckwheat bread	↑LSV in millet bread with some *Lactobacillus spp.* strains; no changes were observed in buckwheat bread	Porosity was satisfactory in all buckwheat sourdough breads, while dissimilarities in structure and pores were evident in millet sourdough breads	NA	NA	Bender et al. (2018)
White and brown teff flour (size <150 μm)	*Lactobacillus fermentum*	Fermentation at 30 °C – 85% RH for 19.5 h until the pH was 3.9–4.1 Teff sourdough was added at 10, 20 and 30%	NR	NA	↓ hardness, springiness and chewiness of crumb bread with 30% of sourdough addition	LSV was not affected (1.8–1.9 mL/g)	NA	NA	NA	Shumoy et al. (2018)

(continued)

Table 5.2 (continued)

Main flour in sourdough	Starter culture of sourdough and initial inoculum size	Fermentation conditions, dough yield and proportion of sourdough addition in a bread recipe	Dominate microorganism at the end of the fermentation	Effect of sourdough addition on:						Author
				Dough rheology	Crumb texture	Specific loaf volume (LSV)	Alveolar structure	Sensorial characteristics	Shelf life	
Pearl millet flour	*L. sanfranciscensi*, *L. brevis*, *L. paralimentarius* and *L. plantarum* isolated and combination of strains (initial inoculum size 10^7 CFU/g of LAB strains)	Fermentation at 30 °C for 24 h. Sourdough was added at 15% DY = 189	The sourdough inoculated simultaneously with *L. sanfranciscensis*, *L. brevis* and *L. paralimentarius* strains reached to 10.14 log CFU/g after a 48 h fermentation	↑ phase angle with a fall in G*, giving as result dough less elastic and softer	Sourdough breads prepared with *L. brevis* and *L. paralimentarius* presented the lowest firmness in crumb	↑ LSV (2.7–3.1 mL/g) in sourdough bread inoculated with a single starter	The sourdough bread with *L. paralimentarius* showed the best performance in porosity (30.13%)	Sourdough breads with different *Lactobacillus* strains presented notable differences in texture and taste according to the judgment of a trained panel (n = 12)	Sourdough with *L. sanfranciscensis*, *L. paralimentarius* and *L. plantarum* retained major content of moisture (45.4%) at the end of storage, meanwhile the sourdough bread with *L. brevis* presented the softer crumb during storage	Nami et al. (2019)
Chia and flaxseed flour	*W. cibaria* CH28, *L. lactis* CH179, *L. plantarum* FUA3171 and *L. fermentum* FUA3165 (initial cell density 7 log CFU/g dough)	Fermentation at 30 °C for 24 h Sourdough was added in a range from 5% to 40% DY = 400	NR	NA	NA	↑ LSV in breads added with 40% of *W. cibaria*-chia sourdough and combination of *L. plantarum* + *L. fermentum*-flaxseed sourdough (2.15 and 2.08 cm^3/g, respectively)	NA	Sorghum-based breads produced with 30 and 40% chia sourdoughs were the most accepted by the panellists (52% and 26%, respectively)	NA	Maidana et al. (2020)

Germinated white sorghum grains (*S. bicolor* (L.) Moench)	*Pediococcus pentosaceus* SA8, *W. confusa* SD8, or *P. pentosaceus* LD7 (initial inoculation 10^8 CFU/mL) isolated from sorghum sponge	Fermentation at 28 °C for 48 h DY = 200	NR	Sourdough with *P. pentosaceus* LD7 had the highest G′ (3.07 Pa) and G″ (6.23 Pa), while sourdough with *P. pentosaceus* SA8 had the least G′ (0.88 Pa) and G″ (2.87 Pa)	↑ hardness, cohesiveness, springiness, gumminess and chewiness	No differences were observed in LSV (average 2.08 cm^3/g) in sourdough bread inoculated with culture starter	NA	NA	All the sourdough bread samples had a shelf-life of 3 days	Olojede et al. (2020)
Germinated and ungerminated pearl millet (*Pennisetum glaucum*) grains	*L. plantarum* MLd27 and *Pichia kudriavzevii* MYd23 (initial inoculum size was 2×10^{10} and 3×10^9 CFU/mL for LAB and yeast, respectively)	Fermentation at 30 °C for 24 h DY = 200	*L. acidophilus*, *L. delbrueckii*, *L. plantarum* and *S. cerevisiae*, *Candida spp.*, *Pichia spp.*	NR	NA	Sourdough bread with unmalted millet grain and *Pichia kudriavzevii* MYd23 ↑ the LSV (3.1 cm^3/g)	NA	Sourdough bread with baker yeast's and *P. kudriavzevii* received the highest score in appearance, crumb, taste, aroma, texture and overall acceptability by a trained panel (n = 12)	Shelf life was extended up to 7–9 days until mould were visible	Banwo et al. (2020)
Rice flour, corn flour and cricket powder	*L. plantarum* 98a, *L. sanfranciscensis* Bb12 and *S. cerevisiae* (10^7 CFU/mL)	Fermentation at 31 °C for 6 h Sourdough was added at 20%	*S. cerevisiae* and LAB	NA	NA	NA	NA	Sourdough received a punctuation >4 in a 7-point scale in colour, taste, smell, aftertaste, appreciation and crispiness	NA	Nissen et al. (2020)

(continued)

Table 5.2 (continued)

Main flour in sourdough	Starter culture of sourdough and initial inoculum size	Fermentation conditions, dough yield and proportion of sourdough addition in a bread recipe	Dominate microorganism at the end of the fermentation	Effect of sourdough addition on:						Author
				Dough rheology	Crumb texture	Specific loaf volume (LSV)	Alveolar structure	Sensorial characteristics	Shelf life	
Amaranth seeds (*Amaranthus spp.*), whole buckwheat (*Fagopyrum esculentum*) and flour and quinoa flour (*Chenopodium quinoa*)	Spontaneous fermentation	Incubation at 30 °C until obtain a mature sourdough by propagation DY = 250	NR	NA	NA	NA	NA	NA	NA	Carbó et al. (2020)
Chia (*Salvia hispanica* L.) flour	Spontaneous fermentation	The mass was incubated at 30 °C for 24 h. Sourdoughs were obtained according to the backslopping, for 10 days DY = 400	*W. cibaria, L. rhamnosus, L. zeae, E. mundtii, E. faecium C. baratii and C. tyrobutyricum*	NA	NA	NA	NA	NA	NA	Maidana et al. (2020)
Sourdough based on whole meal rice (32.5%) and millet flour (7.5%) or wholemeal rice (20%), millet (7.5%) and yellow pea flour (12.5%) (particle size <1120 μm)	*L. reuteri* DSM 20016, *L. fermentum* DSM 20052 or *L. brevis* DSM 20054 (initial inoculum of LAB culture ~10^6 CFU/g)	Fermentation at 37 °C for 16 h Sourdough was added at 20%	NR	NA	NA	NA	NA	NA	NA	Drakula et al. (2021)

Quinoa flour (particle size 0.5 mm)	*Pediococcus pentosaceus* QB17 isolated from quinoa sourdough (initial inoculum of 6 log CFU/g)	Fermentation at 30 °C for 16 h Sourdough was added at 30% DY = 200	Autochthonous *P. pentosaceous* QB17 strain increased in 2.24 log CFU/g after 16 h of fermentation	NA	↓crumb firmness	NA	NA	↑ crust colour, perception of the acid, sourness and aroma attributes ↓ sweet scores (5.4 in a 9 point-hedonic scale)	Shelf life was extended up to 14 days by visible surface moulds	Franco et al. (2021)
White quinoa (*C. quinoa* Wild) and cowpea (*V. unguiculata* (L.) Walp) (The freeze-dried sourdoughs were milled and screened via 500 μm)	Spontaneous fermentation	Incubation at 28 °C for 48 h DY = 200	NR	Antagonist effect was reported in pasting properties of quinoa and cowpea sourdough	NA	NA	NA	NA	NA	Kewuyemi et al. (2022)
Sourdough based on wet grounded chickpea seeds (particle size ~0.5 cm³)	Endogenous microflora (bacilli and clostridia populations)	Chickpea flour fermented at 37 °C for 15 h. Then, a mixture of sourdough and rice flour (1:1 w/w) was fermented at 37 °C for 2 h Sourdough was added at 25%	NA	NA	↓ crumb firmness	↑ LSV	Sourdough increased the number of small pore cells (<4 mm²) respect to the control breads (*S. cerevisae*)	NA	↓ the staling rate and delay the starch retrogradation	Mygdalia et al. (2022)
Rice and quinoa flour	*Limosilactobacillus fermentum* and *L. plantarum* ATCC8014 (10^8 UFC/g) isolated from buckwheat and quinoa sourdough	Incubation at 30 °C for 24 h DY = 200 Sourdough was added at 20%	Supplementary material	NA	No differences were observed in firmness	↑ LSV	NA	NA	NA	Lancetti et al. (2022)

(continued)

Table 5.2 (continued)

Main flour in sourdough	Starter culture of sourdough and initial inoculum size	Fermentation conditions, dough yield and proportion of sourdough addition in a bread recipe	Dominate microorganism at the end of the fermentation	Effect of sourdough addition on:						Author
				Dough rheology	Crumb texture	Specific loaf volume (LSV)	Alveolar structure	Sensorial characteristics	Shelf life	
Refined rice flour, Quinoa (*Chenopodium quinoa*) or buckwheat (*Fagopyrum esculentum*)	Limosilactobacillus fermentum and *L. plantarum* ATCC8014 (10^8 UFC/g). Isolated from buckwheat and quinoa sourdough	Two fermentation processes were evaluated, a single-step process (30 °C, 24 h), and backslopping process for 10 days DY = 200	L. Fermentum (Moreover, homofermentative LAB dominates in spontaneous fermentation processes and heterofermentative sourdough lactobacilli drives sourdough fermentation processes with backslopping)	NA	NA	NA	NA	NA	NA	Lancetti et al. (2022)
Germinated sorghum bicolour flour	*P. pentosaceus* LD7, *P. pentosaceus* SA8 and *W. confusa* SD8 (10^8 UFC/g). Isolated from sorghum sponge	Fermentation at 28 °C for 48 h Sourdough was added at 15% DY = 200	NA	NA	The sourdoughs inoculated with *P. pentosaceus* LD7 and *P. pentosaceus* SA8 exhibited the best attributes. LD7 ↓ hardness, and ↑ cohesiveness and, SA8 ↑ springiness and ↓ stiffness	↑ LSV in sourdough bread with *W. confusa* SD8 (2.50 g/cm^3)	NA	Sourdough bread with *P. pentosaceus* LD7 presented the best qualities for aroma, texture, taste, crumb, and overall acceptability. All sourdough breads received a punctuation 6,4 in a 9-point hedonic scale; except for sourdough bread with *W. confusa*	No differences were observed in the shelf life (extended by 5 days)	Olojede et al. (2022)
Teff flour	*P. acidilactici*, *P. pentosaceus* and *E. durans* (initial inoculum size 5 log UFC/g)	Fermentation at 37 °C for 24 h. Sourdough was added at 20% DY = 280	NA	↓ the dough development time	NA	Sourdough bread with *E. durans* had the ↑ LSV	↑ porosity of the bread	Sourdough bread with *P. pentosaceus* strain received a higher punctuation in taste, aroma and aftetaste (>7 in a 9-hedonic scale) by an untrained panel (n = 25)	Shelf life was prolonged. The addition of sourdough resulted in lower hardness of gluten-free bread crumb during storage	Chochkov et al. (2022)

NA not applicable
NR not reported

The starter maturity is one of the most important key factors to achieve the fulfil quality requirements in leavened baked goods. In practice, qualified bakers determine a starter's maturity by assessing its sensory characteristics (e.g., visual appearance, development and size of bubbles, odour and flavours). Meanwhile, in laboratory scale the starter maturity is generally assessed by the decrease and stability of dough pH, and/or by the enumeration of microorganisms in which certain species of bacteria and yeasts consistently appear at certain times (i.e., youth or maturity) (Calvert et al. 2021).

In general, the sourdough is colonised mainly by homofermentative and heterofermentative lactobacilli and yeasts as dominant microbial flora of the fermentation process. More than 90 different LAB species and more than 40 different yeast species have been isolated from counterpart sourdoughs worldwide. The most common LAB species include *Lactobacillus sanfranciscensis, Lactobacillus brevis* (heterofermentatives), *Lactobacillus plantarum, Pediococcus pentosaceus* (homofermentatives) and *Lactobacillus paralimentarius* (facultative heterofermentative). The most prevalent yeast species are *Saccharomyces cerevisiae* and *Kazachstania humilis*. The symbiotic association between LAB and yeasts is common in food fermentations where LAB are responsible for providing the acid environment for yeast growth, while the yeasts provide vitamins and other growth factors for the LAB development. The ratio LAB:yeast is mostly 10:1 to 100:1. Mature sourdoughs with a stable microbial association are characterized by a cell density >10^8 CFU/g LAB, meanwhile the number of co-existing yeast are usually lower than LAB (Comasio et al. 2020).

From a technological point of view, the use of sourdough inoculated with the isolated or the simultaneous combination of several lactobacilli and/or yeast strains could have an impact on the final quality of GF bread loaves. For instance, the inoculation of teff sourdough with *Enteroccocus durans* significantly increased the loaf specific volume (LSV) (1.70 cm^3/g) compared to *Pediococcus acidilactici* or *Pediococcus pentosaceus* (1.59 and 1.55 cm^3/g, respectively), denoting a strain specificity (Chochkov et al. 2022). Similar results were reported in a study with pearl millet sourdough bread. In this case, the inoculation of sourdough with a single culture starter as *L. brevis* had a greater positive effect on LSV bread (3.1 mL/g). Meanwhile, sourdough inoculated with multiple strains showed a tendency to lower LSV. On the other hand, the highest porosity in crumb bread (30.13%) was observed when sourdough bread was inoculated with *L. paralimentarius* (Nami et al. 2019). Furthermore, the effect of different *Lactobacillus spp.* strains has been studied in millet or buckwheat sourdough GF breads denoting a different performance between them. The simultaneous inoculation of *L. sanfranciscensis*, *L. paralimentarius*, *L. pentosus* and *L. hammesii* in sourdough showed a significant improvement in specific volume, crumb firmness and porosity of breads (Bender et al. 2018). These results highlight that different *Lactobacillus* and/or yeast strains could positively or negatively affect technological quality parameters of GF bread-making according to the raw material and/or de microbial combination.

Over the last years different GF sourdough based on cereals, pseudocereals and legumes have been developed using either spontaneous fermentation or through the addition of culture starters. Among them, the most studied in scientific research are *Lactobacillus plantarum*, *Pediococcus pentosaceus*, *Lactobacillus fermentum*, *Lactobacilus sanfranciscensis*, *Lactobacillus brevis* and *Weisella confuse* (Table 5.2).

5.4 Fermentation Processes: Classification and Characteristics

Depending on the conditions of fermentation process applied, five categories can be described for different types of sourdough:

- **Type 0** sourdough is a type of *pre-dough* or named as mother sponge which is characterised by a short fermentation time at room temperature. This procedure allows the initial propagation of endogenous LAB at higher rate proliferation compared to yeast; therefore, a faster pH reduction (<4) account due to the organic acid synthesis. Typical examples of sourdough type 0 are *biga* to prepare *ciabatta* from Italy, *pâte fermentêe* from France, and *poolish* from Polan. The main difference between these pre-doughs is the level of water hydration (Ramos et al. 2021).
- **Type I** sourdough fermentation is carried out spontaneously by the native yeast and LAB present in raw materials. These yeast and LAB became metabolically active by the addition of water to the flour followed by an incubation period. The grains and/or flour used should not be heat treated, to avoid inactivating the hydrolytic activities from endogenous enzymes and microorganisms. The most competitive organisms will survive and dominate the fermentation process, being mostly LAB and yeasts. In general, in Type I sourdough, the prevalent LAB species are higher than yeast species (Van Kerrebroeck et al. 2017). This baker practice requires longer times to prepare the so-called *pre-dough* or type 0 sourdough, which is added in the appropriate rate (5–50%) to the bread dough. When more often is used the sourdough as an inoculum to propagate the following dough, better it is the adaptation of the microbial association to the fermentation process. In continuously propagated doughs in the same place, only few strains may prevail for years (Hammes et al. 2005).

  The Type I sourdough is characterised as firm dough with a low dough yield (DY <200), fermented at ambient temperature (<30 °C) for 24 h or less time, using the back-slopping method regularly.

  The main disadvantage of this traditional sourdough propagation method is the time- and labour-consuming (e.g. in rye- sourdough bread 24 h, up to three propagation steps). It requires qualified staff, it is not fully controllable from a microbiological point of view, and therefore, it is difficult to scale up.
- **Type II** sourdough fermentation occurs after the addition of specific bacteria (usually LAB, and/or yeast i.e. *Saccharomyces cerevisiae* or bakery yeast) into a flour-water mixture. The sourdough is characterised as liquid doughs with a high

DY (>200), fermented at elevated temperatures (>30 °C) and in one stage for 24–72 h (without the use of back-slopping method). The further addition of baker's yeast to the sourdough could be done at the end of the fermentation process mainly as CO_2 producer and flavour profile of bread. In some cases, specific strain of LAB which are acid tolerant could be added to achieve unique organoleptic properties (i.e., extra sour, lactic taste, strong flavour) and to enhance shelf life (Calvert et al. 2021; Gänzle and Zheng 2019).

It is noteworthy that Type II starters are easier to use at large scales due to their simple standardisation process, giving as result products with better good quality, e.g., homogenous specific loaf, flavour profile and, alveoli structure and crumb texture.

The above classification in Type I and II sourdough allows the specific LAB and yeast strains, i.e., *L. sanfranciscensis* and *C. humilis* are considered typical from Type I; whereas *L. fermentum* which is acid-tolerant LAB specie is prevalent in Type II.

- **Type III** consists of a dehydrated starter version of Type II sourdough employed as acidifier supplement and aroma carrier in bread. The dried format can be easily stored and transported to be used in industrial scale, bakeries or consumers at home-made bread-making.
- **Type IV** is a mixture of Type I and II sourdough, leaving the effects of ecological drift by forcing competition between inoculated microorganisms and those naturally present in the sourdough ecosystem. This bread-making technique is currently produced under controlled fermentation parameters on a laboratory scale (Calvert et al. 2021; Ma et al. 2021; De Vuyst et al. 2017).

5.5 Traditional and Alternative Raw Materials in Sourdough GF Bread

Most of commercial GF baked goods are formulated mainly based on refined flours such as rice and corn, and starch from maize, cassava and potato. These ingredients are generally part of a more complex recipe that includes hydrocolloids, protein from different sources (animal and/or vegetable), and/or emulsifiers. In general, these products are perceived by consumers to have a poor mouth feel, compact and dry crumb, and weak flavour (Roman et al. 2019). Therefore, the study of alternative ingredients could help to develop novel GF sourdough bread, improving technological properties, prolonging the shelf life by retarding the staling, and enhancing either sensorial or nutritional characteristics.

Consumers can buy in minor retails, fresh or dried sourdough as leavening agent to be used alone or in combination with baker's yeast for home-made bread elaboration. In Fig. 5.1 are detailed the flours commercially available for fresh or dried GF sourdough preparation around the world, and those GF flours used for sourdough development recently reported in the scientific bibliography. In both scenarios,

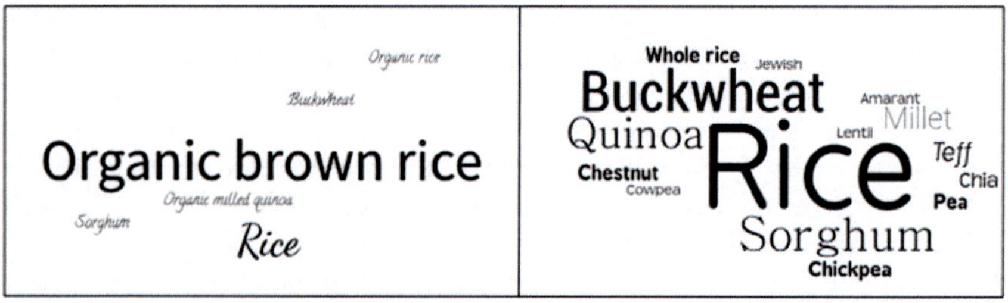

Fig. 5.1 Cloud word of GF flours used for fresh or dried commercial sourdough (n = 11) (left), and GF flours recently reported in scientific bibliography (n = 50) (right)

refined or brown rice, and buckwheat flours are the ingredients most frequently used for sourdough preparation. Nevertheless, the increasing demand of GF sourdough bread by consumers with GRD is driving to the study of other alternatives, as detailed in Tables 5.2 and 5.3. Among them, there are sourdough developed based on cereals such as rice (*Oryza sativa*), millet (*Panicum miliaceum*), sorghum (*Sorghum spp.*), and teff (*Eragrostis tef*); pseudocereals as quinoa (*Chenopodium quinoa*), amaranth (*Amaranthus spp.*) and buckwheat (*Fagopyrum esculentum*); legumes as chickpea (*Cicer arietinum* L.), cowpea (*V. unguiculata* (L.) Walp), pea and lentil; and seeds as chia (*Salvia hispánica*) and flaxseeds.

It is important to highlight that the quality and the composition of the raw materials affect the rheological and sensory properties, nutritional profile, and stability of baked products. In last years, the use of whole-grain flours that contain the starchy endosperm (80–85%), germ (3%) and bran outer layers (including the aleurone and hialine layers, 6–9%) has gained popularity in sourdough wheat breads. The use of whole grain flour or milling fractions such as pericarp and/or germ in the fermentation process could deliver a specific taste, odour and flavour to the bread; in other words, it could produce a completely different sensorial profile in the final product.

5.6 Effect of Sourdough Addition in GF Bread-Making: Rheological and Technological Aspects

The effects of the sourdough technology on the overall quality of GF baked goods in terms of rheological and technological characteristics have been reported recently by several authors. Table 5.2 summarises the main advances reported in these topics.

– ***Rheological sourdough characterisation***

Several devices have been used for the rheological studies of dough, such as the Chopin alveograph, farinograph, visco-analyser, and different types of rheometers, for explaining and complementing the texture and sensory studies of the final bread product.

Table 5.3 Effect of sourdough biotechnology on the nutritional profile of GF bread

Effect of sourdough addition on:			
Macro and micronutrients	Starch hydrolysis/ Glycaemic index	Bioactive compounds	Author
↑ releasing of Ca, Mg and K the inoculation with *S. cerevisae* in comparison with *P. pentosaceus*	NA	NA	Ogunsakin et al. (2015)
↑ the concentration of essential amino acids (Glu, Ala, Arg, Leu, His, Trp and Lys) and γ-amino butyric acid in sourdough based on Italian legume flours ↑ SDF in a range of 33–80% in mostly all sourdough, and ↓ IDF content ↓ the content of raffinose up to 64% in sourdough	NA	↑ extractable total phenols (20–70%) and the radical scavenging activity of all water-soluble extracts; consequently a ↓ in condensed tannins content was observed respect to the control doughs ↑ the phytase activity	Curiel et al. (2015)
NA	↓ the in vitro starch digested in sourdough breads (range value 54.3–56.5%). No changes were observed in RS (1.29–1.89%)	NA	Rinaldi et al. (2017)
↑ the content of SDF (~56%) and glucose (~66%), and ↓ the content of IDF (~16%) in sourdough teff bread. Lipid and protein fractions were not affected by sourdough fermentation	↓ the total content starch (average value 72.6%) in teff sourdough bread	NA	Marti et al. (2017)
NA	↑ the RS as long as sourdough proportion (0–30%) increased in teff bread and during storage time (5 days) ↑ GI in the range of 72–89% as sourdough proportion increase in bread formulation; however, these values were reduced during storage	NA	Shumoy et al. (2018)
↑ the free amino-acids content in chia sourdough; greater accumulation was produced when dough was inoculated simultaneously with *W. cibaria* + *L. lactis*	NA	NA	Maidana et al. (2020)

(continued)

Table 5.3 (continued)

Effect of sourdough addition on:			
Macro and micronutrients	Starch hydrolysis/ Glycaemic index	Bioactive compounds	Author
NA	NA	↑ the phenolic acid content, TPC and antioxidant capacity in sourdough bread Sourdough inoculated with *L. brevis* showed the highest improvement in phenolic acid content (40%), TPC (44%) and antioxidant capacity (30% DPPH, 50% FRAP) compared to control bread	Drakula et al. (2021)
↑ the concentration of free amino acid such as arginine, glutamic acid, leucine, lysine, and phenylalanine in bread added with 30% of quinoa sourdough compared to the control bread	NA	NA	Franco et al. (2021)
↑ the protein content by sourdough addition in bread	↓ the starch hydrolysis and RDS fraction at higher (35%) level of sourdough addition RS was not modified by sourdough addition	No effect was observed in the antioxidant activity in GF bread measured using the DPPH assay	Beltrão Martins et al. (2022)
No differences were observed in proteins and dietary fibre content; meanwhile there was a ↓ in the fat content in fermented breadstick compared to the control	↓ the GI and the estimated hydrolysis index in fermented breadsticks	↑ TPC, DPPH and ABTS of fermented breadsticks compared to the control system	Caponio et al. (2022)
↑ the crude protein, crude fat, crude fibre and ash content The content of Na, K, Cu, Cr and Ca were significantly increased with cowpea sourdough flour; meanwhile Ca, Cr, Cu, Fe, K, Mg, Mn, P and Zn were enhanced with quinoa sourdough flour	NA	↑ TPC, ABTS and DPPH in acetonic extract of cowpea or quinoa sourdough flour	Kewuyemi et al. (2022)

(continued)

Table 5.3 (continued)

Effect of sourdough addition on:			
Macro and micronutrients	Starch hydrolysis/ Glycaemic index	Bioactive compounds	Author
NA	Sourdough process ↓ the *in vitro* starch hydrolysis, which was higher in sourdough based in buckwheat respect to quinoa Sourdough process ↓ the net sugars dialysability	↑ TPC, FRAP and ABTS in quinoa or buckwheat sourdough bread, showing a strain dependence (*Lp. Plantarum*; *Lim fermentum*)	Lancetti et al. (2022)
NA	The inclusion of sourdough chickpea in breads did not significantly alter the in vitro enzymatic starch hydrolysis kinetics	NA	Mygdalia et al. (2022)
No changes were observed in crude protein, carbohydrate, dietary fibre and ash contents in sorghum sourdough bread compared to the control	NA	↑ the tannin and total phenol contents in sorghum sourdough breads inoculated with *P. pentosaceus LD7*, *P pentosaceus* SA8 and *W. confusa* compared to the control sample Total flavonoids and DPPH were not affected by sourdough addition in bread	Olojede et al. (2020, 2022)

NA not applicable, *IDF* insoluble dietary fibre, *SDF* soluble dietary fibre, *RS* resistant starch, *GI* glycaemic index, *TPC* total phenolic content, *DPPH* 2,2-diphenyl-1-picrylhidrazyl free radical, *ABTS* ABTS$^{\bullet+}$ radical cation scavenging activity, *FRAP* ferric ion reducing antioxidant power

- The **Chopin Alveograph** measures flour quality by inflating a bubble in a thin sheet of dough until it bursts. The graphic representation of these steps is known as alveograph from where it can be defined the following dough properties: tenacity, extensibility, elasticity, and baking strength. These characteristics establish the flour suitability for different uses.
- The **farinograph** records the resistance to deformation by mixing flour and water at a specific speed and temperature. During the test, the dough is developed and further broken down. Dough resistance is expressed in dimensionless units known as Farinograph or Brabender Units (BU). The measured parameters are % water absorption, dough development time, dough stability and mixing tolerance (Chochkov et al. 2022)

- The **visco-analyser** is used to determine the starch (and other components) ability to form a viscous paste. The system measures the viscosity by making a temperature cycle (constant at 50 °C- linearly heating up to 90 °C- constant at 90 °C – linearly cooling down to 50 °C) in a 12.5 min test. The results recorded are known as pasting properties and are defined as: peak viscosity and pasting temperature, initial, through and final viscosity, breakdown (it is caused by rupture of swollen starch granules), setback (indicates starch short time retrogradation) (Balet et al. 2019; Genevois et al. 2020).
- The **rheometers** measure the dough response to small oscillatory or rotational deformation. With rotational assays the measuring sample turns in one direction while in an oscillatory test, it oscillates around the axis. The sample provides resistance which is measured very precisely by the torque and the deflection angle. In the rotational test, the user sets the shear rate, and the rheometer determines the required shear stress, or vice versa. The viscosity is then calculated in the rheometer software according to the viscosity law from the value of the shear stress and shear rate. On the other hand, the oscillatory test is used to investigate the viscoelastic behaviour of a dough, and the characterisation of the undestroyed structure at rest. The sample response wave is time-delayed (phase shift) compared to the set oscillation. The values measured by the rheometer (deflection angle, torque, and phase shift) together with the conversion factors for the measuring system give all necessary data to calculate the required rheological parameters such as the storage modulus G′ (related to the solid component) or loss modulus G″ (viscous component).

Taking into account the sourdough technology applied to wheat bread, it has been shown that the gluten network weakens, the viscoelastic properties and gas retention worsen due to the acidification of the dough. In the acid medium the gluten structure is affected by possible acid hydrolysis, by the increased protein solubility and by the higher activity of protease enzymes (Lynch et al. 2018). Although the ingredients and matrix components are quite different, this negative effect on rheological response observed in wheat sourdough might be considered in GF baked goods. Some studies recently reported have been done in sourdough technology analysing how it affects rheology parameters (Table 5.2). Dough elasticity (evaluated by elastic modulus in oscillatory rheology) appeared to have increased by sourdough addition in pearl millet flour (Nami et al. 2019), but it had been reduced in the case of maize flour, (Falade et al. 2014), in rice and chestnut flour (Demirkesen et al. 2016) producing a harder or softer dough depending on the matrix and strain used. Olojede et al. (2020) also found that elastic and loss moduli variation depended on the strain used (G′ and G″ were higher for *P. pentosaceus* LD7 but lower for *P. pentosaceus* SA8 strain).

Furthermore, the dough height and gas retention were increased with corn starch blended with rice flour (Cappa et al. 2016) in an alveograph study. Chochkov et al. (2022) found that sourdough decreased consistency, development time and stability in a teff, corn and rice blend when considering farinographic analysis. While Mariotti et al. 2017 observed an increased dough final height and gas retention in a

GF corn plus rice mix. Although dough consistency is a known parameter in wheat dough (500 BU is the optimal consistency); specifications of consistency levels in GF doughs are not yet available in scientific literature and could have a dependency with the components of the adopted formulation. However, when using the same GF recipe, a higher water levels in the dough (lower consistency) has been found as preferable to achieve a good dough performance during leavening, in particular, when ingredients having a high-water affinity such as dietary fibre are included (Cappa et al. 2013).

On the other hand, using a visco-analyser, the pasting properties of sourdough, showed for teff flour a lower peak viscosity (Marti et al. 2017) as well as for quinoa (lower peak through and final viscosities) but cowpea had higher viscosities than the raw material without fermentation (Kewuyemi et al. 2022). In general, fermentation reduced apparent viscosity of gelatinised bread flour and changed its consistency from a thick sticky gelatinised form into semiliquid/liquid dough (Haydersah et al. 2012).

In conclusion, the interactions between the different ingredients and dough components, the level of acidification, and the strains and concentrations used in the sourdough make it complex to predict the results in the rheology and texture, and in the other bread quality characteristics. Further studies are needed to completely understand the rheology and texture changes during sourdough fermentation.

– ***Synthesis of exopolysaccharides in sourdough***

Considering the rheology aspect, it is important to note that some of the microorganisms from sourdough can produce high molecular weight (Mw) polymers. They may be delivered to the matrix or be generated by enzymes outside the cell (exopolysaccharides –EPs-) modifying the physicochemical properties of the dough in a similar way to commercial gums. These latter gums are long-chain polysaccharides that are widely added to GF products to provide viscoelastic properties similar to the gluten network, improving texture, shelf life and acceptability. The EPs are generated in situ, and therefore, they do not have to be declared on the label. This represents a great advantage when comparing with commercial gums, since consumers demand more and more free additive products. In addition, EPs also add nutritional value to the product, since they are considered soluble fibre sources.

The EPs can contain more than one type of monosaccharide in the carbohydrate chain and therefore, they are named heteropolysaccharides. The latter are produced in very low amounts and their Mw are in the range of 40–900 kDa, being particularly important in fermented dairy products. Other types of EPs are homopolysaccharides that have a single sugar residue (either glucose -glucans- or fructose -fructans-) in all the polymer chains. Their Mw usually are higher than 1000 kDa and they are produced in higher quantities (in the range of 0.1–1.5 g/L of culture), amounts that are economically viable for food applications (De Vuyst and Degeest 1999). Tieking and Gänzle (2005) found that 20% of 140 sourdough *lactobacillus* strains produced EPs from sucrose and that every sourdough will contain at least one EPs producer strain.

In the last few years some EPs have been studied in GF sourdoughs (Bender and Schönlechner 2020). Vogelmann et al. (2009) investigated the adaptability to GF sourdoughs of lactobacilli and found that few strains were competitive. Rühmkorf et al. (2012) showed that for three LAB the flour type (rice, quinoa, buckwheat, and buckwheat core) and sucrose concentration influenced the cell count, the EPs yield, other metabolites and acid (type and quantity) generation. Likewise, oat flour was evaluated for EPs production (Lu et al. 2018). It was observed that β-glucans present in this flour were modified in their Mw, solubility and viscosity by sourdough fermentation, producing more benefits for consumers´ health, and improving texture and overall quality of bread. Depending on fermentation time it was possible to optimise the viscoelastic properties of oat base doughs. Schwab et al. (2008) showed that fermentation with *W. cibaria* decreased bread firmness while increasing the prebiotic content in sorghum sourdoughs. Other authors showed that crumb hardness and shelf life may be improved by the addition of EPs producers' strains in GF sorghum breads (Galle et al. 2010, 2012). These EPs showed great potential for enhancing GF breads quality contrasting the acidification negative effects, retarding or preventing starch retrogradation and thus extending shelf life. In addition, since EPs are not added as additives, products can have clean labels, and also an added value due to the health benefits of sourdough, already mentioned, are increased by EPs as a contribution of prebiotics. On the other hand, the EPs production must be optimised by using the proper raw materials and strains; and other parameters (i.e. acidity, sucrose concentration, fermentation time) should be taken into account within this complex system: GF sourdough.

– ***Technological quality: specific loaf volume, texture, crumb structure and, sensory parameters***

In general, GF baked goods have lower specific volume, dry crumb, poor mouth feel and weak flavour, and a shorter shelf life compared to wheat bread. The use of sourdough addition in an appropriate amount in bread-making could improve the technological stability, safety and prolong the shelf life. Depending on the ingredients used in the bread formulation, different level of sourdough addition in a GF bread-making process are recommended in commercial products (<25%), and in bibliography (<60%). Actually, there is not a consensus to standardise the amount of sourdough addition in bread so far. At laboratory scale, the sourdough addition is dependent on the ingredients used and previous assays that allow establish an optimal proportion to achieve the best performance during proofing, and finally to attain the best quality in the bakery product.

The amount of sourdough addition, the fermentation time and temperature, and back-slopping decrease the pH as consequence of the synthesis and concentration of organic acid in the dough. The acidic medium conditions could have an effect in the main structure-forming components of dough-network as starch and proteins, changing the final quality of the GF breads. Besides, the increase in protein solubility and changes in gelatinised starch granules have an influence in the resulting crumb texture. The GF dough matrix formed by the interaction between proteins-starch is a weak three-dimensional network that is capable to retain the CO_2

produced during proofing stage, resulting in GF breads with compact crumb and non-homogeneous macrostructure with the existing of some large alveoli, possibly due to the coalescence of smaller gas cells (Genevois and de Escalada Pla 2021).

The LSV is one of the most important quality parameters assessed by consumers and is also considered a determining factor for crumb firmness, existing a negative correlation between these parameters (Mygdalia et al. 2022). Thus, a reduction of loaf size volume during the proofing and baking process is undesirable from a consumer acceptance point of view. Volume measurement can be carried out in leavened and unleavened bakery goods using the rapeseed displacement method (American Association for Cereal Chemistry [AACC] 10-05.01, 1998). The results are expressed as cm^3/g or mL/g in order to standardise the procedure with comparison purpose. Detailed information about the methodological procedure is explained in Chap. 6.

Depending on the formulation and the method of baking, wheat LSV presents values between 4 and 5 cm^3/g; whereas GF loaves show lower values: between 1 and 3 cm^3/g (Hager et al. 2012). The increase in LSV in sourdough breads, without the use of extra yeast baker as leavening agent, could be associated with the amylolytic activity of α-amylase present in endogenous microorganisms. The α-amylase activity is associated to the increase of CO_2 production due to the liberation of fermentable sugars, having a positive impact in the LSV of GF breads. In general, the use of sourdough as natural leavening agent in GF bread-making, increases the LSV (Table 5.2). However, depending on ingredients and the type of starter culture, some studies have reported no changes or a negative effect on this parameter (Rinaldi et al. 2017; Mariotti et al. 2017; Cappa et al. 2016; Shumoy et al. 2018). Indeed, the proportion of sourdough addition in bread formulation should also be taken into account since it has been reported in bibliography that lower level (<20%) might enhance the loaf volume; nevertheless, higher percentage of substitution (>40%) might have a detriment effect on LSV (Różyło et al. 2016; Demirkesen et al. 2016).

In general, the development of sourdough with the addition of fresh compressed or dried yeast has showed a positive effect on final quality of GF bread, denoting a synergic between *S. cerevisae* and native lactobacillus and yeast present in flours (Table 5.2). On the other hand, some studies have reported a strain specificity of sourdough over the technological parameters of GF breads, e.g. in the LSV, the structure and texture of crumb bread and, shelf life. For instance, sourdough teff inoculated with *Enterococcus durans* showed the best baking characteristics of GF dough and the highest softness of GF bread during storage compared to inoculation with *Pediococcus acidilactici* and *Pediococcus pentosaceus* strains (Chochkov et al. 2022). A sorghum sourdough inoculated with *Pediococcus pentosaceus* SA8 showed the highest LSV (2.50 cm^3/g) when compared with those inoculated with *Pediococcus pentosaceus* LD7, or *Weissella confuse* WS8 strains (2.17–2.46 cm^3/g) (Olojede et al. 2022).

Therefore, the dominant microorganism in GF sourdough development could enhance or improve the quality parameters of baked goods, and thus satisfy the requirement of consumers with GRD.

Texture and alveoli structure of bread crumb are important indicator of quality that are frequently assessed by consumers at minor retail. Spongy crumb is associated to an aerated and open alveoli structure; meanwhile solid crumb is characterised by a denser and closed alveoli structure. These characteristics give relevant information about the processing conditions, e.g. a non-homogenous and open alveoli structure in crumb could be associated to the use of sourdough as leavening agent. The alveoli are formed due to the generation of CO_2 by yeast during proofing, allowing the dough to arise and retain the air in bubbles.

Digital image analysis can be used to analyse and characterise the crumb structure of GF bread using a software to contrast the two phases, a gas phase represented by the air included in alveoli and, a solid phase denoted by crumb. The crumb images can be scanned from bread slices of ~10 mm thickness with a resolution >300 dpi. Then, a square (25×25 mm^2) from the central crumb zone is selected, and eliminating the crust and excluding the edges, is converted to grey-level image (8-bits image) using the software (ImageJ software, NIH, USA). After that, image is calibrated using a reference measure, the threshold method is used to convert the 8-bit image to binary imagen (gas phase is represented in black and solid phase in white) as is shown in Fig. 5.2 (Gonzales-Barron and Butler 2006; Genevois and de escalada Pla 2021).

Parameters from alveolar structure such as cell area, cell diameter, Dj (mm), average alveoli diameter (mm), cell density (number of alveoli/mm^2) and, crumb air inclusion (%) are measured according to Eqs. 5.2 and 5.3. The crumb uniformity and the equivalent volumetric mean diameter (D [4, 3], mm) can be also evaluated according to Eqs. 5.4 and 5.5, respectively (Corral et al. 2017; Genevois and de Escalada Pla 2021):

$$\text{Alveoli diameter}(\text{mm}) = \sqrt{\frac{4 \text{x} \text{alveoli area}}{\pi}} \tag{5.2}$$

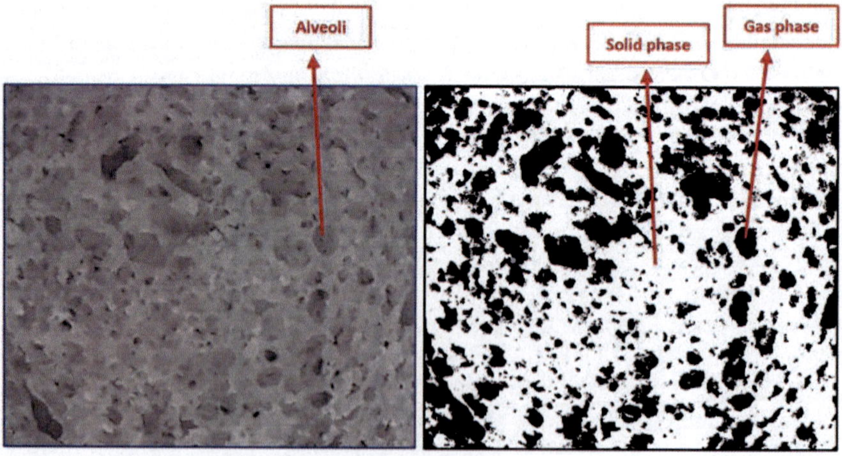

Fig. 5.2 Image of a scanned crumb bread converted, first to grey scale image (left), and then to a binary image (right)

$$\text{Air inclusion}(\%) = \frac{\Sigma\text{alveoli area}}{\text{total area}} * 100 \tag{5.3}$$

$$\text{Uniformity} = \frac{\text{small cells}\left(0.015 \leq \times < 2.000\text{mm}^2\right)}{\text{large cells}\left(2.0 \leq \times < 10.0\text{mm}^2\right)} \tag{5.4}$$

$$D[4,3] = \frac{\sum_{i=1}^{n} D_j^4}{\sum_{i=1}^{n} D_j^3} \tag{5.5}$$

The digital image analysis is a simple, inexpensive and objective method to measure the distribution and size of alveoli in GF bread crumb; consequently, it could be considered as a tool for the quality control in the food industry.

In general, the inclusion of sourdough in leavened GF bread reduces the number of alveoli with higher size and, increases the number of smaller alveoli giving as result crumbs with a homogenous and denser structure. Several studies have reported that a denser alveoli structure is, generally, associated with a softer and resilient crumb sourdough bread (Table 5.2).

Sensorial evaluation of GF sourdough bread is a valuable tool for the product innovation, quality control, assessing the shelf life, and to have a deep quality characterisation, and/or the consumer perceptions (Rizzello et al. 2016). There are analytical methods (objective) and also consumer hedonic studies (subjective) as are detailed in Chap. 9.

Over the las years, the per capita consumption of bread has decline in some developed countries, partially, due to the negative perception associated to a detriment of sensory quality of bread with the industrialisation process; and to the changes in diet habits reducing the intake of carbohydrates (García-Gómez et al. 2022). In this context, the sensorial evaluation of GF sourdough bread has gained importance due to the synthesis of different aromatic compounds that can enhance the flavour and aroma. For instance, the study of different *Lactobacillus* strains in the development of pearl millet sourdough has presented notable differences in bread texture and taste according to the judgment of a trained panel (Nami et al. 2019). In addition, the use of *Pichia kudriavzevii* and baker's yeast as starter culture in millet sourdough bread has received better scores in attributes such appearance, crumbs, taste, aroma, texture and overall acceptability by a trained panel; denoting that the simultaneous presence of microorganism culture could have a synergic effect on sensorial and textural characteristics (Olojede et al. 2020).

In hedonic studies carried out in regular consumers, the use of sourdough based on flours from rice, sorghum, buckwheat, teff, quinoa, chia, flaxseed, or millet in leavened GF bread has shown, in general, good overall acceptability compared to the control breads (Table 5.2). However, the sensorial consumer perception of sourdough GF bread could be influenced by the starter culture used to inoculate the sourdough (Ogunsakin et al. 2015; Ua-Arak et al. 2017) and, the level of addition in the bread formulation (Różyło et al. 2016; Maidana et al. 2020; Olojede et al. 2022; Chochkov et al. 2022).

It is noteworthy that sensorial assessment reported in bibliography, in general, have been carried out in regular consumers so far, highlighting the needed to perform these evaluations in panellist with GRD. These consumers are familiarised with the characteristics of GF baked goods which could be perceived totally different compared to the wheat counterpart.

On the other hand, the application of dried technology to obtain freeze-dried sourdough has also recently been studied, denoting that crumb structure and texture, and/or sensorial profile of bread could be significantly affected. The application of freeze-drying technology at 20 °C and 40 °C to obtain sourdough rice reduced its performance when was added at different levels (10–40%) in GF bread recipe compared to the fresh sourdough. The LSV and alveoli structure were negatively affected by freeze-drying, showing better results when sourdough was freeze-dried at 20 °C respect to 40 °C. In addition, sensorial attributes as taste, aroma texture and overall acceptability where not perceived as different ($p > 0.05$) by consumers in breads with 20% of fresh or freeze-dried sourdough, receiving a punctuation >5 in a 9-point hedonic scale. These sensorial attributes received a lower punctuation (<5 point in a 9-point hedonic scale) when higher percentage of sourdough rice was included in GF bread. Furthermore, the development of buckwheat and amaranth sourdough freeze-dried was studied at different levels of addition (20–30%) in a GF bread, showing that volume, textural and sensorial profile of bread was improved. However, the freeze-dried amaranth sourdough should not be used in an amount > 10% in bread-making according to the responses of consumers in the sensorial evaluation (Różyło et al. 2015a, b, 2016). These results denote that the units operations and the raw material used to develop GF sourdough could have an impact on the final quality of GF bread.

5.7 Commercial Aspects. Cost and Shelf-Life Analysis

Baked goods go through several physical, physicochemical, sensory and microbial changes during storage. Wheat breads are products with a very short shelf-life, in general few days. Meanwhile, GF bread are characterised with a higher staling rate and, therefore a shorter shelf-life, in general hours. The staling of bread is responsible for the disposal of large quantities of bread (8–10%), resulting in considerable economical losses (Katsi et al. 2021).

Staling of bread is a very complex phenomenon that involves physicochemical changes in the moisture content, glass transition, starch crystallisation and, microbiological spoilage, having an impact either in textural or sensorial properties. These modifications are characterised by a significant hardening of crumb, mainly due to the retrogradation of the starch polymers and, the increase in the interaction between starch and proteins molecules. Starch retrogradation is defined as the reassociation of amylose and amylopectin chains into a partially crystalline structure. The changes in amylose fraction are the primary cause for crumb hardening during storage (Farhat and Blanshard 2000). Since amylopectin has a slow crystallisation that requires several days, most staling models analyse the changes in this starch fraction. The retrogradation process of amylopectin occurs above the glass transition involving a nucleation-limited growth in a mobile viscoelastic network (Ronda and Roos 2011).

In addition, during the staling of bread there is a softening of crust with significant loss of crispiness due to the water migration from the crumb to crust and, a moisture exchange between crust and the surrounding environment. Meanwhile at molecular level, there is also water mobility from starch to protein components, favouring the retrogradation of starch gelatinised during baking and, decreasing the amount of free water in bread crumb with a removal of aromatic compounds (Katsi et al. 2021).

Furthermore, high levels of moisture (~30–40%, wet basis) and water activity (~0.90) of baked goods favour the microbial spoilage, especially of *Penicillium*, *Aspergillus* and *Bacillus* genera. The synthesis of organic acid and dough acidification by LAB during the fermentation process delay the growth of spoilage microorganisms and, therefore prolong the shelf-life of bread (Ogunsakin et al. 2015, 2017; Mygdalia et al. 2022). The LAB are also responsible of proteins proteolysis and partial hydrolysis of starch, which may affect physicochemical changes throughout bread storage (Cappa et al. 2016).

The shelf life, in general, is evaluated by the visible growth of mould in bread surface, and through the recording of changes in crumb firmness and starch retrogradation using a texturometer and differential scanning calorimetry (DSC), respectively.

From the isothermal DSC plots, it can be calculated the crystalline fraction (α) by integrating the endothermal peak determining the area related to heat of fusion. Crystallisation kinetics can be analysed plotting the α parameter determined for each time, according to the Avrami model Eq. 5.6 (Avrami 1939):

$$1 - \alpha = \exp\left(-k.t^{n}\right) \tag{5.6}$$

Where α represents the fraction of the crystalline fraction at time t (α = 1 corresponds to the total peak area); *k* is the rate constant of isothermal crystallisation [$(\text{time})^{-n}$] which depends primarily on the crystallisation temperature, and n is known as the Avrami index, a parameter characteristic of nucleation and growth mechanisms of the starch retrogradation.

Several authors have applied Avrami model to explain the hardening process of bread crumb, since this process highly depends on the formation of starch crystals due to retrogradation phenomena (de Escalada Pla et al. 2013; Nieto-Calvache et al. 2022). Therefore, the equation can be re-written as Eq. (5.7):

$$\varphi = \frac{F_\infty - F_t}{F_0 - F_t} = \exp\left(-k.t^n\right) \tag{5.7}$$

Where the crumb firmness is registered using a texturometer, in Newton, at 30% deformation as described in AACC, Method 74.09. F_∞ represents the crumb limiting firmness; F_t is the crumb firmness at time t; and F_0 is the crumb firmness at zero time or initial firmness.

The beneficial effect of sourdough fermentation in retarding the GF bread staling has been study considering culture strains and alternative flours as is detailed in Table 5.2. For instance, the addition of sourdough based on sorghum with *P. pentosaceus* in GF bread has prolonged up to 6 days the shelf-life compared to sourdough with *S. cerevisae* (Ogunsakin et al. 2015). Similar results have been reported with quinoa, white sorghum, pearl millet and teff sourdough (Axel et al. 2015; Olojede et al. 2020; Banwo et al. 2020; Franco et al. 2021; Chochkov et al. 2022). These anti-staling effects of sourdough are attributed, in part, to the amylolytic activity of α-amylases that hydrolyse the molecules starch into dextrins; and consequently, reducing retrogradation (Rinaldi et al. 2017; Mygdalia et al. 2022). Additionally, the type of starter culture could have also a significant positive effect on delaying the crumb hardening. The EPs produced by certain LAB strains, can improve the crumb moisture retention (Nami et al. 2019).

5.8 Nutritional Perspective

Bread is a basic food and due to its energy contribution is considered an important part of the human diet. The nutritional composition of bread is mainly based on carbohydrates (~60%) and protein (~8%).

The changes in diet habits have led to increase the consumer demand of GF baked goods including health claims. Therefore, the development of products with better nutritional profile becomes a challenge for the food industry and the scientific community. In this scenario, the use of whole grains flours or alternative flour in GF bread formulation can significantly enhance the intake of dietary fibre, proteins, vitamins and/or minerals that are deficient in a GF diet (Vici et al. 2016). There is scientific evidence that supports that addition of sourdough in bread making improve either functional properties or nutritional value of leavened baked goods. In particular, sourdough fermentation improves the levels and bioaccesibility of proteins, bioactive compounds and minerals; and decreases the level of anti-nutritional factors and the value of the glycaemic response (Gobbetti et al. 2014; Poutanen et al. 2009).

Carbohydrates are biomolecules that represent the main fraction of flour (~75%) and are present as simple sugars (monosaccharides and disaccharides) and polysaccharides such as starch, cellulose and fibre. A recent study showed that commercially available GF baked goods are characterised by low protein and high fat content. Furthermore, a high proportion of these commercial products (~81%) have presented the addition of refined sugars in their formulation, favouring the intake of foods with a high caloric content (Roman et al. 2019). It is important to highlight that GF bakery goods are characterised by a high glycaemic index (GI) since they are formulated mainly by refined flours and starches.

The concept of GI was proposed by Jenkins et al. 1981 to differentiate the carbohydrates of a consumed meal, according to the way in which they are metabolised. Briefly, the glucose level in blood is recorded within 2 h after the meal intake at different intervals. The curve glucose level versus time is plotted and compared with a standard curve of a reference food (a glucose solution or a white bread). The GI is calculated as the incremental area under the curve (AUC) respect the reference (ISO method 26642:2010) (Eq. 5.8).

$$\text{GI}(\%) = \frac{\text{AUC of food}}{\text{average AUC of reference food}} \times 100 \tag{5.8}$$

Based on the GI values, foods can be categorised as low (<55%), medium (55–69%) or high (>70%) (Li and Hu 2022).

Different in vitro approaches were proposed by several authors and validated with the above GI in vivo method (Goñi et al. 1997; Li and Hu 2022). Nevertheless, a standardised methodology is not available by the moment.

In this scenario, the slow-digestible carbohydrates have a relevant role in food design, since these macromolecules are incompletely or not absorbed in the small intestine, and/or are partly fermented by the microbiota in the large intestine. Dietary fibre carbohydrates, resistant starch (RS), and sugar alcohols are some examples of low-digestible carbohydrates (Grabitske and Slavin 2008).

The rate of starch digestion and, the values of free glucose and starch fractions [rapidly digested starch (RDS), slowly digestible starch (SDS) and RS] can be determined, as well as the predicted GI trough an in vitro static digestion models. These analytical methods are carried out simulating the biochemical, temperature and pH conditions of human gastrointestinal tract, involving oral, stomach and intestinal phase (Mulet-Cabero et al. 2020; Li and Hu 2022). It is important to consider that food composition could affect the starch digestion rate (e.g. phosphorylated starch, RS, dietary fibre, phytonutrients, protein, and fat content) (Ho and wong 2019; Goñi et al. 1997).

The study of the starch fraction digestibility could be a good in vitro indicator when it is complemented with the GI assay. Some studies in sourdough bread have reported a positive correlation (Pearson's product-moment correlations, r) between RDS and GI ($r = >0.79$), while the SDS and RS have been negatively correlated ($r = -0.67$; $r = -0.52$, respectively) (Table 5.3) (Haydersah et al. 2012; Shumoy et al. 2018).

The use of sourdough for GF bread-making has showed a significant reduction either in starch content or GI. For instance, fermentation process allowed reduce 7–11% the digested starch in GF bread (Marti et al. 2017; Rinaldi et al. 2017) and, the GI in a fermented breadstick (Caponio et al. 2022), giving as results starchy foods with higher content of SDS and RS. The synthesis of organic acids such as acetic acid during the fermentation process is associated with a delay in gastric emptying; meanwhile lactic acid induces interactions between starch and proteins during dough baking reducing the starch availability (Shumoy et al. 2018; Caponio et al. 2022). Moreover, during the first stage of sourdough fermentation, the LAB and yeast are responsible for starch hydrolysis, giving as result an increase in the content of rapid-digestible carbohydrates. These latter are used by the microorganisms, firstly as a carbon source for cell growth and, secondly, they convert the glucose into lactic acid through anaerobic glycolysis. Thus, at the end of the fermentation process there is a decrease in carbohydrate content in the food with an impact in the GI value (Chiş et al. 2020). The latest advances in this field are summarised in Table 5.3.

Besides, the flour type used to develop the sourdough could also have an impact in the total starch content after in vitro digestion. A higher reduction of the total starch hydrolysis was reported in sourdough based on buckwheat flour compared to quinoa flour (starch reduction of 17% and 39%, respectively) (Lancetti et al. 2022).

In addition, other carbohydrates, such as sucrose, raffinose, fructose, and soluble fibre can diminish during the fermentation process, probably due to the simultaneous action of the endogenous enzymes produced by LAB (Marti et al. 2017; Baye et al. 2013).

On the other hand, the use of sourdough as leavening agent in bread-making could also increase the levels of RS. Some studies have reported a relationship between the increase of RS content and the level of sourdough addition. This effect could be attributed to several factors like, the formation of free dextrins by action of α-amylase on amylopectin (Shumoy et al. 2018; Marti et al. 2017), the decrease of the dough pH (<4.0) (Gobbetti et al. 2019; Canesin and Cazarin 2021) and due to the starch retrogradation and formation of type 3 RS as it is explained in Chap. 3. Furthermore, the addition of flours rich in dietary fibre and RS content in GF bread formulation has a direct effect on the reduction of starch hydrolysis, and consequently on GI values (Beltrão Martins et al. 2022).

After bread baking, the RS content increases because the other components of the dough were affected by the fermentation process, altering its behaviour during heating (Lancetti et al. 2022; Hefni et al. 2021). A complete or incomplete starch gelatinisation occurs during baking, followed by the starch solubilisation, rendering the polymeric chains more susceptible to amylolytic enzymes. As long as starch chain reordering occurs, the RS increases reducing the susceptibility to enzymatic hydrolysis. During the cooling of bread, an increase of RS levels and SDS may also occur, along with a decrease of rapid-digestible carbohydrates content. The staling of bread could diminish the content of RDS, while the levels of SDS and RS increase (Mygdalia et al. 2022; Horstmann et al. 2017; Shumoy et al. 2018).

It is important to highlight that fermented foods with high RS levels are associated with products with prebiotic properties since RS increase the production of short-chain fatty acids stimulating the microbiota of the human gastrointestinal tract (Markowiak-Kopeć and Śliżewska 2020).

Roman et al. (2019) recorded the nutritional label from n = 228 GF bread and they reported that they presented lower protein compared to a gluten-containing counterpart. The protein content of baked goods is dependent on the raw materials used to formulate them. For instance, the protein content of flours based in cereals is ~11%, pseudocereals ~10% (Franco et al. 2021), in legumes ranges from 15.4% to 24.3% (Curiel et al. 2015) and, in chia and flaxseeds ~24% and ~30%, respectively (Maidana et al. 2020). Therefore, the addition of sourdough developed on alternative flours could be a good strategy to improve not only the technological and sensorial characteristics, but also the nutritional profile of baked goods. Indeed, the design of novel sourdough bread considering the protein complementation between cereal and legume flours could help to fulfil the nutritional deficiencies of vulnerable population groups (Angioloni and Collar 2012).

The sourdough acidification favours the activity of several enzymes with optimal pH between 4.2 and 5.5 (Gänzle et al. 2008; Nionelli and Rizzello 2016). The reduction of pH in the dough could also be achieved by addition of acetic, lactic, tartaric, phosphoric, or citric acid. However, LABs in sourdough exert complex biochemical activities, besides to those linked to lactic acid production (Di Cagno et al. 2002). The proteolysis associated with the metabolic activity of LAB is a key factor that affects the overall quality of bread (Nionelli and Rizzello 2016; Olojede et al. 2020).

The proteolysis has extensively been studied by the indirect determination of free amino acids and peptides accumulation after fermentation period in wheat-based sourdoughs (Reale et al. 2021; Capuani et al. 2013). The first stage is related to the microbial acidification and the reduction of disulphide bonds of proteins by LAB, promoting the primary activity of proteases. The endogenous enzymes in flours, e.g. aminopeptidase, carboxypeptidase, and endopeptidase, are responsible for hydrolysing proteins into oligopeptides (Gänzle et al. 2008; Gobbetti et al. 2014). The second stage occurs due to the proteolytic activity of the enzymes present in the LAB, intracellular peptidase, which cause the release of amino acids (Chavan and Chavan 2011).

Several studies have shown a higher amino acid release when sourdough is used in GF bread-making. For instance, the concentration of essential amino acids (Glutamine, Alanine, Arginine, Leucine, Histidine, Tryptophan and Lysine) and γ-amino butyric acid were increased in sourdough based on Italian legume flours (Curiel et al. 2015). Similar results were reported in GF bread added with 30% of quinoa sourdough, enhancing the concentration of arginine, glutamic acid, leucine, lysine and, phenylalanine (Franco et al. 2021). Besides, a higher release of amino acids was reported in sourdough from chia when it was simultaneously inoculated with *W. cibaria* and *L. lactis* (Maidana et al. 2020).

The amino acids contribute to improve the sensorial properties of leavened baked goods since they are precursors of aromatic compounds such as lactic and acetic acid, diacetyls, acetaldehydes, hexanal, alcohols and, aldehydes (Wu et al. 2022; Nionelli and Rizzello 2016). There are other factors that also have a strong contribution to the flavour of sourdough bread, e.g. the microbial diversity of LAB (homofermentative or heterofermentative), the type of flour used for sourdough development, the time and temperature of fermentation to achieve a mature sourdough, the sourdough proportion used in bread formulation, the content of low Mw sugars, and the cooking temperature and time (Suo et al. 2021; Pétel et al. 2017; Hansen and Schieberle 2005). In general, the sensorial hedonic evaluation of GF sourdough bread in consumers has received high scores in attributes such as taste, aroma, and odour (Table 5.2).

In addition, in vitro assays showed that protein digestibility increases due to the proteolytic activity of LAB present in the sourdough, therefore the nutritional value of the baked good is improved (Nionelli and Rizzello 2016; Zhou et al. 2022).

On the other hand, the proteolytic activity that occurs during sourdough fermentation could made changes at structural level of gluten proteins, in wheat bread, at different degree of depolymerisation and diminish the content of allergenic compounds as gliadins and glutenins which are involved in the etiopathogenesis of GRD (Vermeulen et al. 2007; Nutte et al. 2019). The peptidases of LAB strains present in the sourdough, by themselves, would not produce the complete degradation of gluten, but the strategic combination of several strains could act synergistically (Scherf et al. 2018; Nutte et al. 2019).

As regards the antioxidant compounds in GF bread, several studies have reported that sourdough biotechnology facilitates the extractability and increases its concentration (Table 5.3). Fermentation process can contribute to the release of bound phenolics prior to extraction by pH reduction and the activation of flour endogenous enzymes. Among enzymes, carbohydrases, especially pectinases, are found to be the most effective in breaking covalent bonds and releasing bound phenolic compounds. Besides, proteolytic enzymes of *Lactobacillus* strains are also responsible for hydrolysing phenolic complexes into free soluble phenols (Lancetti et al. 2022).

However, some works have not found any effect of sourdough addition in GF bread on the antioxidant activity using the DPPH assay (Beltrão Martins et al. 2022; Olojede et al. 2020). Possibly, total phenolic compounds released by sourdough fermentation, would not be acting as antioxidants or their antioxidant activity could be lost during bread-making stages. Therefore, the fermentation process and/or metabolism of native LAB strains present in sourdough could affect the antioxidant activity of phenolic compounds, either increasing or decreasing it, due to the association with other compounds that influence the antioxidant activity.

Phytic acid, saponins, condensed tannins and trypsin inhibitors are the main antinutritional factors in cereals, pseudocereals and legumes. In addition, raffinose, stachyose and other oligosaccharides are compounds that could give abdominal discomfort in sensible persons. The presence and content of these compounds depend on the raw material used in manufacturing the bakery product. Up to date, there are few works where these aspects have been deeply analysed in GF sourdough (Table 5.3). For instance, in different flours from Italian legumes, the content of raffinose was diminished up to 64% by sourdough fermentation.

The mineral content of cereals, pseudocereals and legumes ranges between 1.5% and 2.1% (Ogunsakin et al. 2015; Udomkun et al. 2019). However, the bioaccesibility and bioavailability could be affected due to the presence of phytates (Chiş et al. 2020). The production of lactic acid and the pH decreasing would increase the enzymatic activity capable of hydrolysing the phytic acid; and thus enhancing the

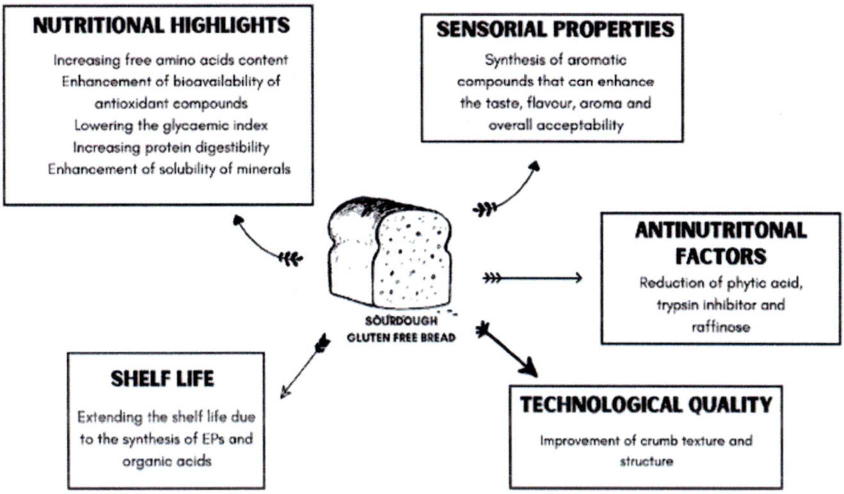

Fig. 5.3 Impact of sourdough biotechnology on the technological properties and nutritional profile of GF bread

solubility of minerals such as Fe, K, Ca, Zn, P, Mg and Cu (Kewuyemi et al. 2022). In addition, some yeast or LAB strains could have a greater impact in the mineral release and/or the reduction of phytic acid and trypsin inhibitor during the fermentation process (Ogunsakin et al. 2015; Starzyńska-Janiszewska and Stodolak 2011). Moreover, the sourdough addition could also significantly reduce the content of raffinose in GF bread (Curiel et al. 2015).

The use of sourdough in GF bread could be a good strategy to improve either technological or nutritional characteristics when it is used in an appropriate proportion. There are several parameters to consider, e.g. the compositions of flour, the native microorganism, or the type and size of culture starter, fermentation conditions, etc. Understanding the main changes occurred in dough and crumb structure, and the biochemical mechanism activated can help to select the optimal conditions to study in future works.

In Fig. 5.3, the main effects of sourdough biotechnology on sensorial, technological, and nutritional properties of GF bread, are summarised.

5.9 Conclusion

Most of the research available to improve GF baked goods has been driven to substitute or imitate the gluten network. The fermentation is a key process in which several biochemical reactions occur, producing physicochemical changes in dough, becoming in an enhancement in overall bread quality. According to the microorganism involved, traditional baker yeast and/or sourdough microbioma, breads with different characteristics are obtained.

Understanding the microbial composition during sourdough fermentation is important to achieve products with good global quality. Parameters such as temperature, inoculum type and size, dough yield and time of sourdough fermentation will determine the rheological behaviour of dough, and structure and texture of crumb bread. From a nutritional point of view, the fermentation process using sourdough enhances the amino acid, mineral and bioactive compounds release, and diminish some anti-nutritional factors and the GI. Sourdough offers a biotechnological tool for producing, in situ, metabolites (EPs) that can act as natural bread improvers reducing the incorporation of additives in GF breads.

Acknowledgments This work was supported by the Universidad Nacional de Entre Ríos (PID UNER 9112; PID UNER 9122), the Universidad de Buenos Aires (UBACYT-20020170100092BA), the National Agency of Scientific and Technical Research (PICT 2018-01019), and the National Scientific and Technical Research Council of Argentina (CONICET). The authors want to acknowledge ACELA Entre Ríos (Asistencia al Celíaco de la Argentina), Gualeguaychú, for their valuable participation and contribution in our projects.

References

AACC (1998) Method 10-05.01 guidelines for measurement of volume by rapeseed displacement. Approved methods of analysis, 10th edn. AACC International, St Paul

Angioloni A, Collar C (2012) Suitability of oat, millet and sorghum in breadmaking. Food Bioprocess Technol 6(6):1486–1493. https://doi.org/10.1007/s11947-012-0786-9

Aparicio-García N, Martínez-Villaluenga C, Frias J et al (2020) Changes in protein profile, bioactive potential and enzymatic activities of gluten-free flours obtained from hulled and dehulled oat varieties as affected by germination conditions. LWT Food Sci Technol 134:109955. https://doi.org/10.1016/j.lwt.2020.109955

Avrami M (1939) Kinetics of phase change. I general theory. J Chem Phys 7(12):1103–1112. https://doi.org/10.1063/1.1750380

Axel C, Röcker B, Brosnan B et al (2015) Application of Lactobacillus amylovorus DSM19280 in gluten-free sourdough bread to improve the microbial shelf life. Int J Food Microbiol 47:36–44. https://doi.org/10.1016/j.fm.2014.10.005

Balet S, Guelpa A, Fox G et al (2019) Rapid Visco Analyser (RVA) as a tool for measuring starch-related physiochemical properties in cereals: a review. Food Anal Methods 12(3):1–17. https://doi.org/10.1007/s12161-019-0581-w

Banwo K, Fasuyi TO, Olojede AO (2020) Potentials of Lactobacillus plantarum and Pichia kudriavzevii in co-fermentation of sourdough from millet. Int J Food Sci 56:857–864. https://doi.org/10.1111/ijfs.14729

Baye K, Mouquet-Rivier C, Icard-Vernière C et al (2013) Influence of flour blend composition on fermentation kinetics and phytate hydrolysis of sourdough used to make injera. Food Chem 138(1):430–436. https://doi.org/10.1016/j.foodchem.2012.10.075

Beltrão Martins R, Garzón R, Peres JA et al (2022) Acorn flour and sourdough: an innovative combination to improve gluten free bread characteristics. Eur Food Res Technol 248:1691–1702. https://doi.org/10.1007/s00217-022-03996-y

Bender D, Schönlechner R (2020) Innovative approaches towards improved gluten-free bread properties. J Cereal Sci 91:102904. https://doi.org/10.1016/j.jcs.2019.102904

Bender D, Fraberger V, Szepasvári P et al (2018) Effects of selected lactobacilli on the functional properties and stability of gluten-free sourdough bread. Eur Food Res Technol 244(6):1037–1046. https://doi.org/10.1007/s00217-017-3020-1

Cabanillas B (2019) Gluten-related disorders: celiac disease, wheat allergy, and nonceliac gluten sensitivity. Crit Rev Food Sci Nutr 60(15):2606–2621. https://doi.org/10.1080/10408398.2019.1651689

Calvert MD, Madden AA, Nichols LM et al (2021) A review of sourdough starters: ecology, practices, and sensory quality with applications for baking and recommendations for future research. PeerJ 9:e11389. https://doi.org/10.7717/peerj.11389

Canesin MR, Cazarin CBB (2021) Nutritional quality and nutrient bioaccessibility in sourdough bread. Curr Opin Food Sci 40:81–86. https://doi.org/10.1016/j.cofs.2021.02.007

Caponio GR, Difonzo G, de Gennaro G et al (2022) Nutritional improvement of gluten-free breadsticks by olive cake addition and sourdough fermentation: how texture, sensory, and aromatic profile were affected? Front Nutr 9:830932. https://doi.org/10.3389/fnut.2022.830932

Cappa C, Lucisano M, Mariotti M (2013) Influence of Psyllium, sugar beet fibre and water on gluten-free dough properties and bread quality. Carbohydr Polym 98(2):1657–1666. https://doi.org/10.1016/j.carbpol.2013.08.007

Cappa C, Lucisano M, Raineri A et al (2016) Gluten-free bread: influence of sourdough and compressed yeast on proofing and baking properties. Foods 5(4):69. https://doi.org/10.3390/foods5040069

Capuani A, Behr J, Vogel RF (2013) Influence of lactic acid bacteria on redox status and on proteolytic activity of buckwheat (Fagopyrum esculentum Moench) sourdoughs. Int J Food Microbiol 165(2):148–155. https://doi.org/10.1016/j.ijfoodmicro.2013.04.020

Carbó R, Gordún E, Fernández A et al (2020) Elaboration of a spontaneous gluten-free sourdough with a mixture of amaranth, buckwheat, and quinoa flours analyzing microbial load, acidity, and pH. Food Sci Technol Int 26(4):344–352. https://doi.org/10.1177/1082013219895357

Chavan RS, Chavan SR (2011) Sourdough technology-a traditional way for wholesome foods: a review. Compr Rev Food Sci Food Saf 10(3):169–182. https://doi.org/10.1111/j.1541-4337.2011.00148.x

Chiş MS, Păucean A, Man SM et al (2020) Quinoa sourdough fermented with Lactobacillus plantarum ATCC 8014 designed for gluten-free muffins—a powerful tool to enhance bioactive compounds. Appl Sci 10(20):7140. https://doi.org/10.3390/app10207140

Chochkov R, Savova-Stoyanova D, Papageorgiou M et al (2022) Effects of teff-based sourdoughs on dough rheology and gluten-free bread quality. Foods 11(7):1012. https://doi.org/10.3390/foods11071012

Cizeikiene D, Jagelaviciute J, Stankevicius M et al (2020) Thermophilic lactic acid bacteria affect the characteristics of sourdough and whole-grain wheat bread. Food Biosci 38(2):100791. https://doi.org/10.1016/j.fbio.2020.100791

Comasio A, Verce M, Van Kerrebroeck S et al (2020) Diverse microbial composition of sourdoughs from different origins. Front Microbiol 11:1212. https://doi.org/10.3389/fmicb.2020.01212

Corral ML, Cerrutti P, Vázquez A et al (2017) Bacterial nanocellulose as a potential additive for wheat bread. Food Hydrocoll 67:189–196. https://doi.org/10.1016/j.foodhyd.2016.11.037

Curiel JA, Coda R, Centomani I et al (2015) Exploitation of the nutritional and functional characteristics of traditional Italian legumes: the potential of sourdough fermentation. Int J Food Microbiol 196:51–61. https://doi.org/10.1016/j.ijfoodmicro.2014.11.032

de Escalada Pla M, Rojas AM, Gerschenson LN (2013) Effect of butternut (Cucurbita moschata Duchesne ex Poiret) fibres on bread making, quality and staling. Food Bioprocess Technol 6(3):828–838. https://doi.org/10.1007/s11947-011-0744-y

De Vuyst L, Degeest B (1999) Heteropolysaccharides from lactic acid bacteria. FEMS Microbiol Rev 23(2):153–177. https://doi.org/10.1111/j.1574-6976.1999.tb00395.x

De Vuyst L, Vancanneyt M (2007) Biodiversity and identification of sourdough lactic acid bacteria. Food Microbiol 24(2):120–127. https://doi.org/10.1016/j.fm.2006.07.005

De Vuyst L, Van Kerrebroeck S, Leroy F (2017) Chapter two -microbial ecology and process technology of sourdough fermentation. Adv Appl Microbiol 100:49–160. https://doi.org/10.1016/bs.aambs.2017.02.003

Debonne E, Van Schoors F, Maene P et al (2020) Comparison of the antifungal effect of undissociated lactic and acetic acid in sourdough bread and in chemically acidified wheat bread. Int J Food Microbiol 321:108551. https://doi.org/10.1016/j.ijfoodmicro.2020.108551

Demirkesen I, Puchulu-Campanella E, Kelkar S (2016) Production and characterization of gluten-free chestnut sourdough breads. Qual Assur Saf Crop Foods 8(3):349–358. https://doi.org/10.3920/QAS2014.0580

Di Cagno R, De Angelis M, Lavermicocca P et al (2002) Proteolysis by sourdough lactic acid bacteria: effects on wheat flour protein fractions and gliadin peptides involved in human cereal intolerance. Appl Environ Microbiol 68(2):623–633. https://doi.org/10.1128/AEM.68.2.623-633.2002

Drakula S, Novotni D, Mustač NC et al (2021) Alteration of phenolics and antioxidant capacity of gluten-free bread by yellow pea flour addition and sourdough fermentation. Food Biosci 44:101424. https://doi.org/10.1016/j.fbio.2021.101424

Dubrovskaya N, Savkina O, Kuznetsova L et al (2018) The development of gluten-free sourdough bread technology with rowan powder. Agron Res 16(2):1360–1372. https://doi.org/10.15159/AR.18.044

Falade AT, Emmambux MN, Buys EM et al (2014) Improvement of maize bread quality through modification of dough rheological properties by lactic acid bacteria fermentation. J Cereal Sci 60(3):471–476. https://doi.org/10.1016/j.jcs.2014.08.010

Farhat I, Blanshard J (2000) Bread staling. In: Chinachoti P, Vodovotz Y (eds) Modeling the kinetics of starch retrogradation, 1st edn. CRC Press, Boca Raton, pp 163–172

Franco W, Evert K, Van Nieuwenhove C (2021) Quinoa flour, the germinated grain flour, and sourdough as alternative sources for gluten-free bread formulation: impact on chemical, textural and sensorial characteristics. Ferment 7(3):115. https://doi.org/10.3390/fermentation7030115

Galle S, Schwab C, Arendt E et al (2010) Exopolysaccharide-forming Weissella strains as starter cultures for sorghum and wheat sourdoughs. J Agric Food Chem 58(9):5834–5841. https://doi.org/10.1021/jf1002683

Galle S, Schwab C, Dal Bello F et al (2012) Influence of in-situ synthesized exopolysaccharides on the quality of gluten-free sorghum sourdough bread. Int J Food Microbiol 155(3):105–112. https://doi.org/10.1016/j.ijfoodmicro.2012.01.009

Gänzle MG, Zheng J (2019) Lifestyles of sourdough lactobacilli – do they matter for microbial ecology and bread quality? Int J Food Microbiol 302:15–23. https://doi.org/10.1016/j.ijfoodmicro.2018.08.019

Gänzle MG, Loponen J, Gobbetti M (2008) Proteolysis in sourdough fermentations: mechanisms and potential for improved bread quality. Trends Food Sci Technol 19(10):513–521. https://doi.org/10.1016/j.tifs.2008.04.002

García-Gómez B, Fernández-Canto N, Vázquez-Odériz ML et al (2022) Sensory descriptive analysis and hedonic consumer test for Galician type breads. Food Control 134:108765. https://doi.org/10.1016/j.foodcont.2021.108765

Genevois CE, de Escalada Pla MF (2021) Soybean by-products and modified cassava starch for improving alveolar structure and quality characteristics of gluten-free bread. Eur Food Res Technol 247:1477–1488. https://doi.org/10.1007/s00217-021-03725-x

Genevois CE, Grenóvero MS, de Escalada Pla MF (2020) Use of different proportions of rice milling fractions as strategy for improving quality parameters and nutritional profile of gluten-free bread. J Food Sci Technol 58(10):3913–3923. https://doi.org/10.1007/s13197-020-04852-1

Gobbetti M, Rizzello CG, Di Cagno R et al (2014) How the sourdough may affect the functional features of leavened baked goods. Food Microbiol 37:30–40. https://doi.org/10.1016/j.fm.2013.04.012

Gobbetti M, De Angelis M, Di Cagno R et al (2019) Novel insights on the functional/nutritional features of the sourdough fermentation. Int J Food Microbiol 302:103–113. https://doi.org/10.1016/j.ijfoodmicro.2018.05

Goñi I, Garcia-Alonso A, Saura-Calixto F (1997) A starch hydrolysis procedure to estimate glycemic index. Nutr Res Rev 17:427–437. https://doi.org/10.1016/S0271-5317(97)00010-9

Gonzales-Barron U, Butler F (2006) A comparison of seven thresholding techniques with the k-means clustering algorithm for measurement of bread-crumb features by digital image analysis. J Food Eng 74(2):268–278. https://doi.org/10.1016/j.jfoodeng.2005.03.00

Grabitske HA, Slavin JL (2008) Low-digestible carbohydrates in practice. J Am Diet Assoc 108(10):1677–1681. https://doi.org/10.1016/j.jada.2008.07.010

Hager AS, Wolter A, Czerny M et al (2012) Investigation of product quality, sensory profile and ultrastructure of breads made from a range of commercial gluten-free flours compared to their wheat counterparts. Eur Food Res Technol 235(2):333–344. https://doi.org/10.1007/s00217-012-1763-2

Hammes WP, Brandt MJ, Francis KL et al (2005) Microbial ecology of cereal fermentations. Trends Food Sci Technol 16(1–3):4–11. https://doi.org/10.1016/j.tifs.2004.02.010

Hansen A, Schieberle P (2005) Generation of aroma compounds during sourdough fermentation: applied and fundamental aspects. Trends Food Sci Technol 16(1–3):85–94. https://doi.org/10.1016/j.tifs.2004.03.007

Haydersah J, Chevallier I, Rochette I et al (2012) Fermentation by amylolytic lactic acid bacteria and consequences for starch digestibility of plantain, breadfruit, and sweet potato flours. J Food Sci 77(8):M466–M472. https://doi.org/10.1111/j.1750-3841.2012.02811.x

Heberle T, Ávila BP, do Nascimento LÁ et al (2022) Consumer perception of breads made with germinated rice flour and its nutritional and technological properties. Appl Food Res 2:100142. https://doi.org/10.1016/j.afres.2022.100142

Hefni ME, Thomsson A, Witthöft CM (2021) Bread making with sourdough and intact cereal and legume grains – effect on glycaemic index and glycaemic load. Int J Food Sci Nutr 72(1):134–142. https://doi.org/10.1080/09637486.2020.1769568

Ho LH, Wong SY (2019) Chemical properties of starch. In: Emeje M (ed) Resistant starch from exotic fruit and its functional properties: a review of recent research. IntechOpen, London, pp 1–21

Horstmann S, Lynch K, Arendt E (2017) Starch characteristics linked to gluten-free products. Foods 6(4):29. https://doi.org/10.3390/foods6040029

ISO (2010) 26642:2010 food products- determination of the glyceamic index (GI) and recommendation for food classification, 1st edn. International Organization for Standardization, Geneva

Jenkins DJ, Wolever TM, Taylor RH et al (1981) Glycemic index of foods: a physiological basis for carbohydrate exchange. Am J Clin Nutr 34(3):362–366. https://doi.org/10.1093/ajcn/34.3.362

Katsi P, Kosma IS, Michailidou S et al (2021) Characterization of artisanal spontaneous sourdough wheat bread from Central Greece: evaluation of physico-chemical, microbiological, and sensory properties in relation to conventional yeast leavened wheat bread. Foods 10(3):635. https://doi.org/10.3390/foods10030635

Kewuyemi YO, Kesa H, Adebo OA (2022) Biochemical properties, nutritional quality, colour profile and techno-functional properties of whole grain sourdough and malted cowpea and quinoa flours. Int J Food Sci Technol 57:1527–1543. https://doi.org/10.1111/ijfs.15512

Lancetti RP, Salvucci E, Paesani C et al (2022) Sourdough on quinoa and buckwheat gluten-free breads: evaluation of autochthonous starter fermentation on bread nutritional and technological properties. Int J Food Sci Technol 57:4804–4815. https://doi.org/10.1111/ijfs.15661

Lattanzi A, Minervini F, Gobbetti M (2014) Assessment of comparative methods for storing type-I wheat sourdough. LWT Food Sci Technol 59(2):948–955. https://doi.org/10.1016/j.lwt.2014.06.032

Li C, Hu Y (2022) In vitro and animal models to predict the glycemic index value of carbohydrate-containing foods. Trends Food Sci Technol 120:16–24. https://doi.org/10.1016/j.tifs.2021.12.031

Lu J, Shan L, Xie Y et al (2018) Effect of fermentation on content, molecule weight distribution and viscosity of β-glucans in oat sourdough. Int J Food Sci Technol 54:62–67. https://doi.org/10.1111/ijfs.13902

Luo W, Sun DW, Zhu Z et al (2018) Improving freeze tolerance of yeast and dough properties for enhancing frozen dough quality – a review of effective methods. Trends Food Sci Technol 72:25–33. https://doi.org/10.1016/j.tifs.2017.11.017

Lynch KM, Coffey A, Arendt EK (2018) Exopolysaccharide producing lactic acid bacteria: their techno-functional role and potential application in gluten-free bread products. Food Res Int 110:52–61. https://doi.org/10.1016/j.foodres.2017.03.012

Ma S, Wang Z, Guo X et al (2021) Sourdough improves the quality of whole-wheat flour products: mechanisms and challenges—a review. Food Chem 360:130038. https://doi.org/10.1016/j.foodchem.2021.13003

Maidana SD, Finch S, Garro M et al (2020) Development of gluten-free breads started with chia and flaxseed sourdoughs fermented by selected lactic acid bacteria. LWT 125(8):109189. https://doi.org/10.1016/j.lwt.2020.109189

Mariotti M, Cappa C, Picozzi C et al (2017) Compressed yeast and type I gluten-free sourdough in gluten-free breadmaking. Food Bioprocess Technol 10(5):962–972. https://doi.org/10.1007/s11947-017-1861-z

Markowiak-Kopeć P, Śliżewska K (2020) The effect of probiotics on the production of short-chain fatty acids by human intestinal microbiome. Nutrients 12(4):1107. https://doi.org/10.3390/nu12041107

Marti A, Marengo M, Bonomi F et al (2017) Molecular features of fermented teff flour relate to its suitability for the production of enriched gluten-free bread. LWT Food Sci Technol 78:296–302. https://doi.org/10.1016/j.lwt.2016.12.042

Mulet-Cabero AI, Egger L, Portmann R et al (2020) A standardised semi-dynamic in vitro digestion method suitable for food – an international consensus. Food Funct 11(2):1702–1720. https://doi.org/10.1039/c9fo01293a

Mygdalia A, Nouska C, Hatzikamari M et al (2022) A sourdough process based on fermented chickpea extract as leavening and anti-staling agent for improving the quality of gluten-free breads. Food Res Int 159:111593. https://doi.org/10.1016/j.foodres.2022.111593

Nami Y, Gharekhani M, Aalami M et al (2019) Lactobacillus-fermented sourdoughs improve the quality of gluten-free bread made from pearl millet flour. J Food Sci Technol 56:4057–4067. https://doi.org/10.1007/s13197-019-03874-8

Nieto-Calvache J, Lorenzo G, Califano A et al (2022) Papaya dietary fiber concentrates for providing functionality to muffin formulations. J Sci Food Agric 103:1326–1333. https://doi.org/10.1002/jsfa.12226

Nionelli L, Rizzello CG (2016) Sourdough-based biotechnologies for the production of gluten-free foods. Foods 5(3):65. https://doi.org/10.3390/foods5030065

Nissen L, Samaei SP, Babini E et al (2020) Gluten free sourdough bread enriched with cricket flour for protein fortification: antioxidant improvement and Volatilome characterization. Food Chem 333:127410. https://doi.org/10.1016/j.foodchem.2020.127410

Nutte J, Saiz AI, Iurlina MO (2019) Microstructural and conformational changes of gluten proteins in wheat-rye sourdough. J Cereal Sci 87:91–97. https://doi.org/10.1016/j.jcs.2019.03.006

Ogunsakin OA, Banwo K, Ogunremi OR et al (2015) Microbiological and physicochemical properties of sourdough bread from sorghum flour. Int Food Res J 22(6):2610–2618. http://www.ifrj.upm.edu.my/22%20(06)%202015/(48).pdf

Ogunsakin AO, Vanajakshi V, Anu-Appaiah KA et al (2017) Evaluation of functionally important lactic acid bacteria and yeasts from Nigerian sorghum as starter cultures for gluten-free sourdough preparation. LWT Food Sci Technol 82:326–334. https://doi.org/10.1016/j.lwt.2017.04.048

Olojede AO, Sanni AI, Banwo K (2020) Rheological, textural and nutritional properties of gluten-free sourdough made with functionally important lactic acid bacteria and yeast from Nigerian sorghum. LWT 120:108875. https://doi.org/10.1016/j.lwt.2019.108875

Olojede AO, Sanni AI, Banwo K et al (2022) Improvement of texture, nutritional qualities, and consumers' perceptions of sorghum-based sourdough bread made with pediococcus pentosaceus and Weissella confusa strains. Fermentation 8(1):32. https://doi.org/10.3390/fermentation8010032

Ortiz C, Valenzuela R, Lucero AY (2017) Celiac disease, nonceliac gluten sensitivity and wheat allergy: comparison of 3 different diseases triggered by the same food. Rev Chil Pediatr 88(3):417–423. https://doi.org/10.4067/S0370-41062017000300017

Pétel C, Onno B, Prost C (2017) Sourdough volatile compounds and their contribution to bread: a review. Trends Food Sci Technol 59:105–123. https://doi.org/10.1016/j.tifs.2016.10.015

Picozzi C, Mariotti M, Cappa C et al (2016) Development of a Type I gluten-free sourdough. Lett Appl Microbiol 62(2):119–125. https://doi.org/10.1111/lam.12525

Poutanen K, Flander L, Katina K (2009) Sourdough and cereal fermentation in a nutritional perspective. Food Microbiol 26(7):693–699. https://doi.org/10.1016/j.fm.2009.07.011

Qian M, Liu D, Zhang X et al (2021) A review of active packaging in bakery products: applications and future trends. Trends Food Sci Technol 114:459–471. https://doi.org/10.1016/j.tifs.2021.06.009

Ramos L, Alonso-Hernando A, Martínez-Castro M et al (2021) Sourdough biotechnology applied to gluten-free baked goods: rescuing the tradition. Foods 10(7):1498. https://doi.org/10.3390/foods10071498

Reale A, Di Stasio L, Di Renzo T et al (2021) Bacteria do it better! Proteomics suggests the molecular basis for improved digestibility of sourdough products. Food Chem 359:129955. https://doi.org/10.1016/j.foodchem.2021.129955

Rinaldi M, Paciulli M, Caligiani A et al (2017) Sourdough fermentation and chestnut flour in gluten-free bread: a shelf-life evaluation. Food Chem 224:144–152. https://doi.org/10.1016/j.foodchem.2016.12.05

Rizzello CG, Lorusso A, Montemurro M et al (2016) Use of sourdough made with quinoa (Chenopodium quinoa) flour and autochthonous selected lactic acid bacteria for enhancing the nutritional, textural and sensory features of white bread. Food Microbiol 56:1–13. https://doi.org/10.1016/j.fm.2015.11.018

Rodríguez-España M, Figueroa-Hernández CY, Figueroa-Cárdenas JD et al (2022) Effects of germination and lactic acid fermentation on nutritional and rheological properties of sorghum: a graphical review. Curr Res Food Sci 5:807–812. https://doi.org/10.1016/j.crfs.2022.04.014

Roman L, Belorio M, Gomez M (2019) Gluten-free breads: the gap between research and commercial reality. Compr Rev Food Sci Food Saf 18:690–702. https://doi.org/10.1111/1541-4337.12437

Ronda F, Roos YH (2011) Staling of fresh and frozen gluten-free bread. J Cereal Sci 53(3):340–346. https://doi.org/10.1016/j.jcs.2011.02.004

Różyło R, Rudy S, Krzykowski A et al (2015a) Effect of adding fresh and freeze-dried buckwheat sourdough on gluten-free bread quality. Int J Food Sci Technol 50(2):313–322. https://doi.org/10.1111/ijfs.12622

Różyło R, Rudy S, Krzykowski A et al (2015b) Novel application of freeze-dried amaranth sourdough in gluten-free bread production. J Food Process Eng 38(2):135–143. https://doi.org/10.1111/jfpe.12152

Różyło R, Rudy S, Krzykowski A et al (2016) Gluten-free bread prepared with fresh and freeze-dried rice sourdough-texture and sensory evaluation. J Texture Stud 47(5):443–453. https://doi.org/10.1111/jtxs.12180

Rühmkorf C, Rübsam H, Becker T (2012) Effect of structurally different microbial homoexopolysaccharides on the quality of gluten-free bread. Eur Food Res Technol 235(1):139–146. https://doi.org/10.1007/s00217-012-1746-3

Sahagún M, Gómez M (2018) Assessing influence of protein source on characteristics of gluten-free breads optimising their hydration level. Food Bioprocess Technol 11(9):1686–1694. https://doi.org/10.1007/s11947-018-2135-0

Scherf KA, Wieser H, Koehler P (2018) Novel approaches for enzymatic gluten degradation to create high-quality gluten-free products. Food Res Int 110:62–72. https://doi.org/10.1016/j.foodres.2016.11.021

Schwab C, Mastrangelo M, Corsetti A et al (2008) Formation of oligosaccharides and polysaccharides by Lactobacillus reuteri LTH5448 and Weissella cibaria 10M in sorghum sourdoughs. Cereal Chem 85(5):679–684. https://doi.org/10.1094/CCHEM-85-5-0679

Shumoy H, Van Bockstaele F, Devecioglu D et al (2018) Effect of sourdough addition and storage time on in vitro starch digestibility and estimated glycemic index of tef bread. Food Chem 264:34–40. https://doi.org/10.1016/j.foodchem.2018.05.019

Starzyńska-Janiszewska A, Stodolak B (2011) Effect of inoculated lactic acid fermentation on antinutritional and antiradical properties of grass pea (Lathyrus sativus "Krab") flour. Pol J Food Nutr Sci 61(4):245–249. https://doi.org/10.2478/v10222-011-0027-3

Suo B, Chen X, Wang Y (2021) Recent research advances of lactic acid bacteria in sourdough: origin, diversity, and function. Curr Opin Food Sci 37:66–75. https://doi.org/10.1016/j.cofs.2020.09.007

Taraghikhah N, Ashtari S, Asri N et al (2020) An updated overview of spectrum of gluten-related disorders: clinical and diagnostic aspects. BMC Gastroenterol 20(1):258. https://doi.org/10.1186/s12876-020-01390-0

Tieking M, Gänzle MG (2005) Exopolysaccharides from cereal-associated lactobacilli. Trends Food Sci Technol 16(1–3):79–84. https://doi.org/10.1016/j.tifs.2004.02.015

Ua-Arak T, Jakob F, Vogel RF (2016) Characterization of growth and exopolysaccharide production of selected acetic acid bacteria in buckwheat sourdoughs. Int J Food Microbiol 23:103–112. https://doi.org/10.1016/j.ijfoodmicro.2016.04.009

Ua-Arak T, Jakob F, Vogel RF (2017) Influence of levan-producing acetic acid bacteria on buckwheat-sourdough breads. Food Microbiol 65:95–104. https://doi.org/10.1016/j.fm.2017.02.002

Udomkun P, Tirawattanawanich C, Ilukor J et al (2019) Promoting the use of locally produced crops in making cereal-legume-based composite flours: an assessment of nutrient, antinutrient, mineral molar ratios, and aflatoxin content. Food Chem 286:651–658. https://doi.org/10.1016/j.foodchem.2019.02.055

Van Kerrebroeck S, Bastos FC, Harth H et al (2016) A low pH does not determine the community dynamics of spontaneously developed backslopped liquid wheat sourdoughs but does influence their metabolite kinetics. Int J Food Microbiol 239:54–64. https://doi.org/10.1016/j.ijfoodmicro.2016.07

Van Kerrebroeck S, Maes D, De Vuyst L (2017) Sourdoughs as a function of their species diversity and process conditions, a meta-analysis. Trends Food Sci Technol 68:152–159. https://doi.org/10.1016/j.tifs.2017.08.016

Vermeulen N, Gänzle MG, Vogel RF (2007) Glutamine deamidation by cereal-associated lactic acid bacteria. J Appl Microbiol 103(4):1197–1205. https://doi.org/10.1111/j.1365-2672.2007.03333.x

Vici G, Belli L, Biondi M et al (2016) Gluten free diet and nutrient deficiencies: a review. Clin Nutr 35(6):1236–1241. https://doi.org/10.1016/j.clnu.2016.05.002

Vogelmann SA, Hertel C (2011) Impact of ecological factors on the stability of microbial associations in sourdough fermentation. Food Microbiol 28(3):583–589. https://doi.org/10.1016/j.fm.2010.11.010

Vogelmann SA, Seitter M, Singer U et al (2009) Adaptability of lactic acid bacteria and yeasts to sourdoughs prepared from cereals, pseudocereals and cassava and use of competitive strains as starters. Int J Food Microbiol 130(3):205–212. https://doi.org/10.1016/j.ijfoodmicro.2009.01.020

Wu S, Peng Y, Xi J et al (2022) Effect of sourdough fermented with corn oil and lactic acid bacteria on bread flavor. LWT 155:112935. https://doi.org/10.1016/j.lwt.2021.112935

Zand E, Bender D, D'Amico S (2018) Improving gluten-free buckwheat bread by sourdough fermentation and addition of arabinoxylan and pyranose 2-oxidase. Bodenkultur 69:227–237. https://doi.org/10.2478/boku-2018-0019

Zhou Y, Ouyang B, Duan M et al (2022) Biological characteristics of the gluten-free sourdough system fermented by Lactobacillus plantarum ST-III and its effect on dough quality and nutritional value during freezing. Food Chem X 14:100350. https://doi.org/10.1016/j.fochx.2022.100350

Chapter 6
Gluten Free Non-Fermented Bakery

Marina F. de Escalada Pla, Noelia E. Silva, Adriana P. Castellanos-Fuentes, Demian A. Molina, and Carolina E. Genevois

Abbreviations

AED	acoustic envelope detector
G′	storage or elastic modulus
G″	viscous or loss modulus
GF	gluten free
GF-NFB	gluten free – non fermented bakery
GI	glycaemic index
LA	leavening acid
LVR	linear viscoelastic range
MAP	modified atmosphere packaging
NFB	non fermented bakery
NV	neutralising values
ROR	rate of reaction
RS	resistance starch
SR	spread ratio

M. F. de Escalada Pla (✉) · N. E. Silva · A. P. Castellanos-Fuentes · D. A. Molina
Facultad de Ciencias Exactas y Naturales. Departamento de Industrias, Universidad de Buenos Aires, Buenos Aires, Argentina

CONICET – Universidad de Buenos Aires, Instituto de Tecnología de Alimentos y Procesos Químicos (ITAPROQ), Buenos Aires, Argentina
e-mail: marina@di.fcen.uba.ar

C. E. Genevois
Instituto de Ciencia y Tecnología de Alimentos Entre Ríos (ICTAER), CONICET-UNER, Entre Ríos, Argentina

Facultad de Bromatología, UNER. Gualeguaychú, Entre Ríos, Argentina
e-mail: carolina.genevois@uner.edu.ar

M. F. de Escalada Pla, C. E. Genevois (eds.), *Designing Gluten Free Bakery and Pasta Products*, https://doi.org/10.1007/978-3-031-28344-4_6

6.1 Introduction

Non-fermented bakery (NFB) comprises a width range of products which are characterised by extended shelf life when comparing with fermented bakery like bread or pizza. Depending on the formulation, shelf life, at room temperature, can vary from 1 week to several months. It can be possible due to the lower water content in the final products and/or the presence of food preservatives like sorbic, benzoic and propionic acids or their potassium salts, as it was stated in Chap. 4. While fresh bread presents moisture contents more than 75% (Genevois et al. 2021; Genevois and de Escalada Pla 2021), in cakes and muffins this value can range between 18–28% (Xu et al. 2020; Wilderjans et al. 2010) and can be even lower in cookies ≈ 8–15% (Nhouchi et al. 2018; Ostermann-Porcel et al. 2016). In NFB like biscuits, crackers, cookies, cakes and muffins, fat, sugar and, in some cases, eggs and milk were incorporated to the formulation, reducing water content of the mix. In general, dough or batters with more solid content, render products with lower moisture content.

Of course, the other difference between bread and NFB is the leavening process. Bread, usually achieve biologically by means of baker's yeast which produces the carbon dioxide (CO_2) gas, necessary for rising the characteristics alveolus. Instead, the spongy structure in muffins and cakes are produced by a chemical reaction in which baking soda (sodium bicarbonate) is neutralised by acid salts. In addition, physical processes can help to incorporate air into the batter by means of the mechanical mixing that contributes to the bubble formation.

According to the batter or dough consistency of NFB, as well as to the shape and the size of the final product, different baking alternatives and cooking times must be performed.

Therefore, the incorporation of more solids in the mix, different leavening as well as baking processes, produce bakery products with a reduced moisture content compared with bread.

In addition, the incorporation of other ingredients in batters of NFB, dilutes the flour compounds in the whole mixture. For this reason, in traditional wheat based NFB, soft wheat flour, or wheat flour with lower gluten content is preferred. It may lead to infer that GF-NFB formulation and processes could be easier to solve than GF bread, and it may be the reason because fewer revisions can be found in bibliography in this aspect. Nevertheless, there are some issues and challenges that remain without being solved in this field.

The aim of the chapter is to provide a review of the function of these ingredients in the formulation as well as the different process steps in order to aid understanding the main topics to focus when searching for new alternatives in this field. For this purpose, a review of the function of the ingredients that were not covered in the other chapters is presented in the first part. The different processes and characteristics for NFB products are described in a second part, ordering the information according to the water content in the formulation. On one hand, those with low moisture content, american biscuits, crackers and cookies are summarised; on the other hand, those with higher moisture content, spongy bakery: cakes and muffins are explained. A summarise of the main topics for cereal bars preparation is also included. Finally, the main aspects that should be in mind for future studies are shared with the reader in the conclusion part.

6.2 Function of Different Ingredients in NFB

The main ingredients in NFB are flour, lipids (fat or oil), sugar and when corresponding, water, eggs or alternative proteins, and baking powder or leavening agents. Additives as emulsifiers and or preservatives can also be added when required. Since specific chapters were dedicated to flours and additives (Chaps. 2, 3, 4 and 5), in this section the description is focused on the other ingredients.

6.2.1 Sugar and Fat Roles in a NFB Mixing

Sucrose contributes to the sweet taste but also acts as a bulking agent in the batter, helping in moisture retention and air entrapment rendering a fine crumb structure. Sucrose also promotes fat crystal aggregates, which enhances air entrapment in the batter as well as the stabilisation of air bubbles during baking. Sucrose contributes to crumb and crust colour formation; in addition, it helps to inhibit microbial spoilage. Starch gelatinization and protein denaturation temperatures raise during the baking process due to the sucrose presence, achieving the desired final crumb structure. In general, granulated sugar, because it is larger in crystal size, incorporates more air into a batter than confectioner's sugar with smaller particle size, which, in addition, can be dissolved quicker in the batter than granulated sugar (O'Sullivan 2017). Partially dissolved sugar can contribute to the liquid phase as dough viscosity during baking (Xu. et al. 2020). Reducing sugars modify the dough consistency and hardness, depending on the physical form in which these sugars are used. Syrups have a greater effect on dough rheology and on the final biscuit colour than those which are added in solid form. Generally, doughs made with syrups are more cohesive, adhesive and sticky (Fiszman et al. 2013).

Fats are used in bakery because they provide tenderness, flavour compounds, eating quality, and gluten structure reduction (Delicato et al. 2020). In high fat and sugar traditional bakery formulations, these ingredients interfere in gluten development due to the low water content during kneading. While, in cake batter, fat contributes with the incorporation of air, due to its emulsifying properties increasing the cake softness. The presence of fat contributes to the appearance, promotes lubricity of baked goods, and increases the feeling of satiety (O'Sullivan 2017). Fats are composed of high amounts of saturated fatty acids which take a solid form at room temperature whereas oils are composed of mainly unsaturated fatty acids which take a liquid form at room temperature. In the recent past hydrogenated vegetable oils, with their higher melting points were commonly used as shortening for biscuit manufacture, but this practice is in disused because of the inevitable presence of trans fats. Trans fat consumption has been related to an increased risk of coronary heart disease and therefore, restriction of these compounds is being applied by regulatory bodies around the world. Palm oil has a high melting point (36 °C) and has been used for replacing hydrogenated vegetable oils in current biscuit manufacture. It must be highlighted that from a nutritional point of view, polyunsaturated oils like rapeseed and sunflower oils are considered healthier than high saturated fat (O'Sullivan 2017).

6.2.2 *Other Ingredients. Eggs and Other Proteins Alternatives*

The role of whole egg in sweet bakery products consists in giving colour, flavour and functional properties, like emulsifying, foaming and gelation to contribute to the spongy structure of the crumb (Marcet et al. 2015). Regarding the muffin's quality, egg white protein increases the height and specific volume (Matos et al. 2014). At the same time, egg yolk allows bakery products to obtain an optimal crumb, increasing the batter volume and the sponginess of the final product (Kamat et al. 1973). In order to reduce cholesterol content, granular fraction of egg yolk was separated from plasmatic fraction and was tested in a GF muffin formulation by Marcet et al. 2015. This granular fraction was mainly constituted by proteins (64%) and lipids (31%) and had a low cholesterol content, maintaining good emulsifying properties. Nevertheless, Marcet et al. 2015 reported that the cooked muffin exhibited more hardness and some colour differences in comparison to the whole egg yolk recipe. Matos et al. 2014 studied different protein sources: soy protein isolate, pea protein isolate, egg white protein and casein, on rheological and quality properties of rice-based gluten free muffins and they concluded that in general, muffins with the best visual appearance were those containing egg white protein or casein. Plant protein and animal protein led to completely opposite effects on the texture of the cakes. While egg white and whey protein increased hardness, cohesiveness and springiness; pea and rice protein reduced the hardness and cohesiveness of the cakes (Sahagún et al. 2018). Plant protein reduces the density of cake batter and increases the bubble size due to the coalescence phenomena, whereas animal protein reduces the bubble size due to its intrinsic foaming properties (Sahagún et al. 2018). A more detailed explanation about these characteristics was presented in the Chap. 4 of this book.

6.2.3 *Chemical Leavening Agents*

Chemical leavening agents were developed as an alternative to yeast fermentation. At the beginning of the nineteenth century, there was a very short supply in grain and grain products. Yeast fermentation resulted in a carbohydrate reduction of up to

3%, therefore, the search of a chemical alternative to provide CO_2 bubbles, could be a possible solution for avoiding this carbohydrate lost. Justus von Liebig (1803–1873) was the first chemist to assay sodium bicarbonate, while Horsford and Liebig (1856) developed the idea and applied for the first patent in this field (Brose et al. 1996). Nowadays, chemical leavening is usually used for biscuits, cookies and spongy bakery while biologically leavening with baker's yeast continues to be that preferred for the bread production. The tendency in the news developments is focused on searching sodium salt substitutes in order to reduce sodium content in food formulation (van der Sman 2021). In NFB products HCO_3^-, is the carrier of carbon dioxide, CO_2, for providing crumb structure. The sequence of the reactions involved based on sodium and ammonium bicarbonate leavening are summarised below and the detailed thermodynamic properties can be deepened in the study reported by van der Sman (2021).

Where NH_2COO^- is the carbamate ion usually formed in NH_3-H_2O-CO_2 systems (Wang et al. 2011). Carbon dioxide releases from these salt carriers when dissolving in the liquid phase of the mixing and in the baking process about 60 °C. Sometimes this realising is not complete, producing undesirable taste in the bakery. For this reason, the basic salt is usually neutralised by an acid or acid salt leavening acids (LA). Then, it can be considered the baking powder as a mix of two salts: one is a CO_2 carrier and the other one, a neutralising salt (LA).

Simplifying, in general, $HCO_3^- + H^+ \rightarrow H_2O + CO_2$ can be considered and depending on the acid salts selected, neutralising value (NV), (Eq. 6.1) and the rate of reaction (ROR) are defined for practical purpose

$$NV = \frac{grams\,of\,CO_2\,carriers}{grams\,of\,leavening\,acids} \cdot 100 \tag{6.1}$$

The rate of reaction (ROR) is the amount of CO_2 (%) released from a defined amount of $NaHCO_3$ under standard conditions within the first 8 min through reaction with the relevant leavening acid (Brose et al. 1996). In Table 6.1, some examples of the most commercially available leavening options were summarised to provide a tool for selecting a convenient alternative. As it can be observed in the first three files, the carriers of CO_2, can be used without addition of LA. Nevertheless, as it was stated before, only few applications are found for this. In general, a mixture of both salts, CO_2 carrier and LA are used as baking powder.

6.3 Different Pastry Productions and Characteristics

Among the wide range of NFB products the study can be grouped in two main families: those with low moisture content, and those with higher moisture content. Therefore, after mixing the ingredients, it can be obtained from a hard dried dough to a low viscous batter. A general flow sheet is presented in Fig. 6.1 to provide a

Table 6.1 Examples of the most commercially available leavening options

Name	Common Name/E number	Function	NV	ROR	Reactions involved	Consideration and possible applications
Sodium bicarbonate	Baking Soda [E500]	CO_2 carrier	–	–	$2NaHCO_3 \rightarrow Na_2CO_3 + CO_2 + H_2O$	Considering low surplus LA: waffle batters.
Potassium Bicarbonate	[E501]	CO_2 carrier	–	–	$2KHCO_3 \rightarrow K_2CO_3 + CO_2 + H_2O$	Low sodium or sodium-free baked goods.
Ammonium Bicarbonate ABC	[E503]	CO_2 carrier	–	–	$(NH_4)_2CO_3 \rightarrow 2NH_3 + CO_2 + H_2O$ $NH_4HCO_3 \rightarrow NH_3 + CO_2 + H_2O$ $NH_4NH_2CO_2 \rightarrow 2NH_3 + CO_2$	Considering only heat realising without LA. Dry baked goods. Cookies and biscuits.
Acidic Potassium tartrate	Cream of Tartar [E336]	LA	45	65–67	$C_4H_5O_6K + NaHCO_3 \rightarrow C_4H_4O_6KNa + CO_2 + H_2O$	Very fast reaction. Cookies, angel food.
Sodium acid pyrophosphate	SAPP [E450]	LA	73	34–37[a]	$Na_2H_2P_2O_7 + 2NaHCO_3 \rightarrow Na_4P_2O_7 + 2CO_2 + 2H_2O$	Medium reaction. House-hold use. Baking mixtures. Cakes, doughnuts and muffins.
Monocalcium phosphate monohydrate	MCPM [E341]	LA	80	59–62	$3Ca(H_2PO_4)_2H_2O + 8NaHCO_3 \rightarrow Ca_3(PO_4)_2 + 4Na_2HPO_4 + 8CO_2 + 11H_2O$	Very fast reaction. Cookies, biscuits and crackers.
Anhydrous monocalcium phosphate coated form	AMPC [E341]	LA	83	57–59	$3Ca(H_2PO_4)_2 + 8NaHCO_3 \rightarrow Ca_3(PO_4)_2 + 4Na_2HPO_4 + 8CO_2 + 8H_2O$	Retarded at start, then fast reaction. Cookies, whipped batters.
Sodium aluminium phosphate acidic	SALP [E541]	LA	100	20–24	$2NaH_{14}Al_3(PO_4)_8.4H_2O + 23NaHCO_3 \rightarrow Na_5Al_6(PO_4)_6(OH)_5.12H_2O + 10Na_2HPO_4 + 14H_2O + 23CO_2$	Retarded reaction. Only permitted in sponge cakes EFSA (2018)

NV Neutralising Value, respect to $NaHCO_3$, according to Brose et al. (1996)
ROR Rate of reaction, according to Brose et al. (1996)
[a]According to the type and manufacturer

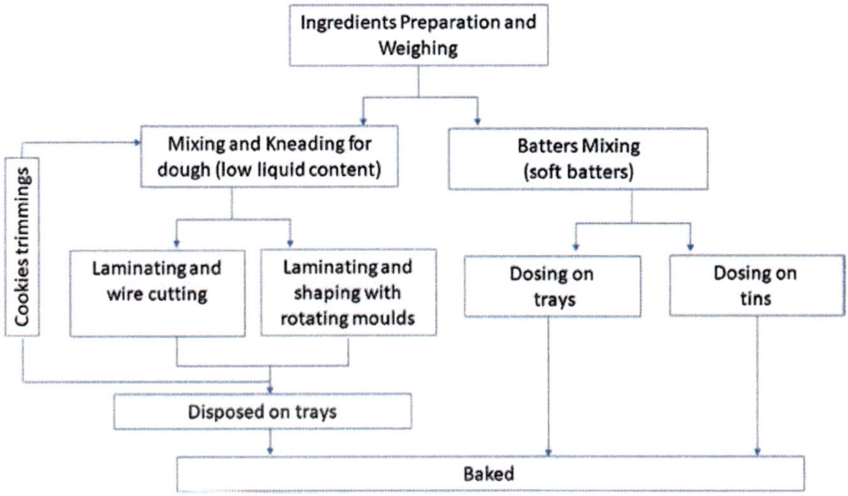

Fig. 6.1 Processes to produce different NFB products

scheme for showing the main differences and also the common unit operations. Characteristics of the products before and after being baked are described in this section.

6.3.1 Biscuits, Crackers and Cookies

"Biscuit" proceeds from latin word *Panis biscoctus* that referred to bread rusks developed during the Middle Ages to provide a very long shelf-life product that could sustain sailors on long sea voyages. At the beginning biscuits were made with flour and water, baked in an oven and dried in a cooler oven to produce a low moisture food product. Nowadays, sugar, fat and salt are added to the flour-water mix for obtaining a more appetising food (O'Sullivan 2017). Regarding cookies, they are widely consumed throughout the world representing one of the largest food categories. They are the complementary snack during a long day of work or study. Versatility, convenience, and attractive sensory attributes and the long shelf life are the most important reasons for the constant growing of the cookies market (Pestorić et al. 2017).

In this point it is worth to highlight that in the United Kingdom and Asia, biscuits are termed interchangeably with cookies (Xu et al. 2020), while in this chapter biscuit is related to American biscuit, small quick leavened dense bread.

6.3.1.1 Dough Characteristics and Process

As it can be observed in Fig. 6.1, biscuits and short dough cookies are submitted to kneading and laminating since the quantity of water in the formulation is low. The mixing time and the dough temperature could be optimised for obtaining adequate sheeting properties. Moreover, it will depend on the type and quantity of the fat/shortening added. Water molecules intervene in the conformational state of biopolymers, interfering with the interactions between the different components of the formulation and therefore, contributing to dough structuring. The limited water content used in biscuit dough, interferes with proteins hydration and aggregation as well as delays or prevents starch gelatinization/pasting during baking (Fiszman et al. 2013). After baking, interaction between the molecular chains of starch and its helical structure causes formation of starch crystals. The formation of starch crystals in the cookies would lead to the resistance of the cookies against enzyme hydrolysis, therefore, it increases the resistant starch (RS) fraction. In this sense, it was reported that a combine effect of low temperature and high baking time is more effective in increasing the RS of the GF cookies than a high temperature and low baking time (Olawoye et al. 2020). In these conditions, Olawoye et al. (2020) also reported lower glycaemic indexes. Therefore, these results have nutritional relevance. From technological point of view, limited water content coupled with the low baking temperature, gives a crisp texture in the final product (Baltsavias et al. 1999).

6.3.1.2 Characteristics of Final Product

The main properties to determine on biscuits, crackers and cookies can be classified in:

6.3.1.3 Physical Attributes

The baked dimensions are defined depending on the shape and size: thickness/diameter, or thickness/width/length; and they are measured with a calliper. From these values Spread Ratio (SR), can be calculated by dividing the width or diameter and thickness of cookies (Paesani et al. 2020). During baking the biscuit dough is transformed into a cellular solid. The CO_2 gases produced by baking powders and water evaporation expands early in baking. The degree of spread is controlled by the spread rate and the biscuit set time which, in turn, depend on the dough characteristics and the level of free water in the dough (Fiszman et al. 2013). SR also depend on baking temperature, since expansion increases with baking temperature, but too high oven temperature leads to early gelatinization of starch and protein coagulation impeding the spread of cookies (Nasser et al. 2021). When hydrocolloids are added in GF cookies formulation, dough consistency change and therefore SR is modified. Reduction in dough viscosity leads to higher SR (Hamdani et al. 2020). Another important indicator partially related to SR, is the puffiness, that is defined as the ratio of the difference of baked product size before and after baking to the thickness of cracker dough (Xu et al. 2020). Analogous, other authors preferer to measure the relative volume increase by comparing the volume of the baked product to the initial dough volume. In this sense, the apparent density of the product is also usually reported and can be estimated by dividing their mass determined by an analytical balance by their volume calculated from their dimensions. While the particle (solid) density of baked products can be determined by means of a helium stereopycnometer (Gondek et al. 2013). For all these determinations, the pieces have to be completely cooled before measurements.

6.3.1.4 Textural Properties

In general, a "three-point bending" test is used to characterise the texture of biscuit, crackers and cookies by means of a Texture analyser. For instance, with a texturometer (TA-XT2, StableMicro Systems, UK), it must be attached with a 3-point bending rig (HDP/M3PB). Maximum peak force required for breaking the pieces is recorded as hardness (Hamdani et al. 2020; Paesani et al. 2020). A penetration test can also be applied for texture characterisation, using a cylindrical probe. In this case, the deformation test is carried out up to 80% strain. From the force-deformation curve, the maximum force (N) and the area under the force-deformation curve (N mm), are recorded. Other parameters that have been used to describe crispness of products with a porous structure are the number of force peaks (drop in force higher than 0.8 N), average drop off (the average drop in force between consecutive peaks and troughs, N) and linear distance (the length of a line joining all points in the force-deformation curve). In addition, the sound generated by the deformed material can be registered by means of an Acoustic Envelope Detector AED (Stable Micro Systems Godalming, Surrey, UK) with a free-field microphone. The detector is mounted to the TA-HD plus texturometer and works under the Texture Exponent 32 software (Stable Micro Systems Godalming, Surrey, UK), which simultaneously registers the sound signal and changes of force during penetration (Gondek et al. 2013). The AED operates by integrating all the frequencies within the band pass range, generating a voltage proportional to the sound pressure level (Fiszman et al. 2013). The following characteristics are determined from the sound signal: number of AED sound peaks, total AE energy, number of AE events, and maximum of AED sound peaks. Each sound graph is simultaneously displayed with the corresponding force-deformation curves. In general, the mechanical characteristics correlated with acoustic parameters in crispy baked products like crackers and biscuits. In addition, the acoustic parameters of texture have demonstrated to be stronger correlated with the sensory perception of texture, compared to the mechanical parameters (Gondek et al. 2013).

6.3.2 *Spongy Bakery: Muffins and Cakes*

Muffins and cakes are among the products most highly appreciated by consumers of all age groups for their convenience, soft texture and taste (de Kock and Magano 2020; Xu et al. 2020; Rodríguez et al. 2022). Muffin is a popular breakfast or afternoon snack food, being incorporated by consumers in their eating habits, therefore they can serve as vehicles for important nutrients delivery (Alpaslan and Hayta 2006).

The matrix of muffins or cakes can be seen as a solid foam. Its characteristic aerated structure is achieved by incorporating bubbles into the batter that, during baking they become interconnected gas cells in the crumb of the final product (Fiszman et al. 2013). In fact, muffin and cake batters are a complex fat-in-water emulsions composed of an egg-sugar-water-fat homogenous mixture as the continuous phase and bubbles as the discontinuous phase in which flour particles are dispersed. Minute air bubbles are trapped in the batter by the surface-active egg proteins, fat, and/or a suitable emulsifier to form an emulsified foam that becomes a sponge after baking (O'Sullivan 2017). Therefore, a large number of small cells provides high volume baked goods if the continuous phase of the batter is capable of retaining these bubbles during the baking process (Matos et al. 2014).

Traditionally, muffins are made from wheat flour, oil/fat, egg, sugar, and milk. They are chemically leavened, rendering high volume pieces with moist spongy, and tender crumb, chewy texture, flat tops (Xu et al. 2020).

Cakes can be formulated without fat, with different sugar:flour ratio, and with whole egg or just white egg. According to the formulation, different cake categories are described in Fig. 6.2.

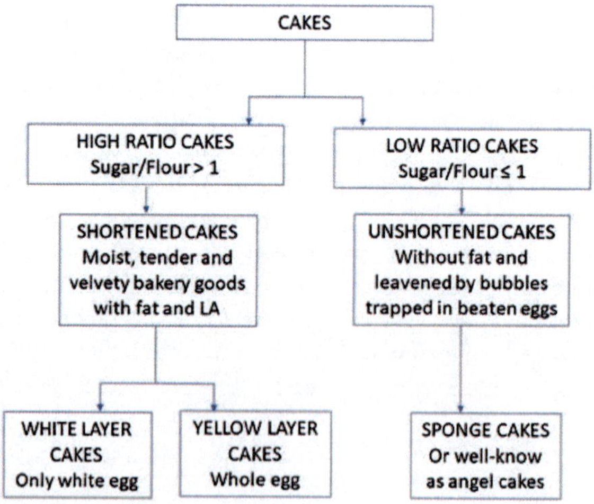

Fig. 6.2 Cake classification

6.3.2.1 Batter Characteristics and Process

The quality of cakes and muffins mainly depends on its crumb texture and final volume. The aeration begins during the mixing of ingredients when bubbles are incorporated into the batter. In the oven, while temperature increases the gelatinization of starch and denaturation of proteins occur. These effects provoke rising in the batter viscosity that aid to trap bubbles. At the end of the baking process, the combined effect of the gelled starch granules and the continuous network of coagulated egg proteins, result in a foam solid structure which is strong enough to be self-supporting when the cake or muffin is taken out of the oven. The starch is responsible for transforming a liquid, flowing batter into a solid, porous structure. The starch granules swell binding the excess water in the system and form the 'building bricks' for the final crumb structure (Donovan 1977).

Baking consists of a transfer of heat by conduction from the mould to the product and by radiation and convection from the oven and the air surrounding the surface of the baked goods. The temperature profile into the cold batter depends on the differences in temperature in the surface and the centre of the product. Simultaneously, a transfer of moisture and loss of water from the product happens during baking. Therefore, both temperature and concentration gradient are responsible, in part, for the development of the final crumb structure and, consequently, for its texture. On the other hand, the generation of carbon dioxide (from the baking powders) also contributes to the crumb structure. The small air bubbles that are incorporated into the batter during the mixing step act as nuclei and grow in size due to the CO_2 and water vapour and the normal process of gas diffusion through the product during baking. This aerated system is thermodynamically unstable since the bubbles tend to escape from batter due to their lower density. Therefore, the number of bubbles into the batter depends not only on the mixing stage, but also on the viscosity of the batter and on how efficient it is for retaining the bubbles. Some ingredients may act as emulsifiers stabilising the bubbles in the batters (Fiszman et al. 2013). The presence of dietary fibre (cellulose and hemicellulose) can strengthen the batter network during baking, preventing them from collapsing (Lau et al. 2022).

Heat transfer in oven is also a key step in the crumb structure setting. In the centre of the piece the temperature rises at first and then remains around 100 °C because the availability of water is high. It is normal for all the starch in this region to gelatinise. Small, evenly distributed crumb cells can be found in the centre rendering a fine final structure. The structure of the top zone is coarser because some starch granules in this zone are still gelatinising up to the final minutes of baking, so the gas cell walls are not rigid and continue to expand. In the bottom zone the temperature rises fastest and then, the water migrates rapidly to colder zones. In this zone, the availability of water falls in a short time and the starch gelatinises at the start of the baking process. The mean gas cell size is larger than in the rest of the product and the range of cell sizes is greater (Fiszman et al. 2013). When microwave baking is applied, the whole sample volume receives the heating energy at the same time instead of, from the outside to the inside, as in conventional heating. This rapid heat transfer increases the internal pressure and enhances mass transfer and the evaporation of water expanding the muffins. In addition, the crust formation in microwave baking is retarded due to the low surface temperature and the muffin can expand for a longer period (Megahey et al. 2005). Therefore, the use of microwave baking could be even more relevant for developing higher muffins, than other physicochemical characteristics related to batter formulation (Rodríguez et al. 2022).

The quality of batters is highly dependent on the air incorporated and retained, and mainly affects the crumb development and structure and the final volume of cakes and muffins. The batter density can be calculated by dividing the weight of the batter by the weight of an equal volume of water (Jyotsna et al. 2004). This density is reduced when air bubbles increase (Xu et al. 2020).

The batter viscosity is the other important property in muffin and cake baking. During baking, the velocity gradient in the batter induces convection current at a given moment that depends on its viscosity. Low batter viscosity resulting in more convection flow (Frye and Setser 1991). Retention of air and leavening gases depends on batters' density and also on batter viscosity (Bath et al. 1992). On one hand low-viscosity batters does not have enough capacity to retain the bubbles rendering low cake or muffins volumes. On the other hand, an excessive viscosity could impede the correct expansion of the batter, and consequently low volume would be obtained in the baked good. The batter viscosity is also relevant in the production process, since changes in viscosity could lead to problems in handling the batter, in mould filling (metering) and in cleaning the machinery, or to greater energy expenditure on pumping in the case of high-viscosity batters (Fiszman et al. 2013).

Batter is a non-Newtonian system, which means that its viscosity depends on their shear rate. For this reason, viscosity needs to be measured at different shear rates and a batter viscosity value should be reported along with the shear rate value at which it was measured. In general, share rate of 160 min^{-1} is selected, when Rapid Viscoelastic Analyser (RVA) at 30 °C is used (Paesani et al. 2021; Sahagún et al. 2018). Flow curves can also be recorded at different shear rates to observe the dependence of the shear stress with the shear rate. In general, muffin and cakes batters presented a pseudoplastic behaviour and, therefore, the recorded data can be fitted to the Ostwald de Waele model or power law model (Eq. 6.2) (Masoodi et al. 2002; Marcet et al. 2015).

$$\tau = k \cdot \dot{\gamma}^n \tag{6.2}$$

Where k is the consistency index and n, is the power law index. If n = 1, the system presents Newtonian behaviour and therefore consistency, k is equivalent to viscosity, μ. For cake batters n < 1 represents a pseudoplastic system (Marcet et al. 2015). Herschel–Bulkley model is another empirical equation that can define the rheological behaviour of batters. This model includes a term, τ_0, that represents the yield stress, or the minimum stress that should be applied before the sample starts to flow (Eq. 6.3).

$$\tau = \tau_0 + k \cdot \dot{\gamma}^n \tag{6.3}$$

Batter consistency changes when heating and also when starch granules begin to swell and gelatinase. Gluten free cereal blendings are being studied permanently for finding alternatives for new formulations. In this sense, the pasting assay is a useful tool for recording the viscosity changes when the hydrated flours were heated. The assay can be performed in the RVA or with a rheometer where viscosity can be recorded at constant shear rate and simultaneously the sample is heated, and temperature profile is registered (Genevois et al. 2021). From the pasting curves recorded, the following parameters can be determined: pasting temperature (°C), peak viscosity (cp), holding strength (cp), breakdown (cp), final viscosity (cp) and setback from trough (cp). Figure 6.3 shows how change the pasting curves when rice flour was replaced by rice bran. Pasting properties are considered an indicator of the processing quality that let understanding the batter behaviour helping to optimise the ingredient concentrations and temperature pressure-shear limits (Dang and Copeland 2004, Genevois et al. 2021).

Linear viscoelastic properties of muffin and cake batters and for biscuit dough are studied summiting the dough or batter sample to small amplitude oscillatory shear strain. In this level of strain, termed "linear viscoelasticity range" (LVR), the sample response is recorded without producing irreversible alteration of its structure. Sample response to different frequencies in the LVR, is called the mechanical spectra, where the storage or elastic modulus, G', and the viscous or loss modulus, G'' can be registered as a function of the frequency. G' represents the energy that the system stores temporarily and can later recover and G'' represents the energy that the system needs for starting to flow, which is irreversibly lost in the form of heat. The mechanical spectra are directly related to the molecular interactions and structure of the systems studied. Depending on the frequency- dependence of the elastic

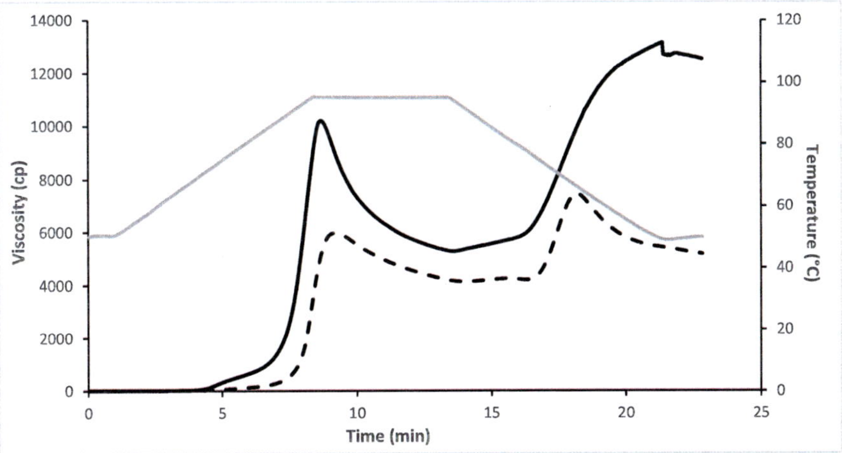

Fig. 6.3 Pasting curves obtained for: rice flour mixture containing 5% rice bran (continuous black line); rice flour mixture containing 20% rice bran (discontinuous black line); temperature profile (grey line) (Genevois et al. 2021)

modulus (G′) and the loss modulus (G″), three types of system can be described: macromolecular solutions (G″ < G′), where both parameters are highly frequency-dependent; weak gels (G′ <10 G″), both parameters are frequency-dependent; and strong gels (G′ >10 G″), where G′ is independent of the frequency (Fiszman et al. 2013). It must be considered that the small strain used in these tests do not simulate the real mixing, beating, or kneading, and baking processes, where the samples are submitted to larger deformations. However, these tests provide information on the structure of the sample in an unaltered state, which could be correlated to the behaviour of the sample when greater deformations are applied. Lower batter densities, due to higher air content, have been associated with higher viscosity and elastic component values, that in turn, have been related to higher bubble stability in the batter, rendering muffins with a greater height, volume and number of air bubbles (Fiszman et al. 2013; Nieto-Calvache et al. 2022). However, these relationships have not always been observed, which indicates that many other factors apart from the rheological properties of the batter contribute to appropriate baking performance (Sanz et al. 2008).

6.3.2.2 Characteristics of Final Product

Physical Attributes

The muffins are cooled at room temperature after removing from the mould and weighed. The muffin height is measured from the highest part of the muffin to the bottom part using a calliper. Muffin volume is determined by the rapeseed displacement method. The specific volume is calculated by dividing volume by weight (Genevois et al. 2021; Kaur and Kaur 2018; Rodriguez et al. 2022).

Regarding cakes characteristics, the weight is recorded after cooling and the volume can be determined by a laser sensor with a BVM-L 370 vol analyser (TexVol Instruments, Viken, Sweden). The cake specific volume is calculated as the ratio between cake volume and its weight (Paesani et al. 2021).

In both cases, muffins and cakes, weight loss is determined as the difference between the weight of the batter and the weight of the baked good obtained after baking, and in general, it is expressed as a percentage (Genevois et al. 2021).

6.3.2.3 Crumb Structure

The muffin or cake slices are scanned (1200 dpi), from the central zone eliminating the crust. The scanned field is converted to 8-bit binary image using the ImageJ software (Bethesda, Maryland, USA) and subsequently analysed. The following parameters are determined: number of alveolus, the size of alveolus as diameter of the equivalent area ($d_{3,2}$) (Eq. 6.4), cell density (alveoli/mm^2), the alveolar percentage on the total area were obtained from the software.

$$d_{3,2} = \frac{\sum ni * di^3}{\sum ni * di^2} \tag{6.4}$$

The ratio of small cells $(0.015 \le x < 2.000)$ mm^2 to large cells $(2.0 \le x < 10.0)$ mm^2 are also calculated as a measure of the crumb uniformity (Lau et al. 2022; Genevois and de Escalada Pla 2021).

6.3.2.4 Textural Properties

The instrumental texture measurement of the muffins and cake is carried out by means of Texture profile analysis (TPA), using a texture analyser (TAX Plus, Stable Micro System), or an Instron Universal testing machine. Crumb slices of ≈ 15 mm thickness and 36 mm diameter are compressed twice (the first and second "bite") up to 30–50%, of deformation, giving a curve (Fig. 6.4). From this curve, three primary textural parameters are obtained: hardness, as the maximum force recorded in the first compression cycle; springiness, as the height ratio recovered by the sample during the time between the end of the first compression and the beginning of the second one (dimensionless parameter) and cohesiveness, which represents the relationship between the area of positive force during the second compression and the area of positive force during the first compression (dimensionless parameter) (Lau et al. 2022; Irigoytia et al. 2022). In addition, the resilience and the chewiness are also interesting parameters to analyse. The resilience is the area during the withdrawal of the first compression divided by the area of the first compression (dimensionless parameter). This parameter is related to the crumb capacity to setback to the

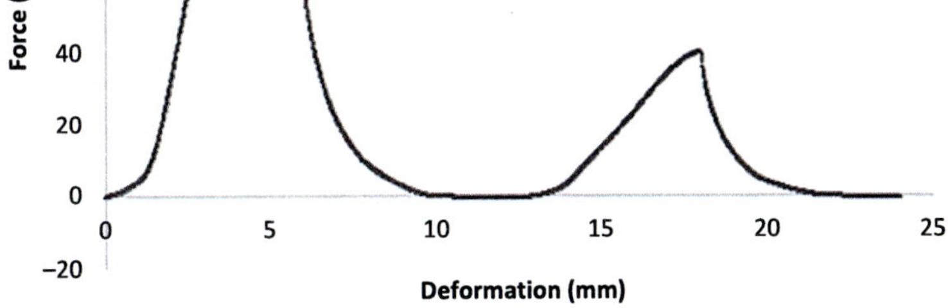

Fig. 6.4 Characteristic TPA profile for crumb of a baked goods from a rice blending (flour, coarse and rice bran)

initial height, and it is associated with the freshness of baked goods when touching them (Genevois and de Escalada Pla 2021). The chewiness is the result of the product: (hardness x springiness x cohesiveness). The product with higher chewiness should be kept in the mouth longer to achieve better wetting before swallowing (Nieto-Calvache et al. 2022).

6.3.3 Colour

Colour is an important quality parameter in NFB. During baking, Maillard and caramelisation reactions can occur giving from a browning colour to a caramel-like colour. During storage, the intensity of colour can also change due to oxidation and spoilage. In some cases, the colour changes cannot be perceived by human visual inspection. Instrumental techniques by means of colorimeters are strongly recommended for measuring food colour in industry and research institutes (Nhouchi et al. 2018; Fiszman et al. 2013).

In general, the results are expressed in accordance with the CIELAB system, where the parameters measured are L* [indicates lightness and ranges from 0 (for black) to 100 (for white)], a* [ranges from -a* (for greenness) to + a* (for redness)], and b* [ranges from -b* (for blueness) to +b* (for yellowness)]. From these parameters the following characteristics can be calculated:

- Hue angle: is the angle for a point calculated from a* and b* coordinates in the colour

$$\text{space} h = \arctan\left(\frac{b^*}{a^*}\right) \tag{6.5}$$

$$\text{Intensity of colour : Chroma : } Chr = \sqrt{\left(a^*\right)^2 + \left(b^*\right)^2} \tag{6.6}$$

The colour difference ΔE* between samples can be determined as:

$$\Delta E^* = \sqrt{\left(\Delta L^*\right)^2 + \left(\Delta a^*\right)^2 + \left(\Delta b^*\right)^2} \tag{6.7}$$

Where, $\Delta L^* = \left(L_1^* - L_2^*\right)^2 ; \Delta a^* = \left(a_1^* - a_2^*\right)^2 ; \Delta b^* = \left(b_1^* - b_2^*\right)^2$; and subscript 1 and 2 represents the values corresponding to the sample 1 and sample 2, respectively. According to Goswami et al. (2015), ΔE* > 3 are totally perceptible to human eyes. As for a 1 < ΔE* < 3, the colour difference could be perceived and ΔE* < 1, are not perceptible to human eyes. Crust and crumb colour in baked goods are mainly dependent on the ingredients of formulation and on the baking process. For instance, when dietary fibre is incorporated to the formula, colour changes could occur according to the fibre source (Irigoytia et al. 2022; Lau et al. 2022; Nieto-Calvache et al. 2022). On the other hand, the baking condition can mainly affect crust colour, due to the occurrence of Maillard reaction. This reaction occurs when proteins react with reducing sugars developing the characteristic brown colour as well as flavour (Michalska et al. 2008). The increase in temperature during baking causes the degradation of sugar that favours the occurrence of Maillard as well as caramelisation reactions (Nhouchi et al. 2018). Nevertheless, the water losses in the crumb are slower, delaying the progress of the Maillard reaction and, therefore, crumb is only slightly coloured (González-Mateo et al. 2009). When microwave baking is applied, the temperatures in the surface of the product and in the surrounding are low, and therefore the Maillard reaction is restricted. In these cases, microwave should be combined with infrared baking in order to develop the characteristic brown colour (Rodriguez et al. 2022).

6.3.4 Nutritional Aspects

Baked goods have been blamed for their high carbohydrates and fat content, that goes hand in hand with the problem of over-nutrition, the cardiovascular diseases, the obesity and the type-2 diabetes (Nhouchi et al. 2018). In addition, for formulating GF bakery, several raw materials selected (maize, pseudo-cereal, sorghum, etc.) belong to the classes of medium-to-high glycaemic index (GI) food. Starch is the main component in raw materials used in the formulation of GF food, it is digested and hydrolysed in the gastrointestinal tract, till glucose molecules. This glucose provides the energy needed to carry out daily activities in human beings. However, the rate at which glucose is released into the bloodstream is of concern in the management of some degenerating diseases (Olawoye et al. 2020). Therefore, some food research institutes and industries aim at finding replacers for fat and oil ingredients as well as lowering sugars or a combination of replacers for providing bakeries with optimal characteristics, easy to process without deteriorating their quality (Nhouchi et al. 2018).

Nevertheless, modifications to the quantities of fat used in conjunction with a concurrent lowering of sugar, will affect significant aspects of the products., e.g. dough rheology, texture of the baked product, distribution and migration on the flavour (O'Sullivan 2017). In this sense, strategies for reducing/replacing the fat type and/or the lipid content were reviewed by Nhouchi et al. 2018. Regarding sugar reduction, it must be considered its role in the cookie structure and texture development due to sugar recrystallization and amorphous glass formation when cookies are cooled down after baking. Some alternatives for calorie reduction options in cookie production are summarised by Xu et al. (2020). On the other hand, Olawoye et al. 2020 could demonstrate that GI could be regulated adjusting the temperature and the time of the baking process for cookies produced with cardaba banana flour, since resistance starch (RS) content increases according to these baking conditions. The slow digestive starch and the RS have been reported to have a low GI and to help in the prevention of metabolic disorder. RS belongs to the starch fraction that is not digested in the small intestine but fermented by the colon microorganism producing short-chain fatty acid and additional energy. Short-chain fatty acid as butyric acid is beneficial in the reduction of colon cancer. Hence, it has been suggested that starch-baked food high in slowly digestible starch and RS should be consumed for health benefits (Olawoye and Gbadamosi 2020).

On the other aspect, flour and starches can be replaced by legumes flours. Dry beans can easily be milled to flour, and contrary to cereal flours, they present higher proteins, fibre and mineral content. Therefore, it must be considered that additionally of improving nutritional profile of baked goods, changes in dough/batters properties as well as in the baked goods characteristics can be occur. Therefore, the incorporation of these flours should be optimised; for example, Schmelter et al. (2021) formulated cookies with *Vicia faba* beans flour and they reported an increasing in hardness and a dark colour of the cookies, as well as significant flavour and taste changes. Cappa et al. (2020) evaluated the baking performance of 25 kidney bean (*Phaseolus vulgaris* L.) varieties when mixing with corn starch in a ratio of 7:3. The authors reported a reduction in pasting properties as well as significant changes on hydration properties and on oil holding capacity.

In addition, the increasing importance of bakery products in today's eating habits means that these food products are being readily accepted by consumers and thus, they can serve as vehicles for important nutrients delivery (Kaur and Kaur 2018; Jnawali et al. 2016). Food products enriched with nutrients and biologically active compounds are often more expensive. On the other hand, fruit and vegetable by-products are very good sources of dietary fibre and phytochemicals and therefore, they may represent cheaper alternatives as additional sources of nutrients and functional ingredients (Drabińska et al. 2018). The studies for converting this by products in new food ingredients have been showed an increasing tendency (de Escalada Pla et al. 2007; Gupta et al. 2015; Nieto-Calvache et al. 2019, O'Shea et al. 2014, Ostermann-Porcel et al. 2017). In this sense the application of these food ingredients in bakery have been and are being widely studied (de Escalada Pla et al. 2013; Drabińska et al. 2018; Lau et al. 2022; Irigoytia et al. 2022, Nieto-Calvache et al. 2022).

6.3.5 Shelf Life and Commercial Aspects

Bakery market growth had been estimated about 1.5% yearly worldwide by Nashat and Abdullah (2016). More recently market estimations showed, a global market for cookies of around USD 30.6 billion in 2018 with an expecting growth of 5.3% each year for (2019–2025) period. While the global cake market is expected to grow by an annual rate of 3.3%, reaching USD 75 billion by 2023 (Xu et al. 2020). Regarding muffins market, it is expected to grow by USD 1.19 billion at an annual rate of 3% in 2021–2025 period, driven by for the growing demand for portioned snack, gluten-free and healthy bakery products (Rodríguez et al. 2022).

In the case of gluten-free products market (bakery goods, snacks ready-to-eat products, pizza and pasta, condiments, and dressing) it is increasing from USD

4.18 billion in 2017 to an expected USD 6.47 billion in 2023 (Xu et al. 2020). Bread and cookies are considered as the most globally consumed cereal-based gluten-free foods. The market of gluten-free bakery products is considerably growing since better diagnostic methods allow identifying an increasing number of people suffering coeliac disease and other gluten-related disorders. In addition, healthy consumers, family members and friends of coeliac patients, can also eat gluten-free products as a lifestyle. All these factors promote the gluten-free market and its continuing growth (Foschia et al. 2016).

Puerta et al. (2020) have gathered information from social networks such as Twitter to analyse the co-occurrence networks emerged from spontaneous and direct opinions of Spanish consumers about "gluten free" or "libre de gluten". This strategy allows exploration of topics concerning a certain group of consumers. Five categories of products were identified: bread, cake, cookie, beer, and pizza; and also, the context of consumption and purchasing. Tweets were posted to share eating or preparing food situations and to recommend in relation to brands, supermarkets and restaurants. The most frequent sub-themes were related to products (cake-pastry, bread, cookie and pizza-dough-patty), culinary preparations (recipe), places (city, bakery and restaurant), and product associated characteristics (brand). Therefore, the quality and the freshness of the final bakeries became a challenge for baker industries since they are decisive for satisfying consumers. The success for the attraction of consumers and satisfying them, are tightly related to the: (i) formulation; (ii) processing; and (iii) storage (Nhouchi, et al. 2018).

6.3.5.1 NFB Shelf Life

The sensory evaluation of changes occurring during NFB storage, is an essential measure for perceiving the quality loss. However, it is still an expensive and time-consuming tool to perform. Therefore, physicochemical parameters have a crucial role in measuring stability. They can be used either to predict the endpoint of NFB shelf life, or to confirm the results obtained by a sensory panel (Pestorić et al. 2017). The major critical points that should be controlled in bakery products during storage, are related to: (1) spoilage, (2) staling and (3) off-flavour development due to oxidative rancidity.

As higher water activity in the baked goods increases the risk of microbial spoilage, susceptibility to find deterioration can be consider in the following order: breads > cakes and muffins > other confectionary products. When all baked products leave the oven, their surfaces are sterile. The microbial contamination occurs during cooling (handling, slicing) (Cauvain 2011; O'Sullivan 2017). Occasionally, heat-resistant spores of the organism *Bacillus subtilis* contaminate the baker's flour, surviving the baking process and then germinating in the bread as it cools producing an unacceptable fruity odour and ropey crumb texture. Nevertheless, the main spoilage is generally related to mould that contaminates the surface of the pieces during cooling (O'Sullivan 2017). Of course, when it happens, the main steps to take are the implementation of a good manufacturing process that includes sanitising of equipment, tools, and the surrounding area. In the case of heat resistance spores, acidifying the dough with acetic acid could be necessary till to be sure that contamination could be controlled. Instead, surface contamination of baked goods can be controlled in the packaging step, for instance with modified atmosphere packaging (MAP). Active ethanol emitters, sachets containing 3 mL of alcohol gel, as well as ethanol spraying on sample surface (Hempel et al. 2013) have been reported as a good technique to extend shelf life in baked goods packed in low density polyethylene bags, since it delays the onset of inevitable mould growth (O'Sullivan 2017).

The staling is a complex physicochemical process occurring during storage of baked goods, being responsible for huge economic losses to the baking and retail sectors every year (Nhouchi et al. 2018; O'Sullivan 2017). The dynamic redistribution of water in the alveolar products produces multiple physical-chemical processes, independent of microbial spoilage, like the starch recrystallization, changes in the glass transition temperature and the decrease in the plasticity of the protein network (Monteau et al. 2017; Nhouchi et al. 2018).

Water migration affects the structural properties of cereal-based products during storage. In high or medium moisture content bakery products, like breads and cakes, moisture migration from the interior to the exterior of the product, produces firming of the crumb and a softening of the crust. From the consumer perspective, crumb firmness during staling is of greater concern than the softening of the crust. For this reason, traditionally, staling has been monitored recording crumb firmness during storage by means of compressibility methods (de Escalada Pla et al. 2013; Nhouchi et al. 2018; O'Sullivan 2017). Emulsifier additives as explained in Chap. 4 can be used in NFB for controlled staling, while in fermented bakery sourdough technology is also proposed as it was stated in Chap. 5. Instead, in biscuits and crackers, the moisture contents are so low that moisture migrates from the atmosphere into the product, rather than from product to atmosphere as with bread and cakes. Therefore, these products become soft when staling (Cauvain 2011, O'Sullivan 2017). Nevertheless, in cookies that are high in sugar and low moisture, sucrose recrystallization occurs because of this water migration producing the contrary effect in the first storage period while in long storage period (more than two months) the peak force decreased (Belcourt and Labuza 2007; Pestorić et al. 2017).

Because of the low water activity and high sugar content, biscuits and cookies have shown resistance to microbial spoilage. Nevertheless, oxidation issues can occur producing off-flavours that can be the limiting factor to shelf life in the absence of microbial spoilage and staling (O'Sullivan 2017). Non enzymatic browning reactions can also appear in some kinds of cookies depending on the sugar type, aw, temperature, pH. This colour development occurs largely during later stages of storage. Therefore, its measurement can be used to predict the completion of shelf life. In general, colour difference, ΔE, is calculated as it was explained previously, and is recorded during storage taking as reference the colour parameters (L^*, a^* and b^*) determined at time 0 of storage. For prolonged storage time, the colour differences can be appreciated by the human eye ($3 < \Delta E < 6$) or can be obvious $\Delta E > 6$ (Pestorić et al. 2017). As regards, lipid oxidation, it can be monitored by fluorescence spectroscopy coupled with chemometric tools (Botosoa et al. 2013; Nhouchi et al. 2018) and it can be controlled, in part, applying the correct MAP packaging with intelligent oxygen sensors (O'Sullivan 2017).

Empirical models for fitting to experimental data independent variables like different storage conditions, as well as dependent or response variables like physico-chemical properties of baked goods, can be a useful predictive stability tool and in the recent years has become a plentiful area for research (Pestorić et al. 2017).

6.4 Cereal Bars

Changes in the daily routine of a large part of the world's population have driven the growing demand of ready-to-eat convenience products (Popkin et al. 2020). In this context, cereal bars were introduced in the market nearly two decades ago. They are considered fast snacks containing a wide range of nutrients; which are available in small packaging; they are convenient to carry to be eaten anywhere and anytime (Ribeiro Rodrigues de Barros Vinhal et al. 2022; Samakradhamrongthai et al. 2021; Yadav and Bhatnagar 2015).

Cereal bars formulation comprises a wide range of alternatives to fit consumer's needs. From high energy cereal bars to light or diet options (Bizerra-Brito et al. 2013; Ribeiro Rodrigues de Barros Vinhal 2022; Samakradhamrongthai et al. 2021; Srebernich et al. 2016). In general, in regular cereal bars formulation, corn syrup and/or honey are used in different proportions (20–30%) as binding agent of a mixture where the main components are cereal and nuts (35–60%) with addition of minor ingredients (≈15%) of dried fruits (apples, pineapple, raisin, etc) and seeds (pumpkin seeds, sesame seeds, sunflower seeds, quinoa, etc.). Peanut butter or palm oil can be incorporated in certain cases; while for reducing sugar incorporation, concentrate apple juice, acacia gum, inulin, sorbitol has been also proposed (Puangjinda et al. 2016; Ribeiro Rodrigues de Barros Vinhal 2022; Samakradhamrongthai et al. 2021; Srebernich et al. 2016).

Basically, the process consists in mixing all the ingredients. According to the consistence heating may be necessary for improving the mixing step. In turn, the mixture is pressed in a mould, cooled, and depending on the formula it is also dried. Finally, bars are cut and packed. In general, the cereals to be incorporated in the formulation have been previously extruded to obtain puffing or popping grains (like puffed rice) or flakes (like corn or oat flakes), since there is not a baking step in the cereal bars process. Therefore, most of the reactions previously explained during baking in baked goods, can proceed during extrusion-cooking through different mechanism.

Extrusion-cooking is a green technology that provides a convenient, and efficient manufacturing process to obtained expanded snacks (Brennan et al. 2008). Unlike conventional hydrothermal cooking (such as dough baking), which occurs under mild processing conditions (high water content, long residence time and moderate temperatures), extrusion-cooking typically operates under severe processing conditions (low water content and high temperature) and short residence times. In addition to the thermal energy, extrusion-cooking also delivers mechanical energy to the material. Under these extreme processing conditions, biopolymers (starch, fibre, and proteins) transformation does not follow classic mechanisms such as gelatinization of starches and denaturation of proteins under moderate conditions. Instead, thermomechanical conversion of biopolymers involves more complex mechanisms rendering a cooked biopolymeric melt that contain gelatinized starch, denatured protein, amylose-lipid complexes and also dextrins (from starch dextrinization) and protein aggregations, which are products of the reactions of degradation that happen due to the severe processing conditions (Bouvier and Campanella 2014). In addition, other reactions that occur during extrusion, can enhance nutritional and organoleptic properties of the raw material. For instance, inactivation of anti-nutritional compounds, changes in bioactive compounds and/or their bioaccessibility, changes in antioxidant properties, increase of the RS content and of the *in vitro* protein digestibility, and the improvement of sensory attributes (Nadeesha Dilrukshi et al. 2022).

Considering the range of possibilities in extruded GF cereals along with the multiple combinations for formulating cereal bars, statistical design of experiments is recommended to study the main effects of different ingredients on the product characterisation and to find out the optimal conditions. A review of the application of these designs will be covered in the Chap. 8.

Regarding cereal bars, the main properties determined are water activity and moisture content, as well as textural and colour characteristics. Proximal composition determination is mandatory for nutritional/reglementary reasons. Bioactive compounds, and their change during processing are also reported when necessary. Certainly, the sensory assays are highly recommended (Agbaje et al. 2016; Puangjinda et al. 2016; Ribeiro Rodrigues de Barros Vinhal 2022; Samakradhamrongthai et al. 2021; Srebernich et al. 2016). Sensory aspect of GF products is deepened in the Chap. 9 of this book.

6.5 Conclusion

In contrast to FB like bread and pizza, in NFB several ingredients are incorporated and therefore, the lack of gluten in the food matrix could be in part, counter act with the components from the other added ingredients. Sugar, fat, eggs stabilise the mixing avoiding the bubbles to collapse in aerated NFB. In cookies and biscuits, these ingredients have effect on the colour, flavour and texture. Chemical leavening agents can be selected according to their NV and ROR in order to fit with the specific requirements of the formula. Regarding the process, mixing and baking are the critical steps for assuring batter or dough stability and therefore, the correct crumb development in the aerated NFB. The packaging step should be carefully adjusted for providing the expected prolonged shelf life. Contrary to baked goods, cereal bars are formulated with extruded raw material and therefore, it is not necessary the baking step, being the studies focused on the effect of the raw materials and the mix conditions. A revision of the measurements of the main physicochemical characteristics of NFB has been performed for providing a cheaper and less time-consuming alternative to confirm the sensory evaluation. Nutritional aspects as fat, sugar, and sodium reduction in the formula, as well as incorporation of nutrient and/or bioactive compounds have shown the tendency of the recent studies. Changes in the primary ingredients may provoke modifications on batter or dough consistency that in turn are related to the quality characteristics of the final product. Understanding the role of different components in the matrix of the systems as well as the function of the unit operations involved in the process, can help to select the conditions to study in future works.

Acknowledgments This work was supported by the National Agency of Scientific and Technical Research (PICT-2018-01019), CONICET, the Universidad de Buenos Aires (UBACYT-20020170100092BA), and the National University of Entre Rios (PID-UNER-9112). The authors want to acknowledge ACELA Entre Ríos (Asistencia al Celiaco de la Argentina), Gualeguaychú for their valuable participation and contribution in our projects.

References

Agbaje R, Hassan CZ, Norlelawati A et al (2016) Development and physico-chemical analysis of granola formulated with puffed glutinous rice and selected dried Sunnah foods. Int Food Res J 23(2):498–506

Alpaslan M, Hayta M (2006) The effects of flaxseed, soy and corn flours on the textural and sensory properties of a bakery product. J Food Qual 29:617–627. https://doi.org/10.1111/j.1745-4557.2006.00099.x

Baltsavias A, Jurgens A, Van Vliet T (1999) Fracture properties of short-dough biscuits: effect of composition. J Cereal Sci 29:235–244. https://doi.org/10.1006/jcrs.1999.0249

Bath D, Shelke K, Hoseney R (1992) Fat replacers in high-ratio layer cakes. Cereal Foods World 37(7):495–500

Belcourt L, Labuza T (2007) Effect of raffinose on sucrose recrystallization and textural changes in soft cookies. J Food Sci 72:65–71. https://doi.org/10.1111/j.1750-3841.2006.00218.x

Bizerra Brito AL, Rodrigues Brito L, Araújo Honorato F et al (2013) Classification of cereal bars using near infrared spectroscopy and linear discriminant analysis. Food Res Int 51:924–928. https://doi.org/10.1016/j.foodres.2013.02.014

Botosoa EP, Chèné C, Karoui R (2013) Use of front face fluorescence for monitoring lipid oxidation during ageing of cakes. Food Chem 141:1130–1139. https://doi.org/10.1016/j.foodchem.2013.03.059

Bouvier JM, Campanella OH (2014) Chapter 6. The generic extrusion process III: thermomechanical cooking and food product texturization. In: Bouvier J-M, Campanella OH, Edition F (eds) Extrusion processing technology: food and non-food biomaterials. Wiley, West Sussex, pp 242–306

Brennan MA, Merts I, Monro J et al (2008) Impact of guar gum and wheat bran on the physical and nutritional quality of extruded breakfast cereals. Starch/Staerke 60(5):248–256. https://doi.org/10.1002/star.200700698

Brose E, Becker G, Bouchain W (1996) Chemical leavening agents. Chemische Fabrik Budenhaim, Rudolf A. Oetker. Universitätsdruckerei und Verlag H. Scmidt Mainz, New York, pp 5–84

Cappa C, Kelly JD, Ng PKW (2020) Baking performance of 25 edible dry bean powders: correlation between cookie quality and rapid test indices. Food Chem 302:125338. https://doi.org/10.1016/j.foodchem.2019.125338

Cauvain SP (2011) Chapter 23 The stability and shelf life of bread and other bakery products. In: Kilcast (ed) Food and beverage stability and shelf life. Woodhead Publishing limited, Cambridge, pp 657–682. https://doi.org/10.1533/9780857092540.3.657

Dang JMC, Copeland L (2004) Genotype and environmental influenceson pasting properties of rice flour. Cereal Chem 81:486–489. https://doi.org/10.1094/CCHEM.2004.81.4.486

de Barros GLRR, Ribeiro Sanches M, Teixeira Barcia M et al (2022) Murici (Byrsonima verbascifolia): a high bioactive potential fruit for application in cereal bars. LWT Food Sci Technol 160:113279. https://doi.org/10.1016/j.lwt.2022.113279

de Escalada PM, Ponce N, Stortz C et al (2007) Composition and functional properties of enriched fiber products obtained from pumpkin (*Cucurbita moschata* Duchesne ex Poiret). LWT 40:1176–1185. https://doi.org/10.1016/j.lwt.2006.08.006

de Escalada PM, Rojas AM, Gerschenson L (2013) Effect of butternut (*Cucurbita Moschata* Duchesne ex Poiret) fibres on bread-making, quality and staling. Food Bioprocess Technol 6(3):828–838. https://doi.org/10.1007/s11947-011-0744-y

de Kock HL, Magano NN (2020) Sensory tools for the development of gluten-free bakery foods. J Cereal Sci 94:102990. https://doi.org/10.1016/j.jcs.2020.102990

Delicato C, Schouteten JJ, Dewettinck K et al (2020) Consumers' perception of bakery products with insect fat as partial butter replacement. Food Qual Prefer 79:103755. https://doi.org/10.1016/j.foodqual.2019.103755

Donovan JW (1977) A study of the baking process by differential scanning calorimetry. J Sci Food Agric 28:571–578. https://doi.org/10.1002/jsfa.2740280616

Drabińska N, Ciska E, Szmatowicz B et al (2018) Broccoli by-products improve the nutraceutical potential of gluten-free mini sponge cakes. Food Chem 267:170–177. https://doi.org/10.1016/j.foodchem.2017.08.119

EFSA Panel on Food Additives and Nutrient Sources added to Food (ANS) (2018) Re-evaluation of aluminium sulphates (E 520–523) and sodium aluminium phosphate (E 541) as food additives. EFSA J 16(7):e05372. https://doi.org/10.2903/j.efsa.2018.5372

Fiszman SM, Sanz T, Salvador A (2013) Chapter 13- instrumental assessment of the sensory quality of baked goods in D. In: Kilcast (ed) Instrumental assessment of food sensory quality, IATA-CSIC, Spain. Woodhead Publishing Limited, Sawston, pp 374–402. https://doi.org/10.1533/9780857098856.3.374

Foschia M, Horstmann S, Arendt EK et al (2016) Nutritional therapy – facing the gap between coeliac disease and gluten-free food. Int J Food Microbiol 239:113–124. https://doi.org/10.1016/j.ijfoodmicro.2016.06.014

Frye A, Setser C (1991) Optimising texture of reduced-calorie yellow layer cakes. Cereal Chem 69(3):338–343

Genevois C, de Escalada PM (2021) Soybean by-products and modified cassava starch for improving alveolar structure and quality characteristics of gluten-free bread. Eur Food Res Technol 247:1477–1488. https://doi.org/10.1007/s00217-021-03725-x

Genevois C, Grenóvero MS, de Escalada Pla M (2021) Use of different proportions of rice milling fractions as strategy for improving quality parameters and nutritional profile of gluten-free bread. J Food Sci Technol 58:3913–3923. https://doi.org/10.1007/s13197-020-04852-1

Gondek E, Jakubczyk E, Herremans E et al (2013) Acoustic, mechanical and microstructural properties of extruded crisp bread. J Cereal Sci 58:132–139. https://doi.org/10.1016/j.jcs.2013.03.010

González-Mateo S, González-San José ML, Muñiz P (2009) Presence of Maillard products in Spanish muffins and evaluation of colour and antioxidant potential. Food Chem Toxicol 47(11):2798–2805. https://doi.org/10.1016/j.fct.2009.08.015

Goswami D, Gupta RK, Mridula D et al (2015) Barnyard millet-based muffins: physical, textural and sensory properties. LWT Food Sci Technol 64:374–380. https://doi.org/10.1016/j.lwt.2015.05.060

Gupta P, Ray J, Aggarwal BK et al (2015) Food processing residue analysis and its functional components as related to human health: recent developments. Austin J Nutr Food Sci 3(3):1068

Hamdani AM, Wani IA, Bhat NA (2020) Gluten free cookies from rice-chickpea composite flour using exudate gums from acacia, apricot and karaya. Food Biosci 35:100541. https://doi.org/10.1016/j.fbio.2020.100541

Hempel A, O'Sullivan MG, Papkovsky D et al (2013) Use of smart packaging technologies for monitoring and extending the shelf-life quality of modified atmosphere packaged (MAP) bread: application of intelligent oxygen sensors and active ethanol emitters. Eur Food Res Technol 237:117–124. https://doi.org/10.1007/s00217-013-1968-z

Irigoytia MB, Irigoytia K, Sosa N et al (2022) Blueberry by-product as a novel food ingredient: physicochemical characterization and study of its application in a bakery product. J Sci Food Agric 102(11):4551–4560. https://doi.org/10.1002/jsfa.11812

Jnawali P, Kumar V, Tanwar B (2016) Celiac disease: overview and considerations for development of gluten-free foods. Food Sci Human Wellness 5:169–176. https://doi.org/10.1016/j.fshw.2016.09.003

Jyotsna R, Prabhasankar P, Indrani D et al (2004) Improvement of rheological and baking properties of cake batters with emulsifier gels. J Food Sci 69(1):16–19. https://doi.org/10.1111/j.1365-2621.2004.tb17880.x

Kamat VB, Lawrence GA, Hart CJ et al (1973) Contribution of egg yolk lipoproteins to cake structure. J Sci Food Agric 24:77–88. https://doi.org/10.1002/jsfa.2740240112

Kaur R, Kaur M (2018) Microstructural, physicochemical, antioxidant, textural and quality characteristics of wheat muffins as influenced by partial replacement with ground flaxseed. LWT Food Sci Technol 91:278–285. https://doi.org/10.1016/j.lwt.2018.01.059

Lau T, Clayton N, Harbourne J et al (2022) Sweet corn cob as a functional ingredient in bakery products. Food Chem X 13:100180. https://doi.org/10.1016/j.fochx.2021.100180

Marcet I, Paredes B, Díaz M (2015) Egg yolk granules as low-cholesterol replacer of whole egg yolk in the preparation of gluten-free muffins. LWT Food Sci Technol 62:613e619. https://doi.org/10.1016/j.lwt.2014.08.031

Masoodi F, Sharma B, Chauhan G (2002) Use of apple pomace as a source of dietary fiber in cakes. Plant Foods Hum Nutr 57:121–128. https://doi.org/10.1023/A:1015264032164

Matos M, Sanz T, Rosell CM (2014) Establishing the function of proteins on the rheological and quality properties of rice-based gluten free muffins. Food Hydrocoll 35:150e158. https://doi.org/10.1016/j.foodhyd.2013.05.007

Megahey EK, McMinn WAM, Magee TRA (2005) Experimental study of microwave baking of Madeira cake batter. Food Bioprod Process 83(4):277–287. https://doi.org/10.1205/fbp.05033

Michalska A, Amigo-Benavent M, Zielinski H et al (2008) Effect of bread making on formation of Maillard reaction products contributing to the overall antioxidant activity of rye bread. J Cereal Sci 48(1):123–132. https://doi.org/10.1016/j.jcs.2007.08.012

Monteau JY, Purlis E, Besbes E et al (2017) Water transfer in bread during staling: physical phenomena and modelling. J Food Eng 211:95–103. https://doi.org/10.1016/j.jfoodeng.2017.04.016

Nadeesha Dilrukshi HN, Torrico DD, Brennan MA et al (2022) Effects of extrusion processing on the bioactive constituents, in vitro digestibility, amino acid composition, and antioxidant potential of novel gluten-free extruded snacks fortified with cowpea and whey protein concentrate. Food Chem 389:133107. https://doi.org/10.1016/j.foodchem.2022.133107

Naseer B, Naik HR, Hussain SZ et al (2021) Effect of carboxymethyl cellulose and baking conditions on in-vitro starch digestibility and physico-textural characteristics of low glycemic index gluten-free rice cookies. LWT Food Sci Technol 141:110885. https://doi.org/10.1016/j.lwt.2021.110885

Nashat S, Abdullah MZ (2016) Chapter 21 quality evaluation of bakery products. In: Da-Wen S (ed) Computer vision technology for food quality evaluation, 2nd edn. Elsevier, Amsterdam, pp 525–589. https://doi.org/10.1016/B978-0-12-802232-0.00021-9

Nhouchi Z, Botosoa EP, Karoui R (2018) Critical assessment of formulation, processing and storage conditions on the quality of alveolar baked products determined by different analytical techniques: a review. Trends Food Sci Technol 81:159–171. https://doi.org/10.1016/j.tifs.2018.09.014

Nieto-Calvache J, de Escalada PM, Gerschenson L (2019) Dietary fiber concentrates produced from papaya by-products for agroindustrial waste valorization. Int J Food Sci Technol 54:1074–1080. https://doi.org/10.1111/ijfs.13962

Nieto-Calvache J, Lorenzo G, Califano A et al (2022) Papaya dietary fiber concentrates for providing functionality to muffin formulations. Jornal of the Science of Food and Agriculture 103(3):1326–1333. https://doi.org/10.1002/jsfa.12226

O'Shea N, Arendt E, Gallagher E (2014) State of art. In gluten-free research. J Food Sci 79(6):R1067–R1075. https://doi.org/10.1111/1750-3841.12479

Olawoye B, Gbadamosi S (2020) Sensory profiling and mapping of gluten-free cookies made from blends Cardaba banana flour and starch. J Food Process Preserv 44:e14643. https://doi.org/10.1111/jfpp.14643

Olawoye B, Gbadamosi SO, Otemuyiwa IO et al (2020) Gluten-free cookies with low glycemic index and glycemic load: optimization of the process variables via response surface methodology and artificial neural network. Heliyon 6:e05117. https://doi.org/10.1016/j.heliyon.2020.e05117

Ostermann-Porcel MV, Rinaldoni AN, Rodríguez Furlan LT et al (2016) Influence of the particle size and level of substitution of okara flour in the development of gluten-free cookies. Int J Res Advent Technol 4(8):82–92. https://doi.org/10.1155/2017/4071585

Ostermann-Porcel MV, Rinaldoni A, Rodriguez-Furlán L et al (2017) Quality assessment of dried okara as a source of production of gluten-free flour. J Sci Food Agric 97:2934–2941. https://doi.org/10.1002/jsfa.8131

O'Sullivan MG (2017) Chapter 14 – sensory properties of bakery and confectionary products. In: A handbook for sensory and consumer-driven new product development. Innovative technologies for the food and beverage industry, Woodhead Publishing series in food science, technology and nutrition. Woodhead Publishing, Duxford, pp 305–324. https://doi.org/10.1016/B978-0-08-100352-7.00014-2

Paesani C, Bravo-Núñez A, Gómez M (2020) Effect of extrusion of whole-grain maize flour on the characteristics of gluten-free cookies. LWT Food Sci Technol 132(2020):109931. https://doi.org/10.1016/j.lwt.2020.109931

Paesani C, Bravo-Núñez A, Gómez M (2021) Effect of stabilized wholegrain maize flours on the quality characteristics of gluten-free layer cakes. LWT Food Sci Technol 135:109959. https://doi.org/10.1016/j.lwt.2020.109959

Pestorić M, Sakač M, Pezo L et al (2017) Physicochemical characteristics as the markers in predicting the selflife of gluten-free cookies. J Cereal Sci 77:172e179–172e179. https://doi.org/10.1016/j.jcs.2017.08.013

Popkin BM, Corvalan C, Grummer-Strawn LM (2020) Dynamics of the double burden of malnutrition and the changing nutrition reality. Lancet 395:65–74. https://doi.org/10.1016/S0140-6736(19)32497-3

Puangjinda K, Matan N, Nisoa M (2016) Development of a snack bar containing popped rice (Khai Mod Rin) for pre-school children. Int Food Res J 23(1):237–242

Puerta P, Laguna L, Vidal L et al (2020) Co-occurrence networks of Twitter content after manual or automatic processing. A case-study on "gluten-free". Food Qual Prefer 86:103993. https://doi.org/10.1016/j.foodqual.2020.103993

Rodríguez R, Alvarez-Sabatel S, Ríos Y et al (2022) Effect of microwave technology and upcycled orange fibre on the quality of gluten-free muffins. LWT Food Sci Technol 158:113148. https://doi.org/10.1016/j.lwt.2022.113148

Sahagún M, Bravo-Núñez A, Báscones G et al (2018) Influence of protein source on the characteristics of gluten-free layer cakes. LWT Food Sci Technol 94:50–56. https://doi.org/10.1016/j.lwt.2018.04.014

Samakradhamrongthai RS, Jannu T, Renaldi G (2021) Physicochemical properties and sensory evaluation of high energy cereal bar and its consumer acceptability. Heliyon 7:e07776. https://doi.org/10.1016/j.heliyon.2021.e07776

Sanz T, Salvador A, Fiszman SM (2008) Evaluation of four types of resistant starch in muffin baking performance and relationship with batter rheology. Eur Food Res Technol 227:813–819. https://doi.org/10.1007/s00217-007-0791-9

Schmelter L, Rohm H, Struck S (2021) Gluten-free bakery products: cookies made from different Vicia faba bean varieties. Future Foods 4:100038. https://doi.org/10.1016/j.fufo.2021.100038

Srebernich SM, Gonçalves GMS, Ormenese RCSC et al (2016) Physico chemical, sensory and nutritional characteristics of cereal bars with addition of acacia gum, inulin, and sorbitol. Food Sci Technol 36(3):555–562. https://doi.org/10.1590/1678-457X.05416

Van der Sman RGM (2021) Thermodynamic description of the chemical leavening in biscuits. Curr Res Food Sci 4:191–199. https://doi.org/10.1016/j.crfs.2021.03.006

Wang X, Conway W, Fernandes D et al (2011) Kinetics of the reversible reaction of CO2 (aq) with ammonia in aqueous solution. J Phys Chem 115(24):6405–6412. https://doi.org/10.1021/jp108491a

Wilderjans E, Luyts A, Goesaert H et al (2010) A model approach to starch and protein functionality in a pound cake system. Food Chemistry 120(1):44–51. https://doi.org/10.1016/j.foodchem.2009.09.067

Xu J, Zhang Y, Wang W et al (2020) Advanced properties of gluten-free cookies, cakes, and crackers: a review. Trends Food Sci Technol 103:200–213. https://doi.org/10.1016/j.tifs.2020.07.017

Yadav L, Bhatnagar V (2015) Optimization of ingredients in cereal bar. J Food Sci Res 6(2):273–278. https://doi.org/10.15740/HAS/FSRJ/6.2/273-278

Chapter 7
Gluten Free Edible Films, Coatings and Toppings

Silvia Flores, María Alejandra García, Lía Gerschenson, María Gabriela Kupervaser, Carola Sosa, María Victoria Traffano-Schiffo, and Florencia Versino

Abbreviations

AFM	Atomic force microscopy
ASTM	American society for testing materials
Tg	Glass transition temperature
GF	Gluten free
HPMC	Hidroxyporpyl methylcellulose
LDPE	Low density polyethylene
MC	Methylcellulose
OPP	Oriented polypropylene
SEM	Scanning electron microscopy

S. Flores (✉) · L. Gerschenson
Universidad de Buenos Aires (UBA), Facultad de Ciencias Exactas y Naturales (FCEN), Departamento de Industrias, Ciudad Autónoma de Buenos Aires, Argentina

CONICET – Universidad de Buenos Aires, Instituto de Tecnología de Alimentos y Procesos Químicos (ITAPROQ), Ciudad Autónoma de Buenos Aires, Argentina
e-mail: sflores@di.fcen.uba.ar; lia@di.fcen.uba.ar

M. A. García · F. Versino
Centro de Investigación y Desarrollo en Criotecnología de Alimentos (CIDCA), Facultad de Ciencias Exactas, UNLP-CONICET-CICPBA, La Plata, Buenos Aires, Argentina
e-mail: magarcia@quimica.unlp.edu.ar; florencia.versino@ing.unlp.edu.ar

M. G. Kupervaser · C. Sosa
Grupo de Investigación en Biotecnología y Alimentos (BIOTEC), Universidad Tecnológica Nacional, Facultad Regional Resistencia, Resistencia, Chaco, Argentina
e-mail: g_kupervaser@ca.frre.utn.edu.ar; departamentoiq@frre.utn.edu.ar

M. V. Traffano-Schiffo
Instituto de Química Básica y Aplicada del Nordeste Argentino, IQUIBA-NEA, UNNE-CONICET, Corrientes, Argentina
e-mail: m.traffanoschiffo@conicet.gov.ar

M. F. de Escalada Pla, C. E. Genevois (eds.), *Designing Gluten Free Bakery and Pasta Products*, https://doi.org/10.1007/978-3-031-28344-4_7

a_w Water activity
WVP Water vapour permeability

7.1 Introduction

The gluten intolerances have determined diet changes based on the elimination of ingredients that contain prolamins and glutenin from wheat, rye and barley being replaced, in part, for alternative grains and tubers that do not induce the disease, for instance, rice, corn, sorghum, and millet (Lebwohl and Green 2021). This has led to an important challenge for the food industry due to the need of developing formulation strategies, generally known as "gluten free" (GF) ones, that include the use of suitable additives linked to this dietary modification, while helping to produce safety and organoleptically adequate food products (Zoumpopoulou and Tsakalidou 2019). According to the Food and Drug Administration (U.S.A.), the GF food is defined as the food that does not contain gluten, or its presence should be lower than 20 ppm (McCabe 2010).

Bread and sweet baked goods (cakes, biscuits, doughnuts, etc.) are an essential constituent of the human daily diet, representing the most important basic food worldwide (Nils-Gerrit Wunsch 2020; Xu et al. 2020). There is a wide assortment of such products and, a possible classification is the one proposed by Smith et al. (2004) who grouped them as follow: unsweetened (bread, rolls, buns, crumpets, muffins, and bagels), sweet (pancakes, doughnuts, waffles, and cookies) and filled (fruit and meat pies, sausage rolls, pastries, sandwiches, cream cakes, pizza, and quiche) goods. In their formulation, these products include complex carbohydrates (mainly wheat flour), proteins, lipids, vitamins, and minerals (Soukoulis et al. 2014).

Another classification proposed is based on the water activity (a_w), one of the most important product properties affecting the physical and microbial deterioration of bakery products. Smith and Simpson (1995) classified bakery products as follow: (a) low moisture bakery products (cookies and crackers, $a_w < 0.6$) in which microbiological spoilage is not a problem, (b) intermediate moisture products (chocolate coated, doughnuts, Danish pastries, cream-filled cake, soft cookies, a_w 0.6–0.85) where osmophilic yeasts and moulds are the predominant spoilage microorganisms, and (c) high moisture products (bread, pita bread, fruit pies, carrot cake, cheesecake, pizza crust, pizza, $a_w > 0.85$ and generally 0.94–0.99), where almost all bacteria, yeasts, and moulds are capable of growth (Smith et al. 2004).

When no preservative additives are added, bread and bakery products are characterised by their limited shelf-life reaching a maximum of 3–5 days at room temperature. After this time, physical, chemical and microbiological changes are produced, resulting in the loss of freshness, texture, taste and microbial spoilage (growth of bacteria, yeast and mould) causing consumer's rejection (Melini and Melini 2018). Those alterations can cause not only economic losses, but also threaten human health. Therefore, to extend bread and bakery products shelf-life and to assure their quality and safety properties, preservation techniques such as the use of preservatives or adequate packaging materials and the application of innovative processing technologies are proposed (Mitelut et al. 2021; Qian et al. 2021).

Over time, one of the most conventional technique applied to extended freshness quality was the use of chemical additives as was previously detailed in Chap. 4. The bakery industry is looking for novel alternatives including the use of antioxidant and antimicrobial compounds obtained from natural sources, new packaging technologies, application of functional coatings, etc. (Klinmalai et al. 2021; Silva et al. 2021; Nallan Chakravartula et al. 2019a).

Traditionally, to select a suitable packaging material for bakery products, the most important properties usually sought are gases and water vapour barrier, UV barrier, thermal stability, mechanical resistance (Roy and Rhim 2020). The most used packaging materials to preserve bread are different types of paper, such as waxed paper or the glazed imitation parchment which is strong and has grease resistance. It is usually impregnated on both sides with paraffin wax containing low density polyethylene (LDPE) and other additives (Martins et al. 2021). One alternative is LDPE bags with a strip of adhesive tape at the end to be twisted and sealed. Cakes and pastry products, which are more susceptible to crushing damage, are usually packed in grease-resistant paperboard bags with transparent cellophane windows and wrap, such as cling film, plastic nests or aluminium foil base plates and double plastic film layers. For long shelf-life products (biscuits and other), cellulose films coated with LDPE are generally used (De Pilli 2020; Galić et al. 2009) or other multi-layered films such as aluminium-coated LDPE, oriented polypropylene (OPP) or acrylic-coated OPP films which represent more effective barriers to oxygen and water vapour. In the case of fresh baked stuff immediately consumed, it is commonly packaged in bags made of polyolefin film, such as LDPE or polypropylene bags, normally micro-perforated to allow moisture to escape and avoid leathery consistency of the crust (Pasqualone 2019).

Regarding packaging methods, the application of new technologies such as vacuum packaging, nitrogen flushing, modified atmosphere, functional or active packaging (with antimicrobial activity) reduce the growth of spoilage microorganisms, extending bakery products shelf-life (Qian et al. 2021).

It is important to highlight that the plastic derived from fossil hydrocarbons comprise 46% of global plastic waste generation, producing a huge impact to the environment, which often end up in landfill sites or oceans, causing a significant pollution due to the poor infrastructure, the lack of recycling options and to the long periods of time required for their degradation (Tiseo 2021; Geyer et al. 2017). Thus, there is a wide interest in the development of new materials for substituting plastic packaging by using renewable resources to reduce polluting residues.

In this framework, biodegradable packaging has emerged as an innovative and promising solution since they decompose after fulfilling their purpose (Chiralt et al. 2020; Tapia-Blácido et al. 2020). New biodegradable materials can be classified in chemically synthesised polymers made from natural or petroleum-based molecules (polylactic acid, polycaprolactone, polyvinyl alcohol, polyglycolic acid, polybutylene succinate, polybutylene adipate-co-terephthalate); directly extracted from biomass (biopolymers such as cellulose, starches, chitosan, alginate, gelatine, collagen, etc.) and biosynthesized via microbial fermentation (polyhydroxyalkanoates, bacterial cellulose) (Zhang et al. 2022; Kamarudin et al. 2022; Birania et al. 2022). These have been used to develop new eco-friendly and active systems that could be applied to protect or improve quality of GF bakery products. In the following sections of this chapter, a special description of biodegradable and edible matrices is performed.

7.2 Edible Films, Coatings and Toppings

7.2.1 Edible Films and Coatings

The named edible films can be defined as standalone materials disposed as thin layers based on eatable components (biopolymers, food additives, etc.) and are generally used in the production of wraps, pouches, bags, capsules and casings. On the contrary, coatings involve slurries that are directly applied (by deposition, adhesion and drying) on the food surface and are considered as an integral part of the food product. They are designed not to be removed from the food item. Usually, they can be classified according to their formulation or the application method used, as will be described in the methodology section. To obtain edible packaging the following main technique stages must be performed: achieving the solubilisation of the biopolymer in a suitable solvent to obtain the slurry (for films and coatings) or mixing solid materials if it is used a thermomechanical process (without solvent addition, for films), solvent evaporation when corresponding and film constitution and stabilisation. There are no differences in the material composition between coatings and films but they are mainly different in relation to their thickness (Aguirre-Joya et al. 2018).

Edible active packaging is an innovative solution due to its capability to carry preservatives compounds, which reduce the microorganism's growth and assure the safety and quality of foods extending their shelf-life (Jafarzadeh et al. 2020; Fang et al. 2017). Certain additives can be incorporated into the edible packaging formulation such as antimicrobials and antioxidants compounds (Qian et al. 2021; Dobrucka and Cierpiszewski 2014).

There are different methods to incorporate those compounds (Qian et al. 2021):

(a) Direct incorporation of preservatives (thermally stable) into the packaging materials produced by solvent casting or extrusion technology (co-extrusion, extrusion or injection moulding);
(b) Surface coating of packaging material with a film containing antimicrobial agents (essential oils derived from plants, such as cinnamon, clove, oregano, thyme, and lemon) entering the headspace through evaporation or migration to the food surface through diffusion (Mani-Lopez et al. 2018; Fang et al. 2017). This method illustrates an additional use of films;

(c) Sachet/pad of antimicrobial packaging (non-volatile or volatile) are designed to hold by adsorbing or embedding the antimicrobial agents to be released inside the package continuously (Ju et al. 2019; Otoni et al. 2016). This type of packaging presents some limitations such as, the risk of accidental ingestion and additional operational steps to place them in each package;
(d) Stimuli-responsive antimicrobial packaging, in which responsive nano-carriers can encapsulate active compounds materials and release them on demand when an external stimulus (light, temperature and pressure) is applied (Qian et al. 2021).

Regarding the materials, as structural material or film matrix, biopolymers are generally used. These might be: (a) hydrocolloids that includes proteins such as collagen, gelatine, mung bean protein, corn zein, whey protein, soy protein, casein and others (Chen et al. 2019); and polysaccharides such as starch, cellulose and its derivatives, pectin, chitosan, alginate, carrageenan, pullulan and gellan gum (Kouhi et al. 2020); (b) lipid-based materials (bee wax, paraffin wax, carnauba wax, polycthylene wax, candelilla wax, rice bran wax, ouricury wax and jojoba oil); and (c) blend of hydrocolloids and lipids (Jeya Jeevahan et al. 2020; Zhong et al. 2019).

Moreover, they have to be aligned with the consciousness growth on celiac disease and gluten intolerance, which represents one-third of the global food intolerance market, added to consumer's choice to follow a GF diet that has had an important impact in the growth of GF products in the last 10 years (Juhász et al. 2020). In this context, the use of ingredients that provide safety characteristics and additionally have favourable nutritional and mechanical profiles to be used as edible packaging materials has become a focus of interest (Vilpoux et al. 2019).

Other hydrocolloids are the most crucial ingredients in edible packaging for GF baking products such as hydroxypropyl methylcellulose (HPMC) and carboxymethylcellulose (CMC), present good barrier properties against oxygen and lipids in film formulation (Roman et al. 2018; Anton and Artfield 2008). Likewise, β-glucan, pectin, carrageenan, xanthan gum, guar gum, locust bean gum, tara gum or agarose are applied in commercially available GF products (Vidaurre Ruiz et al. 2019). CMC, chitosan, ε-poly-L-lysine are natural polymers that present desirable film-forming properties and also antimicrobial activity (Fang et al. 2017).

Regarding starch sources, wheat, rye, and barley are common cereals containing gluten. Besides, contamination of oats with wheat, rye or barley can occur during grain harvesting, transport, storage and processing (Xu et al. 2020). Previous research has been extensively focused on GF edible packaging made from various natural GF starches such as potato, sweet potato, cassava, rice, sorghum. Figure 7.1 summarises main materials used to formulate GF edible films and coatings.

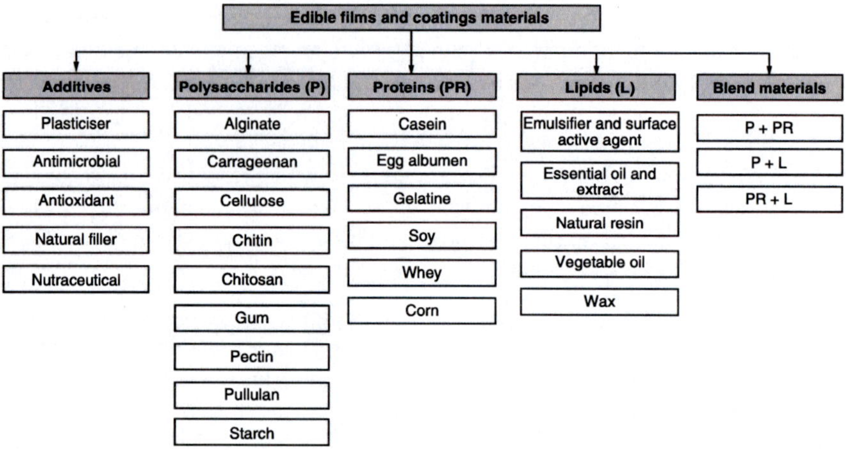

Fig. 7.1 Main materials used to formulate GF edible films and coatings

7.2.2 *Toppings*

To achieve a more attractive appearance and therefore a greater degree of acceptance by consumers, toppings are incorporated into bakery products. They create a decorative quality and provide additional flavour with the addition of small particles (chunky, crisp or chewy bits) contributing different textures, flavours and colours, widening the range of products considerably. Toppings are applied mainly for aesthetic and decorative reasons, however, in some cases they positively contribute by providing also desired technological effects, such as to promote the regulation of water activity at the surface of the product or reduce the risk of microbial growth. Additionally, the access of oxygen can be minimised, preventing the exposure to light and protecting the product mechanically. By combining these positive effects, it is possible to extend the shelf-life of bakery products (Tiefenbacher 2017).

Frequently, toppings consist of dry ingredients, such as seeds, grains, chopped nuts, cereal crisps, fruit pieces (candied or dried), chocolate chips or sprinkles, cocoa (nibs roasted and powder), cookie crumbles, puffed marshmallow, jelly bits, flavoured bits, cheese, herbs, seasonings (spices), toffee (milk caramel) or fudge bits, sugar (powder or crystals), or salt that are sprinkled superficially on the dough or in the final product. When those ingredients in small discrete pieces are added into filling creams, chocolate enrobing or bakery products are called inclusions (Tiefenbacher 2017).

Moreover, wet toppings or wet ingredients can be applied on bakery products by frosting (thick and opaque mixture) covering the surface and sometimes filling the inside of cakes. Some examples are icing, mixture of confectioners powdered sugar and liquid, thin enough to be brushed on with a pastry brush or spread on pastries, rolls, and simple cakes; glaze or enrobing. Other examples are a mixture of sugar and liquid thin enough to be poured – about the consistency of thin corn syrup to coat fruit cakes, cupcakes and pieces of cake; and fillings like a thick mixture which is used between the layers of cake. It may be some of the frosting to which nuts, marshmallows or fruits are added. Whipped cream and custard mixtures are sometimes used for fillings (Tiefenbacher 2017) and natural or untreated cocoa is often used in frostings, icings, and fudge (Ortiz 2016).

In bakery products like muffins, toppings can be as simple as a cinnamon/sugar blend or as complex as a nut streusel. Some toppings are also materials meant to 'sink in' to the muffin creating a 'filling' such as the addition of a sweet cream cheese mixture, creating changes in texture and flavour as the consumer eats the product. In bagels, toppings (seeds, finely chopped onion, or salt) are often coated on the top after boiling and before baking (Ortiz 2016). Table 7.1 shows different sources of ingredients used for bakery toppings.

Table 7.1 Raw and partially processed gluten and GF sources used for bakery toppings

Source	GF food matrix	May contain gluten trace	Gluten
Grains and alternatives	Amaranth, buckwheat, chestnut, corn (maize), millet, cornmeal, quinoa, rice, sago, sorghum, soya, tapioca, teff, uncontaminated oats		Barley, bulgur wheat, couscous, dinkel wheat, durum wheat, einkorn wheat, emmer wheat, Kamut, rye, semolina, spelt, triticale, barley, oats
Milk products, cheese and eggs	Cheese, eggs, and milk (liquid and dried) cream (single, double, whipping, clotted, soured), buttermilk, plain yoghourt	Some soft and spreadable cheeses, coffee and tea whiteners, fruit and flavoured yoghurts, and soya desserts	Yoghourt, or muesli with whole grains
Fruit, vegetables, nuts, seeds, and pulses	Fresh, frozen, canned, dried, baked, and boiled fruit and vegetables. Plain nuts, seeds, and pulses	Fruit pie fillings, processed vegetable products, deep-fried, microwave, and frozen chips, instant mash, potato waffles, roast potatoes. Roasted nuts and pulses in flavoured sauces (baked beans)	Fruit in batter and bread crumbs
Home baking	Arrowroot, artificial sweeteners, corn starch, cream of tartar, food colouring, gelatine, icing sugar, potato starch, ground almonds	Baking powder, cake decoration, marzipan, ready-to-use icing	Batter mixes, bread crumbs, stuffing mix
Confectionary, desserts, and savoury snacks	GF jelly, licorice root, seaside rock, homemade popcorn, plain rice cakes, and crackers	Chocolate, ice cream mousses, sweets, tapioca pudding. Flavoured popcorn, potato and vegetable crisps, flavoured rice cakes, and rice crackers	Made from wheat, rye, and barley, pretzels, wafers, licorice sweets, pudding made using semolina or wheat flour

Adapted from Jones et al. (2016)

7.3 Preparation and Characterization of Edible Films, Coatings and Toppings

Several technologies can be used to produce and study edible films, coatings and toppings. Differences arise basically from food type and form of application on the final product, the materials composition and properties requirements. For instance, edible coatings are usually directly applied on the food product surface, while edible film is separately produced and later used as packaging material. Various biopolymers such as polysaccharides, proteins, lipids and their composites are used in films and coatings formulations, most of which are GF, thus a wide spectrum of properties and processing conditions are possible and need to be studied and optimised regarding the final product requirements. Besides, aiming to further extend the food shelf-life span, many active films and coatings have been developed, most of which contain essential oils (EOs) and other antioxidant or flavonoids rich compounds. These are usually volatile or thermosensitive compounds which limit the film or coating preparation and application technologies.

7.3.1 Processing Technologies

Edible films can be manufactured by two techniques: a *wet route* based on a biopolymer solution (usually water based) with further solvent evaporation, known as *casting;* and a *dry route* in which polymers are processed in low moisture conditions with the presence of plasticisers and other additives (e.g., compression moulding or extrusion). The first is a batch process with some limitations, such as restricted product size and yield, long production times, high energy demand (for solvent evaporation) and large volumes of solvent (since solids do not exceed 10–12% of the suspension total mass). Therefore, it is mainly used at a laboratory scale, still extensively studied for surface coating characterisations. Besides, semi-continuous *tape-casting* and *spread-coating* techniques can also be used for large-scale manufacture of biodegradable and edible films (Oliveira de Moraes et al. 2013). In both techniques the film forming solution (or suspension) is spread over the laminated material to be coated (paper for example) or directly on a non-adherent carrier-tape. The film thickness is adjusted with micrometric screws that regulate the gap left by the spreading blade and depends strongly on the solution's rheological behaviour (Ortega et al. 2021). The suspension is later dried by heat conduction, circulation of hot air (heat convection) or infrared heating, resulting in a bi-layer material (spread-coating) or film that can be easily removed from the tape-carrier surface. Later on, and depending on the film characteristics, it can be rolled, cut, drilled, stamped or laminated. Various GF edible films obtained by casting have been studied as biodegradable or edible packaging for foods based on starches (Bertuzzi et al. 2007; Flores et al. 2007; Müller et al. 2008; Oliveira de Moraes et al. 2013; Pérez-Vergara et al. 2020; Mantovan et al. 2018; López and García 2012; Versino et al. 2016), pectins (Troung and Kobayashi 2020; Nallan Chakravartula et al. 2019b; Fishman et al. 2000; Sucheta et al. 2019; Gouveia et al. 2019), gelatine (Fakhouri et al. 2015; Musso et al. 2017; Wang et al. 2021), chitosan and other marine derived hydrocolloids (Senturk Parreidt et al. 2018a, b; López et al. 2015; Pranoto et al. 2005; Tan et al. 2020; Fu et al. 2021; Morales-Jiménez et al. 2020), soy, whey and pea proteins (Seung and Rhee 2004; Denavi et al. 2009; Nallan Chakravartula et al. 2019b; Seydim et al. 2020; Huntrakul et al. 2020; Sun et al. 2013), among others. Drying conditions are strongly dependent on the biopolymer and solvent used, temperature typically ranges from room temperature to 60 °C with drying times of 5 to over 48 h. In casting method films thickness can be adjusted by controlling the ratio of film suspension weight to plate area. Drying conditions (rate and temperature) determine film characteristics (e.g., water content, crystallinity, etc.), affecting its microstructure and properties (Bader and Göritz 1994)

Larger scale production technologies are needed to produce cost-effective, bio-based edible materials as food packaging. Thus, existing technology for synthetic materials are also used as continuous technologies like extrusion followed by blown, injection or thermo-compression (Mohammadi Nafchi et al. 2013; Flores et al. 2010; Garrido et al. 2016; Huntrakul et al. 2020; Fakhouri et al. 2013). Melt processing requires high temperatures and shear to disrupt the biopolymers' original structure, plasticising it. However, additives, such as plasticisers and antioxidants, are needed to thermally plasticise the polymer mix avoiding its degradation (Ortega et al. 2021).

Thermoplastic starch (TPS) based films are obtained by melt-mixing, though it is highly sensitive to moisture and present stickiness during processing (López et al. 2013b). Therefore, blending the starch with other polymers improves film formability, and mechanical, barrier and thermal properties as has been extensively reported in literature (Dang and Yoksan 2015; Pelissari et al. 2012; Fakhouri et al. 2013; Huntrakul et al. 2020; Ochoa-Yepes et al. 2019; Jebalia et al. 2019; Ferreira et al. 2021; Fishman et al. 2000; Flores et al. 2010). Extrusion can be single, twin or multiple screwed co-rotating or counter rotating (i.e., screws rotate in the same or opposite directions respect to the feed and product flow) or a mixture of both in the case of a multiple screw extruder. Temperature profiles through the extruder are important parameters for polymer processing that facilitate commercial processability and condition the materials properties.

The selected film processing technology influences the film formation mechanism and therefore the resulting physical properties of the material. Casting creates films stabilised largely by non-covalent interactions (hydrogen bonds, hydrophobic and electrostatic interactions) while extrusion and compression moulding may induce covalent interactions among the matrix compounds. Some investigation comparing these technologies indicate that extruded materials result in greater toughness and stiffness while casting films are more flexible, especially when cross linkage was evidenced in thermoformed or extruded materials (Ciannamea et al. 2014; Versino et al. 2016; Ochoa-Yepes et al. 2019).

Active packaging technologies offer new or extra functions such as gases scavengers (O_2, CO_2, and ethylene), moisture regulation, flavours emission control and preservation, microorganism growth prevention, among others, that are aimed to extend the shelf-life of foods maintaining their nutritional quality and safety

(Kechichian et al. 2010; Jamróz and Pavel 2020; Remya et al. 2017). Active films are usually prepared with the same methods previously described, though alternatives for protection and migration control are usually needed when EOs are used. Encapsulation and electrospinning have been reported as successful methods to preserve and modulate the EOs antimicrobial or antioxidant properties (Scaffaro et al. 2020; Varghese et al. 2020; Sharifi and Pirsa 2021; Atarés and Chiralt 2016). Moreover, Oriani et al. (2014) stated that a maximum of 0.1% of EOs into an edible coating minimises their sensory impact; encapsulation can also be used in this regard.

Edible coating can be applied on a food product by four different techniques: *dipping, spraying, fluidized-bed,* and *panning* (Senturk Parreidt et al. 2018a, b; Suhag et al. 2020). Its efficiency is strongly dependent on the selected application procedure, regarding the nature of food that should be coated, such as shape and size, their surface characteristics and the desired coating thickness and the coating material properties such as surface tension, density, and viscosity (Andrade et al. 2012). Dipping is the most widely used method to apply edible coatings on fresh products, particularly in ready to eat fruits and vegetables. In general, they are submerged for 5–30 s in the formulation of edible coatings which commonly can include antimicrobials and/or antioxidant to extend product's shelf-life (Suhag et al. 2020; Guerreiro et al. 2015; Senturk Parreidt et al. 2018a, b). It is a simple and low-cost technique commonly used at laboratory scale. The process consists of three steps: immersion, deposition, and evaporation of solvents (Andrade et al. 2012; Costa et al. 2014). Adhesion of the coating solution relies on the interaction with the food surface. For instance, smooth and uniform adhesion on hydrophobic rough surfaces can be very difficult due to the low surface free energy (Senturk Parreidt et al. 2018a, b). Meanwhile, when the coating affinity for the product surface is high, the time required will be minimal, allowing the coating solution to be applied spontaneously (Park and Seo 2011). Multilayer or layer-by-layer coating techniques are often needed in fresh cut products to achieve good adhesion on the highly hydrophilic surface. In this regard, Guerreiro et al. (2015) applied an edible coating to raspberries by first immersion into alginate or pectin coating solution followed by the immersion in a calcium chloride solution, allowing to form the typical egg-box gel due to the chemical gelation of the hydrocolloid in presence of a bivalent cation salt.

On the other hand, the spraying method is frequently used for industrial applications, in this technique the coating solution is distributed through the formation of droplets over the targeted food surface area with the help of nozzles (Suhag et al. 2020). One of the advantages of the spraying technique is that it needs less amount of coating material to effectively coat the surface product due to the high spraying pressure used (60–80 psi) (Andrade et al. 2012). Additionally, the thickness control as well as the possibility of multilayer applications are also valued characteristics. Spray-flow characteristics are dependent on liquid properties (density, viscosity and surface tension), operating conditions (mainly flow rate and air pressure), and system conditions (nozzle design, spray angle, etc.). Three types of spraying techniques have been used: (i) air spray atomization, where air is used for fine spraying of the droplet on food products; it is a cost effective method used on food products (Valdés et al. 2017), (ii) air assisted airless atomization, when high-viscosity and high-solids coatings formulations are used (Peretto et al. 2017), and (iii) pressure atomization, in this technique, the edible coating is applied to food products by passing it through small size nozzles (Andrade et al. 2012).

Likewise, edible coatings can serve as adhesive for decorative toppings, which are commonly included in bakery products (typically between 12% and 22% volume percentage of the total product) to enhance their attractive sensory characteristics (Tiefenbacher 2017). In this sense, small particulate inclusions or decorative toppings of different texture, flavour and colour can be used. Examples of currently used toppings in bakery products are chopped nuts, cereal crisps, candied fruit or toffee pieces, chocolate chips, cookie crumbles, flavoured bits, sugar or chocolate sprinkles, coarse sugar or spices. These are processed by conventional food processing technologies, such as air drying, extrusion cooking, melt mixing, etc. and are usually GF if cleaning protocols are carefully managed.

Recently, 3D printing of edible inks and pastes have been studied and commercialised, especially as food toppings. This technology expands the food processing alternatives for customizable nutrient content food products (Dankar et al. 2018). Current 3D food printing techniques include paste extrusion, ink-jet printing, powder binding deposition, sheet lamination, melt extrusion of chocolate, and bioprinting (Rowat et al. 2021).

7.3.2 *Characterisation*

The performance of edible films and coatings in extending food products shelf-life depends on the materials light, water vapour and gas permeability and their mechanical properties to resist transport and different ambient conditions. Coating integrity is a critical factor that depends on matrix flexibility, surface tension and adhesion to the food product. Besides, rheological characteristics and surface adherence are of particular importance for edible coating formulations, due to their direct impact on surface covering and durability. Similarly, controlled or slow-release kinetics determine its performance as active material and therefore its effectiveness on the product preservation. Finally, such properties need to be preserved by the film or coating until the food that it wraps is consumed or, in the worst case, disposed of. Consequently, all properties should be evaluated through time, ideally simulating the storage conditions and average time until consumption of the packed or coated food product.

7.3.2.1 Rheological Behaviour and Surface Properties

Rheological properties of film suspension should be tailored to fit the coating process: spraying requires low viscosity while higher viscosity is needed for immersion coating. The thin film formed on food surfaces depends on the viscosity of the coating solutions and can be well controlled with a specific spray-gun application

(Andrade et al. 2012; Suhag et al. 2020). This technology offers consistent coating with uniform thickness, and the possibility for multilayer applications (Martín-Belloso et al. 2009; Ustunol 2009). The highly viscous solution cannot be sprayed very easily on the food products so that only dipping methods can be adapted which results in the higher thickness of the coating material on the surface of food products (Andrade et al. 2012).

Likewise, considering the scale-up of the coating or film production the rheological behaviour of filmogenic solutions or suspensions is critical and conditions the processing operations involved, such as the pumping machine capacity. In general, starch-based filmogenic suspensions, which are widely used in coating formulations, exhibit a pseudoplastic behaviour while other formulations based on polysaccharides such as cellulose derivatives (like methylcellulose (MC) or HPMC) presented a Newtonian behaviour at low concentrations (1%).

On the other hand, coating formulation and mainly, its surface tension as well as food product characteristics determine the adhesion to food substrate and successful coating application. Products with smooth and soft surfaces (such as some vegetables like tomato) require formulations with low surface tensions to ensure coating adherence and uniformity. For products with irregular and rough surfaces (such as strawberries) the formulation must include plasticisers to prevent the appearance of cracks or pores in the coating. An alternative to enhance coating adhesion is the addition of surfactants and lipids to filmogenic suspensions, reducing their surface tension. The more similar the surface tensions of the product surface and that of the coating formulation, the greater the compatibility and the better the adhesion of the coating. Coating compatibility also is related to the hydrophilic-hydrophobic characteristic of both the surface and the formulation, which could be evaluated through contact angle measurements (Ramírez et al. 2012; Rossi et al. 2019).

Film or coating superficial appearance depends on their formulation, since matrices without plasticisers are brittle and rigid due to the strong interactions between the polymer chains that can also lead to aggregate formation. Besides, these structures are incompatible with irregular product surfaces leading to cracks and pores and conditioning coating integrity. The presence of these defects also limits barrier and mechanical properties of films and coatings. Plasticiser addition in the formulations can solve this problem by improving the coating flexibility (García et al. 1998; López et al. 2010). Likewise, the plasticiser/polymer ratio should be optimised since high plasticiser concentrations reduce barrier properties and may cause segregation from the matrix. In starch-based formulations glycerol or sorbitol are commonly used as plasticisers in concentrations between 5 and 50 g/L, depending on starch concentration (García et al. 2009; Versino et al. 2016).

7.3.2.2 Mechanical Properties

Uniaxial tensile tests are usually performed to assess the film's mechanical resistance. From these tests, strain-stress curves are obtained and the Elastic Young Modulus, maximum tensile strength and elongation at break are assessed. The mechanical properties depend on additives-matrix interactions that can also be strongly affected by physical, chemical, and environmental conditions, which influence the material stability and flexibility. Plasticisers are often needed to enhance the materials flexibility, especially in starch-based films and coatings (Versino et al. 2016). The addition of lipids, including essential oils has also been reported to increase extensibility of biopolymers-based materials (Bof et al. 2021; García et al. 2001; Jamróz and Pavel 2020).

On the other hand, dynamic mechanical analysis is a useful tool to study relaxation processes associated with glass transition temperatures (Tg). The Tg corresponds to the temperature at which tanδ and E" (loss moduli) curves presented a maximum peak while E' (storage moduli) curve shows an abrupt fall. It has been widely used especially in starch-based formulations. The knowledge of the Tg is crucial since it is strongly related to mechanical film properties and also, modifications on both film formulations and storage conditioning may affect Tg and consequently the mechanical resistance and flexibility of developed films. In this sense, the inclusion of plasticisers decreases the intermolecular forces between polymer chains and consequently reduces Tg values. Thus, being water the most ubiquitous plasticiser of hydrophilic films and coatings, film water content and relative humidity of storage should be carefully controlled and monitored.

7.3.2.3 Barrier Properties

Water and gas barrier properties are key for food products preservation. Gas permeability is usually tested on films or the coating standing by its own (also as a film). Water vapour permeability (WVP) is often determined gravimetrically according to American Society for Testing Materials (ASTM) standard test method, ASTM E96/E96M or a modification of this norm, thus various relative humidity conditions have been reported (Huntrakul et al. 2020; Nallan Chakravartula et al. 2019b; Musso et al. 2017; Ochoa-Yepes et al. 2019; Fakhouri et al. 2015). The WVP indicates the ability of the film or coating to protect the food from moisture migration from or towards the product. For instance, to prevent pastry from drying which would not be desirable for texture acceptance by the costumer or to prevent an increase in moisture content and water activity, which can promote mould growth and a faster degradation of the product. Unplasticised films often yield significantly higher WVP values than plasticised ones, due to the presence of pores and cracks (Versino et al. 2016). Even though plasticisers used in edible films and coatings are generally hydrophilic, its inclusion generates structural modifications on the biopolymer network leading to a less ordered and compact structure. In general, starch-based films exhibit lower WVP values compared to both protein films and other polysaccharide-based films (García et al. 2001, 2004; Versino and García 2014; Rivero et al. 2010; Tavassoli-Kafrani et al. 2016).

Considering that hydrocolloid-based films are very sensitive to relative humidity, physicochemical characterisation generally includes water sorption isotherms determination, useful for the estimation of film stability under different ambient conditions. In general, sorption isotherms are obtained, being experimental data satisfactorily fitted by GAB model, estimating the monolayer water content values (Mali et al. 2002; Müller et al. 2009).

Regarding film gas permeability most methods use the same principle: a measurement of the gas transmission rate through an edible film located between two compartments. One side of the film is exposed to the gas being studied, and a detector is placed in the other compartment, which is initially free of the permeated compound (Sánchez-Tamayo et al. 2020). These methods were developed for synthetic materials, described in the ASTM procedures, and adapted to edible films and coatings (ASTM D3985, F1927). The manometric and the volumetric methods measure the difference in absolute pressure, and the continuous-flow or isostatic method uses a stream flux of the gas to be measured on one side of the film and a nitrogen stream on the other side to carry the gas to the analyser. Coulometric sensors, infrared sensors, or gas chromatography may be used for gas concentrations analysis. In the case of O_2 permeability the use of specific equipment, the Mocon Oxtran 2/21, is widely used due to its precision and simplicity. Although for CO_2, N_2 and ethylene the determination requires the use of an especially designed cell and in general chromatography measurements. It is well known that polysaccharides films such as starch-based ones exhibit a highly selective gas permeability ratio (CO_2/O_2) compared with conventional synthetic materials. The modified atmosphere created by the coating generates a physical capture of CO_2 inside the fruit or vegetable and partial sealing of the pores, reducing the gas exchange and gas transfer rates; and this is monitored through respiration activity measurements. This selective gas permeability can be attributed to a higher solubility of CO_2 than O_2 in the film matrix. Development of composite edible films and coatings with selective gas permeability could be promising for controlling respiratory exchange and improving the conservation of food products.

7.3.2.4 Microstructure

The materials microstructure is generally studied by microscopy techniques, mainly scanning electron microscopy (SEM) or atomic force microscopy (AFM). Compact and homogeneous matrix of films is an indicator of structural integrity and, consequently, good mechanical properties are expected. To evaluate this, SEM observations of both the surface and the cross-sections are carried out. Figure 7.2 shows the microstructure of an edible coating based on HPMC applied on pumping vegetable tissue.

Topography and roughness of starch films surface can be evaluated by AFM. In the case of nanocomposite films transmission electron microscopy is also conducted to evaluate the nanometric size particles included in the matrices.

Interactions among film-formulation components as well as their compatibility are commonly studied by Fourier transform infrared spectroscopy, being this technique combined with chemometric analysis. In order to evaluate the crystallinity degree of edible films and coatings X-ray diffraction is commonly performed. Film crystallinity depends on the biopolymer source and plasticisers, film drying

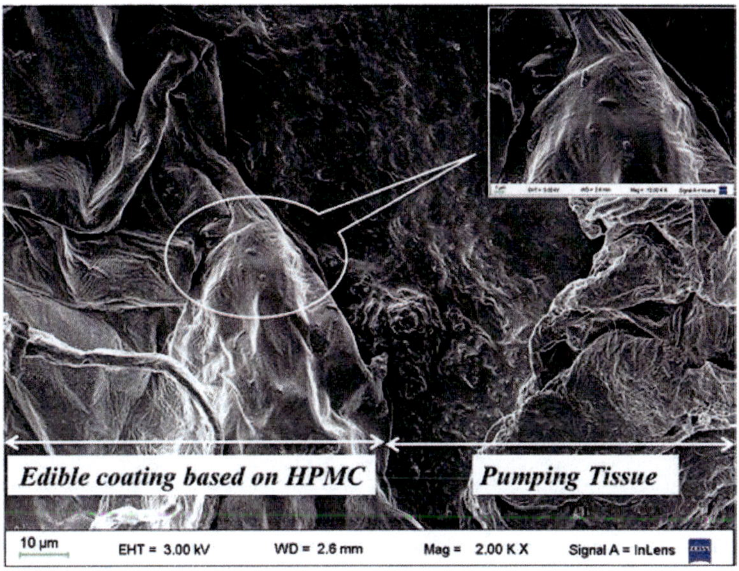

Fig. 7.2 Microstructure of an edible coating based on HPMC supporting *L. casei* cells and applied on pumping vegetable tissue

conditions and their final moisture content (García et al. 2009). Evolution of film matrix crystalline structure during storage can also be evaluated by differential scanning calorimetry, which allows to determine the Tg, being in this case the modulated technique more appropriate since it discriminates between the total heat flux, and the reversible and non-reversible contribution.

7.3.3 Characterisation After Application on Food or Simulated Food Systems

In the case of edible coatings and toppings a complete sensorial analysis is mandatory, showing that the coatings did not influence consumer acceptance, especially when taste is evaluated. In general, sensory panels are performed with both trained and untrained panellists on the basis of a hedonic scale. The selection of panellists includes men and women covering a wide age range to simulate the spectrum of potential consumers of the product being evaluated. In this sense, adhesion properties evaluation should be taken into account, especially for products destined for distant markets or long term storage, since it conditions the coatings' performance (Ncama et al. 2018).

Likewise, the microbiological tests should be conducted to assure the product safety. In this sense, the absence of microorganisms that cause foodborne illness as well as the counts of aerobic mesophilic and psychrophilic bacteria and mould and yeasts are commonly evaluated following standard procedures. This is of particular interest when active films and coatings are applied to extend food shelf-life. In this sense, López et al. (2013a, b) developed films based on blends of native and acetylated corn starches containing glycerol as plasticiser, potassium sorbate and citric acid as antimicrobial agents. The developed active starch films were able to inhibit *Candida spp., Penicillium spp., S. aureus and Salmonella spp.* growth, which are responsible for some foodborne diseases. These active films were effective to extend cheese shelf-life from 14 to 17 days at 4 °C. Besides, sorbate controlled release from the polymeric matrix was studied and diffusion coefficients in aqueous and semisolid media were also determined (López et al. 2013a). Rivero et al. (2013) also studied the controlled release of propionic acid from chitosan films to dough.

7.4 Application as Shelf-Life Improver and as Carriers of Bioactive Compounds, Vitamins or Minerals

Actual challenges faced by the food industry involve the extension of food shelf-life without impairing the nutritious properties of food products and through the use of sustainable techniques (Díaz-Montes and Castro-Muñoz 2021). The food products available in the market for celiac population, particularly bakery stuffs, might have reduced nutritional and organoleptic quality due to the necessary change in formulation. Such nutrient deficiencies promote an unbalanced diet for GF consumers, especially regarding fibre, bioactive compounds, vitamins and minerals (Capriles et al. 2016). As a consequence, important efforts have been focused in diversifying and improving the offer of GF items with better nutritional characteristics (Genevois et al. 2020).

With the purpose of contributing to the development of healthy foods with long shelf-life, many emergent technologies have been explored in the last years. As was previously mentioned, edible films and coatings are one of the hurdles that have been explored. They are produced using polysaccharides, proteins, and lipids, and besides, they can support antioxidants, antimicrobials, vitamins, probiotics, minerals, flavouring, and colouring agents. The use of antioxidants, antimicrobials and other nutraceuticals supported in these edibles layers allows to control their location, their release and the matrix also exerts a physical protection that slows down their destruction. As a consequence, films and coatings can help to improve shelf-life and/or food quality (Gerschenson et al. 2018; Alzate et al. 2021). In particular, in the case of considering the probability of consumer's gluten intolerances, the use of edibles films must be adapted to this restriction, ensuring the absence of harmful proteins in the formulation. In this case, alternative proteins, starches, rice by-products or different hydrocolloids like alginate that have algal origin, can be used for films and coatings production (Senturk Parreidt et al. 2018a, b). In addition, edible films and coatings can contribute to enhance the nutritional properties of foods through the support of vitamins, probiotics, and other compounds.

In the next items and Table 7.2, there will be described some matrices mainly based on polysaccharides that were developed in the last years and that can be used

Table 7.2 Different GF edible films and coatings used in bakery products

Application	GF matrix	Active agent	Bakery stuff	Main effects	Shelf-life (t, T)	References
Coating	Groundnut oil	N.I.	GF flatbread	Slowing of staling rate	8 days 2 °C	Patil et al. (2019)
Coating	Corn starch, MC, soybean oil, glycerol	N.I.	Crackers	Reduction of the hydration kinetic in a high a_w environment	20 days 25 °C	Bravin et al. (2006)
Coating	Egg protein, hydrocolloid component, vegetable oil	N.I.	Sweet baked goods	Reduction of water migration rate between components	85 days 25 °C	De Pilli (2020)
Coating	*Lepidium sativum* seed gum	N.I.	Sorghum GF bread	Improvement of crust and overall quality in comparison with normal glazes	N.R.	Sahraiyan et al. (2020)
Coating	Okra mucilage	N.I.	Soft dough biscuits	Improvement of the crispiness	6 days 25 °C	Senanayake et al. (2021)
Coating	Candelilla wax (in sunflower oil), beeswax (in sunflower oil), HPMC	N.I.	Bread	Reductions of bread weight loss and the crumb firmness	14 days 25 °C	Chen et al. (2021)
Coating	Pectin, alginate and whey protein	N.I.	Mini-buns	Reduction of moisture loss and textural changes	N.R.	Nallan Chakravartula et al. (2019c)
Coating	Sodium alginate, whey, glycerol	Lactic acid bacteria	Bread	Reduction of mesophilic and facultative aerobic bacteria count protection against mycelium fungi of genera *Aspergillus* and *Penicillium*	5 days 28 °C	Gregirchak et al. (2020)
Coating	Egg white protein	Carvacrol, thymol, *trans*-cinnamaldehyde	Bread	High antifungal efficacy of coatings supporting thymol and carvacrol nanocomplexes	7 days 25 °C	Deseta et al. (2021)
Coating	Cassava starch, inverted sugar, sucrose	Soluble coffee, cocoa powder or propolis extract	Muffins	High antimicrobial action against mould and yeast maintenance of the global quality	87 days 25 °C	de Oliveira Melo Naponucena et al. (2019)

(continued)

Table 7.2 (continued)

Application	GF matrix	Active agent	Bakery stuff	Main effects	Shelf-life (t, T)	References
Coating	Sodium alginate or blends sodium alginate and whey protein concentrate	*Lactobacillus rhamnosus* GG	Pan bread	Improvement of the viability of *L. rhamnosus* GG No modification of textural, flavour and thermophysical properties of crust	7 days 25 °C	Soukoulis et al. (2014)
Coating	Potato starch, inverted sugar, sucrose	Potassium sorbate and/or citric acid	Mini panettone	Inhibition of mould/yeast grown	48 days 35 °C	Ferreira Saraiva et al. (2016)
Coating	Sodium alginate, whey protein, glycerol	*L. brevis*	GF cookies	Improvement nutritional quality without modifying physical and sensorial properties	30 days 35 °C	Chávez et al. (2022)
Coating	Mung bean starch, guar gum, sunflower seed oil	Grapefruit seed extract	Non-glutinous rice flour cakes	Improvement stability by retarding starch retrogradation and inhibiting *B. cereus* and *P. citrinum* growth	N.R.	Lee et al. (2020)
Film	Starch-based (tapioca, potato, corn), cellulose nanofiber.	N.I.	Muffin	Good performance as a liner to hold the batter and protect the muffins from sticking to the pan during baking. Film could be consumed	N.R.	Shih and Zhao (2021)
Film	MC, polyethylene glycol	Clove bud or oregano essential oil (Tween 80 addition)	Bread slices	Reduction of yeasts and moulds counts	15 days 25 °C	Otoni et al. (2014)
Film	Cellulose-derivative polymer	Cinnamaldehyde	Pastry dough (P d) and bread (B)	Inhibition of aerobic mesophilic, yeast and mould growth.	P d: 30 days 8 °C. B: 12 days 23 °C	Lopes et al. (2013)
Film	Chitosan	Apricot kernel essential oil	Bread	Inhibition of fungal growth	10 days 25 °C	Priyadarshi et al. (2018)
Film and coating	Chitosan-carboxymethyl cellulose-oleic acid	Zinc oxide nanoparticles	Sliced bread	Reduction of fungal growth and retard the staling rate	35 days 25 °C	Noshirvani et al. (2017)

NI not incorporated, *NR* not reported

in the development of food products that need GF formulation. Many advances have been reported in relation to improve global quality of diverse traditional bakery products based on wheat using active edible films and coatings through the extension of microbial stability during storage (de Oliveira et al. 2019; Qian et al. 2021; Axel et al. 2017; Noshirvani et al. 2017), the maintenance of the crispiness and textural characteristic by reducing staling (Senanayake et al. 2021; Nallan Chakravartula et al. 2019c; Chen et al. 2021) and the increase of nutritional or functional properties, through probiotics or prebiotics incorporation (Zoghi et al. 2020; Fernándes et al. 2020). On the contrary, few studies were performed combining GF edible films or coatings on GF bakery products. Recently, Chavez et al. (2022) covered GF cookies with an edible coating based on sodium alginate (1% w/w), whey of milk protein (2% w/w) and glycerol (5% w/w) water solution supporting probiotics, *L. brevis* strain, improving functional value without affecting sensorial and physical properties. Another research (Lee et al. 2020), reported that cakes made with non-glutinous rice flour and coated with mung bean starch and guar gum slurry containing sunflower seed oil, decreased the hardness by 29% and the crystallisation rate by 24% compared with those of uncoated samples along storage at 25 °C. The authors concluded that edible coating retard the starch retrogradation in coated cakes. In the same study, the addition of 0.8% (w/w) grapefruit seed extract to coating exerted an effective antimicrobial activity against *B. cereus* and *P. citrinum* during rice cake storage. Similarly, Patil et al. (2019) demonstrated that staling rate was successfully retarded with the help of a groundnut oil coating on the surface of the GF flatbread during storage at 4 °C. Finally, Sahraiyan et al. (2020) analysed the effects of traditional glazes (oil, cheese powder, xanthan gum) on the physicochemical and sensory parameters of sorghum GF bread and were compared with *Lepidium sativum* seed gum coating. Results showed that application of novel glaze was better than the usual glazes to improve the crust and overall quality of GF bread.

7.4.1 Films and Coatings and WVP Control

Bravin et al. (2006) studied the development of emulsified edible films constituted by corn starch, MC and soybean oil. The techniques explored for deposition of the film forming solution were spreading or spraying. The presence of oil depressed the WVP. With this formulation, both techniques produced, in general, similar WVP. Atomization pressure of 2 bar and film thickness of 30 μm were identified as optimum for the application of edible coating to bakery products. Edible coating of previously described characteristics was applied for controlling moisture uptake in crackers submitted to RH of 65–85%. Crackers coated with this formulation showed a longer shelf-life due to the control of moisture transfer exerted by the film, confirming its potential for slowing the hydration rate in the RH range studied. In another study, Shih et al. (2011) developed edible films using various ratios of pullulan and rice wax up to 46.4% (w/w). Authors reported that water vapour barrier increased and hydration capacity decreased with a higher addition of rice wax helping to lengthen the shelf-life of food products. Several bio-polymeric matrices were analysed by Cando et al. (2017), who studied the production by casting technique of biodegradable films based on dispersions of a mix (50:50) of cassava, rice or potato starch and bovine gelatine. The total solid concentration of the dispersions was 2% (w/w) and glycerol was used as plasticiser. The films with cassava starch showed the lowest WVP. Nisar et al. (2018) developed antimicrobial films based on citrus pectin with the incorporation of different levels of clove bud essential oil. The inclusion of oil diminished the WVP and increased the deformability and heat stability of the films.

7.4.2 Films and Coatings. Weight Loss and Antimicrobial/Antioxidant Effect

Sadygova and Kozlov (2015) developed an edible foam for coating bakery products, with gram flour (5–15%), ashberry powder (5–10%), table salt (1–3%) and water up to 100%. The film was produced through drying at 55–65 °C for reducing the moisture content to 5–10%. This coating lengthens the shelf-life of bakery products helping to decrease microbiological count. Ferreira Saraiva et al. (2016) studied the application of edible coatings based on potato starch (46 g/kg), inverted sugar (14 g/kg) and sucrose (7 g/kg), with the purpose of reducing the preservatives added to mini panettones. The preservatives added to coating formulations were potassium sorbate (1 g/kg), citric acid (10 g/kg) and both additives (1 g/kg sorbate and 10 g/kg citric acid or 0.5 g/kg sorbate and 5 g/kg citric acid). Panettones without coating and additives showed the growth of mould and yeasts after 24 days of storage. On the contrary, the presence of films with both additives showed fungal growth only after 40 days. The authors concluded that the use as coatings of films with additives in concentrations lower than those normally used for these foods, increased their shelf-life.

Regarding active films added with natural preservatives, Nisar et al. (2018) showed that antimicrobial films based on citrus pectin with the incorporation of different levels of clove bud essential oil were effective against *S. aureus*, *E. coli and L. monocytogenes* when evaluated through the diffusion tests, showing a diameter increase from 18.50 to 30.27 mm, 12.53 to 21.20 mm and 14.67 to 26.43 mm, respectively, with the increase of oil concentration from 0.5% to 1.5%. The most sensible bacteria was *S. aureus*. According to Alzate et al. (2017) the addition of carvacrol, the main component of the oregano essential oil, to edible film formulation based on cassava starch and HPMC, highly improved the antimicrobial barrier action against *Z. bailii*, *L. plantarum*, and *P. fluorescens* in comparison with films containing only potassium sorbate. Recently, Mahcene et al. (2020) studied the use of sodium alginate to constitute films incorporated with essential oils of some medicinal plants (*R. officinalis* L, *A. herba alba Asso*, *O. basilicum* L and *M.*

pulegium L). The films showed a strong antibacterial effect against *Staphylococcus aureus* (ATCC 43300), *Escherichia coli* (ATCC 25922), *Salmonella enterica* (ATCC 14028), *Enterococcus faecium* (ATCC 35667), *Klebsiella pneumoniae* (ATCC 70060) and *Enterococcus faecalis* (ATCC 29212). The antioxidant capacity, reported as DPPH inhibition %, of the different films showed values of 4% for *M. pulegium*'s oil film to 23% for *O. basilicum* oil film in comparison with the control film which revealed no radical scavenging activity. The authors attributed these low values to the destruction of the active principles during film production and/or to the reaction of active principles with alginate.

Utama-ang et al. (2021) studied the microwave-assisted extraction (400 W, 1 min) of phenolic compounds from dried ginger and its incorporation (3.2% w/v) in a rice-based edible film. This edible film showed antioxidant activity due to the presence of 6-gingerol, 6-shogaol, paradol and zingerone. The incorporation to the formulation of 3.2% (w/v) ginger extract determined that the film showed antimicrobial activity against *S. mutans* DMST 18777. Yerramathi et al. (2021) developed a film based on alginate crosslinked with ferulic acid, for extending the shelf-life of different foods. The edible films developed showed an increasing antioxidant effect with the concentration of ferulic acid. Table 7.2 summarises the different GF active edible packaging used to improve the quality or extend the shelf-life of bakery products.

The effectiveness of the methods described in Table 7.2 depend on the food product characteristics (shape and size), the composition of the edible films and coatings, the physical properties (surface tension, density, and viscosity) (Andrade et al. 2012; Debeaufort and Voilley 2009), the processing method used and the sensory compatibility with the food (Restrepo et al. 2018).

7.4.3 Films and Coatings for Supporting Micronutrients/Probiotics

In particular, edible films have been proposed for the support and protection of probiotics. Probiotics are defined as nonpathogenic living microorganisms that have beneficial effects on host health and disease prevention when administered in adequate amounts (Kunes and Kvetina 2016). Soukoulis et al. (2014) studied the application of film forming solutions based on 1% w/w sodium alginate or in blends of 0.5% w/w sodium alginate and 2% whey protein concentrate, to bread. These solutions contained the probiotic *Lactobacillus rhamnosus* GG, and after its application on the surface of the bread, a drying step (60 °C, 10 min or 180 °C, 2 min) gave origin to a film that did not affect visually the crust and did not affect bread staling. The presence of whey protein concentrate improved the viability of the lactobacilli during drying and also during bread storage. The authors reported that films based exclusively on sodium alginate increased the viability of lactobacilli under simulated gastro-intestinal and concluded that a slice of bread (3–40 g) can provide approximately 7 log CFU of lactobacilli, contributing to the development of more healthy foods. In another study, Altamirano-Fortoul et al. (2012) developed functional bread combining *L. acidophilus* encapsulation and starch based edible coating. The results demonstrated the ability of the coating to protect the probiotics during baking, allowing their survival. However, significant physicochemical changes were observed on the crust. Many other GF bio-polymeric matrices have been assays as carriers of probiotics to broaden the offer of functional foods and to improve probiotic viability during processing and storage (Zoghi et al. 2020).

Likewise, edible coatings may also act as carriers of nutrients. Caseins and whey proteins based matrices have been used to control the release or support of calcium, iron, vitamin D, A, E and folic acid in several food stuffs (Daniloski et al. 2021; Mei and Zhao 2003). Genevois et al. (2016) developed a refrigerated ready-to-eat food based on pumpkin and fortified with iron and ascorbic acid supported in a coating matrix, which helped to enhance their bioaccessibility at *in vitro* simulated lumen conditions. Edible folic acid-nanolaminates were obtained by the layer-by-layer technique using alginate and chitosan biopolymers while the vitamin was incorporated by post-diffusion (Acevedo-Fani et al. 2018). These systems were able to protect folic acid from degradation by UV irradiation whereas the release profiles were affected by pH level, being faster in simulated conditions of the small intestine (pH 7). In another work, Behjati and Yazdanpanah (2021) elaborated a nano-emulsion vitamin D_3 fortified edible film based on quince seed gum which promoted high stability of the vitamin. Therefore, the authors concluded that fortified edible films can be used in ready-to-eat food products to improve vitamin intake. Moreover, Vitamin C (L-(+)-ascorbic acid), with important antioxidant activity, could be retained and protected when was supported in an alginate edible coating (De'Nobili et al. 2017) or a high methoxyl pectin edible film (Pérez et al. 2009), constituting an effective strategy for reduce its degradation. The authors demonstrated that the immobilisation of water in the film network modulated vitamin loss.

7.5 Conclusions

GF edible films, coatings and toppings applied to bakery products provide protection against external factors that can alter their quality. Toppings are essential for flavour and determine the appearance of the product, providing certain short-term barrier protection. On the other hand, edible coatings and films are a great barrier that focuses on extending long-term protection and provide a way to incorporate active components, such as antimicrobials or antioxidants to prevent microbial and oxidative impairment. In addition, edible films and coatings also can improve the nutritional quality of GF bakeries, since they can support vitamins, minerals, probiotics, etc. Therefore, actual GF available products can become functional foods offering to consumers with disorders related to gluten intake, higher quality and more diversified foods. Thus, improved GF bakery could help to avoid the risk of a nutritional deficiency and to exert a positive effect on health beyond basic nutrition. Future research must be focused on studying the effects of different GF formulations and processing of edible films, coatings and toppings on the physicochemical, sensorial and nutritional properties of GF bakery products. In addition, the influence of the application methodology on such characteristics should be further explored in order to help the achievement of a greater insertion of these technologies in the food industry while contributing to the generation of healthy foods.

References

Acevedo-Fani A, Soliva-Fortuny R, Martín-Belloso O (2018) Photo-protection and controlled release of folic acid using edible alginate/chitosan nanolaminates. J Food Eng 229:72–82. https://doi.org/10.1016/j.jfoodeng.2017.03.024

Aguirre-Joya JA, De Leon-Zapata MA, Alvarez-Perez OB et al (2018) Basic and applied concepts of edible packaging for foods. In: Grumezescu AM, Holban AM (eds) Food packaging and preservation. Handbook of food bioengineering, vol 9. Academic, Cambridge, MA, pp 1–61. https://doi.org/10.1016/B978-0-12-811516-9.00001-4

Altamirano-Fortoul R, Moreno-Terrazas R, Quezada-Gallo A et al (2012) Viability of some probiotic coatings in bread and its effect on the crust mechanical properties. Food Hydrocoll 29(1):166–174. https://doi.org/10.1016/j.foodhyd.2012.02.015

Alzate P, Miramont S, Flores S et al (2017) Effect of the potassium sorbate and carvacrol addition on the properties and antimicrobial activity of tapioca starch – hydroxypropyl methylcellulose edible films. Starch – Stärke 69(5–6):1600261. https://doi.org/10.1002/star.201600261

Alzate P, Gerschenson L, Flores S (2021) Study of the performance of particles based on modified starches containing potassium sorbate and incorporated into biodegradable films: physicochemical characterization and antimicrobial action. Chemistry 3(2):658–671. https://doi.org/10.3390/chemistry3020046

American Society for Testing Materials – ASTM (2010) D3985-05: standard test method for oxygen gas transmission rate through plastic film and sheeting using coulometric sensor. pp 656–661

American Society for Testing Materials – ASTM (2011) E96/E96M10: standard test methods for water vapour transmission of materials. pp 701–708

American Society for Testing Materials – ASTM (2014) F1927-14: standard test method for determination of oxygen gas transmission rate, permeability and permeance at controlled relative humidity through barrier materials using a coulometric detector. pp 1–6

Andrade RD, Skurtys O, Osorio FA (2012) Atomizing spray systems for application of edible coatings. Compr Rev Food Sci Food Saf 11(3):323–337. https://doi.org/10.1111/j.1541-4337.2012.00186.x

Anton A, Artfield S (2008) Hydrocolloids in gluten-free breads: a review. Int J Food Sci Nutr 59(1):11–23. https://doi.org/10.1080/09637480701625630

Atarés L, Chiralt A (2016) Essential oils as additives in biodegradable films and coatings for active food packaging. Trends Food Sci Technol 48:51–62. https://doi.org/10.1016/j.tifs.2015.12.001

Axel C, Zannini E, Arendt EK (2017) Mold spoilage of bread and its biopreservation: a review of current strategies for bread shelf-life extension. Crit Rev Food Sci Nutr 57(16):3528–3542. https://doi.org/10.1080/10408398.2016.1147417

Bader HG, Göritz D (1994) Investigations on high amylose corn starch films. Part 3: stress strain behaviour. Starch – Stärke 46(11):435–439. https://doi.org/10.1002/star.19940461106

Behjati J, Yazdanpanah S (2021) Nanoemulsion and emulsion vitamin D_3 fortified edible film based on quince seed gum. Carbohydr Polym 262:117948. https://doi.org/10.1016/j.carbpol.2021.117948

Bertuzzi MA, Castro Vidaurre EF, Armada M et al (2007) Water vapor permeability of edible starch based films. J Food Eng 80(3):972–978. https://doi.org/10.1016/j.jfoodeng.2006.07.016

Birania S, Kumar S, Kumar N et al (2022) Advances in development of biodegradable food packaging material from agricultural and agro-industry waste. J Food Process Eng 45(1):e13930. https://doi.org/10.1111/jfpe.13930

Bof MJ, Laurent FE, Massolo F et al (2021) Bio-packaging material impact on blueberries quality attributes under transport and marketing conditions. Polymers 13(4):481. https://doi.org/10.3390/polym13040481

Bravin B, Peressini D, Sensidoni A (2006) Development and application of polysaccharide–lipid edible coating to extend shelf-life of dry bakery products. J Food Eng 76(3):280–290. https://doi.org/10.1016/j.jfoodeng.2005.05.021

Cando E, Moreira C, Acosta S (2017) Characterization and application of biodegradable edible films produced by casting, from combinations of rice, cassava and potato starches with gelatin, in peanuts. In: Global partnerships for development and engineering education: proceedings of the 15th LACCEI international multi-conference for engineering, education and technology, Boca Raton, FL, United States. 19–21 July 2017. https://doi.org/10.18687/LACCEI2017.1.1.272

Capriles VD, dos Santos FG, Arêas JAG (2016) Gluten-free breadmaking: improving nutritional and bioactive compounds. J Cereal Sci 67:83–91. https://doi.org/10.1016/j.jcs.2015.08.005

Chávez S, Rodríguez-Herrera R, Silva S et al (2022) Formulation of a gluten-free cookie with prebiotics and an edible cover enriched with probiotics. Lett Appl NanoBiosci 11(2):3459–3469. https://doi.org/10.33263/LIANBS112.34593469

Chen G, Dong S, Zhao S et al (2019) Improving functional properties of zein film via compositing with chitosan and cold plasma treatment. Ind Crop Prod 129:318–326. https://doi.org/10.1016/j.indcrop.2018.11.072

Chen Y, Gavaliatsis T, Kuster S et al (2021) Crust treatments to reduce bread staling. Curr Res Nutr Food Sci 4:182–190. https://doi.org/10.1016/j.crfs.2021.03.004

Chiralt A, Menzel C, Hernández-García E et al (2020) Use of by-products in edible coatings and biodegradable packaging materials for food preservation. In: Betoret N, Betoret E (eds) Sustainability of the food system. Academic, Cambridge, MA, pp 101–127

Ciannamea EM, Stefani PM, Ruseckaite RA (2014) Physical and mechanical properties of compression molded and solution casting soybean protein concentrate based films. Food Hydrocoll 38:193–204. https://doi.org/10.1016/j.foodhyd.2013.12.013

Costa R, Saraiva A, Carvalho L et al (2014) The use of biodegradable mulch films on strawberry crop in Portugal. Sci Hortic 173:65–70. https://doi.org/10.1016/j.scienta.2014.04.020

Dang KM, Yoksan R (2015) Development of thermoplastic starch blown film by incorporating plasticized chitosan. Carbohydr Polym 115:575–581. https://doi.org/10.1016/j.carbpol.2014.09.005

Daniloski D, Trajkovska Petkoska A, Lee NA et al (2021) Active edible packaging based on milk proteins: a route to carry and deliver nutraceuticals. Trends Food Sci Technol 111:688–705. https://doi.org/10.1016/j.tifs.2021.03.024

Dankar I, Haddarah A, Omar FEL et al (2018) 3D printing technology: the new era for food customization and elaboration. Trends Food Sci Technol 75:231–242. https://doi.org/10.1016/j.tifs.2018.03.018

De Moraes JO, Scheibe AS, Sereno A et al (2013) Scale-up of the production of cassava starch based films using tape-casting. J Food Eng 119(4):800–808. https://doi.org/10.1016/j.jfoodeng.2013.07.009

de Oliveira Melo Naponucena L, Aparecida Souza Machado B, Ferreira Saraiva LE et al (2019) Physicochemical and microbiological stability of muffins packed in actives edible coatings from cassava starch: inverted sugar/sucrose and natural additives. Afr J Biotechnol 18(10):206–219. https://doi.org/10.5897/ajb2018.16741

De Pilli T (2020) Development of a vegetable oil and egg proteins edible film to replace preservatives and primary packaging of sweet baked goods. Food Control 114:107273. https://doi.org/10.1016/j.foodcont.2020.107273

De'Nobili MD, Genevois C, Rojas AM et al (2017) Stabilization of L-(+)-ascorbic acid in an iron fortified vegetable product (*Cucurbita moschata* Duchesne ex Poiret) using an alginate coating. In: Parsons E (ed) Ascorbic acid: properties, synthesis and applications. Nova Science Publishers Inc, New York, pp 105–122

Debeaufort F, Voilley A (2009) Lipid-based edible films and coatings. In: Huber K, Embuscado M (eds) Edible films and coatings for food applications. Springer, New York, pp 135–168. https://doi.org/10.1007/978-0-387-92824-1_5

Denavi G, Tapia-Blácido DR, Añón MC et al (2009) Effects of drying conditions on some physical properties of soy protein films. J Food Eng 90(3):341–349. https://doi.org/10.1016/j.jfoodeng.2008.07.001

Deseta ML, Sponton OE, Erben M et al (2021) Nanocomplexes based on egg white protein nanoparticles and bioactive compounds as antifungal edible coatings to extend bread shelf life. Food Res Int 148:110597. https://doi.org/10.1016/j.foodres.2021.110597

Díaz-Montes E, Castro-Muñoz R (2021) Edible films and coatings as food-quality preservers: an overview. Foods 10:249. https://doi.org/10.3390/foods10020249

Dobrucka R, Cierpiszewski R (2014) Active and intelligent packaging food – research and development – a review. Polish J Food Nutr Sci 64(1):7–15. https://doi.org/10.2478/v10222-012-0091-3

Fakhouri FM, Costa D, Yamashita F et al (2013) Comparative study of processing methods for starch/gelatin films. Carbohydr Polym 95(2):681–689. https://doi.org/10.1016/j.carbpol.2013.03.027

Fakhouri FM, Martelli SM, Caon T et al (2015) Edible films and coatings based on starch/gelatin: film properties and effect of coatings on quality of refrigerated red crimson grapes. Postharvest Biol Technol 109:57–64. https://doi.org/10.1016/j.postharvbio.2015.05.015

Fang Z, Zhao Y, Warner RD et al (2017) Active and intelligent packaging in meat industry. Trends Food Sci Technol 61:60–71. https://doi.org/10.1016/j.tifs.2017.01.002

Fernandes LM, Guimarães JT, Pimentel TC et al (2020) Edible whey protein films and coatings added with prebiotic ingredients. In: Barba FJ, Putnik P, Bursać Kovačević D (eds) Agri-food industry strategies for healthy diets and sustainability. Academic, Cambridge, MA, pp 177–193. https://doi.org/10.1016/B978-0-12-817226-1.00007-2

Ferreira Saraiva LE, Naponucena LOM, da Silva Santos V et al (2016) Development and application of edible film of active potato starch to extend mini panettone shelf life. LWT 73:311–319. https://doi.org/10.1016/j.lwt.2016.05.047

Ferreira LF, Figueiredo LP, Martins MA et al (2021) Active coatings of thermoplastic starch and chitosan with alpha-tocopherol/bentonite for special green coffee beans. Int J Biol Macromol 170:810–819. https://doi.org/10.1016/j.ijbiomac.2020.12.199

Fishman ML, Coffin DR, Konstance RP et al (2000) Extrusion of pectin/starch blends plasticized with glycerol. Carbohydr Polym 41(4):317–325. https://doi.org/10.1016/S0144-8617(99)00117-4

Flores S, Famá L, Rojas AM et al (2007) Physical properties of tapioca-starch edible films: influence of filmmaking and potassium sorbate. Food Res Int 40(2):257–265. https://doi.org/10.1016/j.foodres.2006.02.004

Flores SK, Daryne Costa FY, Gerschenson LN et al (2010) Mixture design for evaluation of potassium sorbate and xanthan gum effect on properties of tapioca starch films obtained by extrusion. Mater Sci Eng C 30:196–202. https://doi.org/10.1016/j.msec.2009.10.001

Fu B, Mei S, Su X et al (2021) Integrating waste fish scale-derived gelatin and chitosan into edible nanocomposite film for perishable fruits. Int J Biol Macromol 191:1164–1174. https://doi.org/10.1016/j.ijbiomac.2021.09.171

Galić K, Ćurić D, Gabrić D (2009) Shelf-life of packaged bakery goods – a review. Crit Rev Food Sci Nutr 49(5):405–426. https://doi.org/10.1080/10408390802067878

García MA, Martino MN, Zaritzky NE (1998) Plasticized starch-based coatings to improve strawberry (Fragaria × Ananassa) quality and stability. J Agric Food Chem 46(9):3758–3767. https://doi.org/10.1021/jf980014c

García MA, Martino MN, Zaritzky NE (2001) Composite starch-based coatings applied to strawberries (Fragaria Ananassa). Nahrung/Food 45(4):267–272. https://doi.org/10.1002/1521-3803(20010801)45:4<267::AID-FOOD267>3.0.CO;2-3

Garcia MA, Pinotti A, Martino MN et al (2004) Characterization of composite hydrocolloid films. Carbohydr Polym 56(3):339–345. https://doi.org/10.1016/j.carbpol.2004.03.003

García NL, Famá L, Dufresne A et al (2009) A comparison between the physico-chemical properties of tuber and cereal starches. Food Res Int 42(8):976–982. https://doi.org/10.1016/j.foodres.2009.05.004

Garrido T, Peñalba M, de la Caba K et al (2016) Injection-manufactured biocomposites from extruded soy protein with algae waste as a filler. Compos Part B Eng 86:197–202. https://doi.org/10.1016/j.compositesb.2015.09.058

Genevois CE, de Escalada Pla MF, Flores SK (2016) Application of edible coatings to improve global quality of fortified pumpkin. Innov Food Sci Emerg Technol 33:506–514. https://doi.org/10.1016/j.ifset.2015.11.001

Genevois C, Grenóvero M, de Escalada PM (2020) Use of different proportions of rice milling fractions as strategy for improving quality parameters and nutritional profile of gluten-free bread. J Food Sci Technol 58(10):3913–3923. https://doi.org/10.1007/s13197-020-04852-1

Gerschenson LN, Flores S, Espinel R et al (2018) Innovations in the development of antimicrobial edible films made from biopolymers and oregano. In: Gross DA (ed) Edible films and coatings: advances in research and application, Food science and technology. Nova Science Publishers, Inc., Hauppauge, pp 127–158

Geyer R, Jambeck JR, Law KL (2017) Production, use, and fate of all plastics ever made. Sci Adv 3(7):e1700782. https://doi.org/10.1126/sciadv.1700782

Gouveia TIA, Biernacki K, Castro MCR et al (2019) A new approach to develop biodegradable films based on thermoplastic pectin. Food Hydrocoll 97:105175. https://doi.org/10.1016/j.foodhyd.2019.105175

Gregirchak N, Stabnikova O, Stabnikov V (2020) Application of lactic acid bacteria for coating of wheat bread to protect it from microbial spoilage. Plant Foods Hum Nutr 75(2):223–229. https://doi.org/10.1007/s11130-020-00803-5

Guerreiro AC, Gago CML, Faleiro ML et al (2015) Raspberry fresh fruit quality as affected by pectin- and alginate-based edible coatings enriched with essential oils. Sci Hortic 194:138–146. https://doi.org/10.1016/j.scienta.2015.08.004

Huntrakul K, Yoksan R, Sane A et al (2020) Effects of pea protein on properties of cassava starch edible films produced by blown-film extrusion for oil packaging. Food Packag Shelf Life 24:100480. https://doi.org/10.1016/j.fpsl.2020.100480

Jafarzadeh S, Jafari SM, Salehabadi A et al (2020) Biodegradable green packaging with antimicrobial functions based on the bioactive compounds from tropical plants and their by-products. Trends Food Sci Technol 100:262–277. https://doi.org/10.1016/j.tifs.2020.04.017

Jamróz E, Pavel K (2020) Polysaccharide and protein films with antimicrobial/antioxidant activity in the food industry: a review. Polymers 12(6). https://doi.org/10.3390/POLYM12061289

Jebalia I, Maigret J-E, Réguerre A-L et al (2019) Morphology and mechanical behaviour of pea-based starch-protein composites obtained by extrusion. Carbohydr Polym 223:115086. https://doi.org/10.1016/j.carbpol.2019.115086

Jeya Jeevahan J, Chandrasekaran M, Venkatesan SP et al (2020) Scaling up difficulties and commercial aspects of edible films for food packaging: a review. Trends Food Sci Technol 100:210–222. https://doi.org/10.1016/j.tifs.2020.04.014

Jones J, Zevallos V, Wrigley C (2016) Appendix 3. Grains, foods, and ingredients suiting gluten-free diets for celiac disease. Reference module in food. Science. https://doi.org/10.1016/b978-0-08-100596-5.00249-3

Ju J, Chen X, Xie Y et al (2019) Application of essential oil as a sustained release preparation in food packaging. Trends Food Sci Technol 92:22–32. https://doi.org/10.1016/j.tifs.2019.08.005

Juhász A, Colgrave ML, Howitt CA (2020) Developing gluten-free cereals and the role of proteomics in product safety. J Cereal Sci 93:102932. https://doi.org/10.1016/j.jcs.2020.102932

Kamarudin SH, Rayung M, Abu F et al (2022) A review on antimicrobial packaging from biodegradable polymer composites. Polymers 14(1):174. https://doi.org/10.3390/polym14010174

Kechichian V, Ditchfield C, Veiga-Santos P et al (2010) Natural antimicrobial ingredients incorporated in biodegradable films based on cassava starch. LWT 43(7):1088–1094. https://doi.org/10.1016/j.lwt.2010.02.014

Klinmalai P, Atcharawan Srisa A, Laorenza Y et al (2021) Antifungal and plasticization effects of carvacrol in biodegradable poly(lactic acid) and poly(butylene adipate terephthalate) blend films for bakery packaging. LWT 152:112356. https://doi.org/10.1016/j.lwt.2021.112356

Kouhi M, Prabhakaran MP, Ramakrishna S (2020) Edible polymers: an insight into its application in food, biomedicine and cosmetics. Trends Food Sci Technol 103:248–263. https://doi.org/10.1016/j.tifs.2020.05.025

Kunes M, Kvetina J (2016) Probiotics: preclinical testing for verification of their gastrointestinal effectiveness. In: Gupta RC (ed) Nutraceuticals. Academic, Cambridge, MA, pp 799–810. https://doi.org/10.1016/B978-0-12-802147-7.00056-5

Lebwohl B, Green PHR (2021) Celiac disease. In: Feldman M, Friedman LS, Brandt LJ (eds) Sleisenger and Fordtran's gastrointestinal and liver disease, 11th edn. Elsevier, Philadelphia, pp 1736–1755

Lee E, Song H, Choi I et al (2020) Effects of mung bean starch/guar gum-based edible emulsion coatings on the staling and safety of rice cakes. Carbohydr Polym 247:116696. https://doi.org/10.1016/j.carbpol.2020.1166

Lopes FA, de Fátima Ferreira Soares N, de Cássia Pires Lopes C et al (2013) Conservation of bakery products through cinnamaldehyde antimicrobial films. Packag Technol Sci 27(4):293–302. https://doi.org/10.1002/pts.2033

López OV, García MA (2012) Starch films from a novel (Pachyrhizus Ahipa) and conventional sources: development and characterization. Mater Sci Eng C 32(7):1931–1940. https://doi.org/10.1016/j.msec.2012.05.035

López OV, Viña SZ, Pachas ANA et al (2010) Composition and food properties of *Pachyrhizus Ahipa* roots and starch. Int J Food Sci Technol 45(2):223–233. https://doi.org/10.1111/j.1365-2621.2009.02125.x

López OV, Giannuzzi L, Zaritzky NE et al (2013a) Potassium sorbate controlled release from corn starch films. Mater Sci Eng C 133(3):1583–1591. https://doi.org/10.1016/j.msec.2012.12.064

López OV, Zaritzky NE, Grossmann MVE et al (2013b) Acetylated and native corn starch blend films produced by blown extrusion. J Food Eng 116(2):286–297. https://doi.org/10.1016/J.JFOODENG.2012.12.03

López OV, Ninago MD, Lencina MMS et al (2015) Thermoplastic starch plasticized with alginate-glycerol mixtures: melt-processing evaluation and film properties. Carbohydr Polym 126:83–90. https://doi.org/10.1016/j.carbpol.2015.03.030

Mahcene Z, Khelil A, Hasni S et al (2020) Development and characterization of sodium alginate based active edible films incorporated with essential oils of some medicinal plants. Int J Biol Macromol 145:124–132. https://doi.org/10.1016/j.ijbiomac.2019.12.093

Mali S, Grossmann MVE, Garcia MA et al (2002) Microstructural characterization of yam starch films. Carbohydr Polym 50(4):379–386. https://doi.org/10.1016/s0144-8617(02)00058-9

Mani-Lopez E, Valle-Vargas GP, Palou E et al (2018) *Penicillium expansum* inhibition on bread by lemongrass essential oil in vapor phase. J Food Prot 81(3):467–471. https://doi.org/10.4315/0362-028x.jfp-17-315

Mantovan J, Bersaneti GT, Faria-Tischer PCS et al (2018) Use of microbial levan in edible films based on cassava starch. Food Packag Shelf Life 18:31–36. https://doi.org/10.1016/j.fpsl.2018.08.003

Martín-Belloso O, Rojas-Graü MA, Soliva-Fortuny R (2009) Delivery of flavor and active ingredients using edible films and coatings. In: Huber K, Embuscado M (eds) Edible films and coatings for food applications. Springer, New York, pp 295–313. https://doi.org/10.1007/978-0-387-92824-1_10

Martins IE, Shittu TA, Onabanjo OO et al (2021) Effect of packaging materials and storage conditions on the microbial quality of pearl millet sourdough bread. J Food Sci Technol 58(1):52–61. https://doi.org/10.1007/s13197-020-04513-3

McCabe MS (2010) Balancing consumer protection and scientific integrity in the face of uncertainty: the example of gluten-free foods. Food Drug Law J 65(2):367–390

Mei Y, Zhao Y (2003) Barrier and mechanical properties of milk protein-based edible films containing nutraceuticals. J Agric Food Chem 51(7):1914–1918. https://doi.org/10.1021/jf025944h

Melini V, Melini F (2018) Strategies to extend bread and GF bread shelf-life: from sourdough to antimicrobial active packaging and nanotechnology. Fermentation 4(1):9. https://doi.org/10.3390/fermentation4010009

Mitelut AC, Popa EE, Popescu PA et al (2021) Trends of innovation in bread and bakery production. In: Galanakis CM (ed) Trends in wheat and bread making. Academic, Cambridge, MA, pp 199–226. https://doi.org/10.1016/B978-0-12-821048-2.00007-6

Mohammadi Nafchi A, Moradpour M, Saeidi M et al (2013) Thermoplastic starches: properties, challenges, and prospects. Starch – Stärke 65(1–2):61–72. https://doi.org/10.1002/star.201200201

Morales-Jiménez M, Gouveia L, Yáñez-Fernández J et al (2020) Production, preparation and characterization of microalgae-based biopolymer as a potential bioactive film. Coatings 10(2):120. https://doi.org/10.3390/coatings10020120

Müller CM, Yamashita F, Laurindo JB (2008) Evaluation of the effects of glycerol and sorbitol concentration and water activity on the water barrier properties of cassava starch films through a solubility approach. Carbohydr Polym 72(1):82–87. https://doi.org/10.1016/j.carbpol.2007.07.026

Müller CM, Laurindo JB, Yamashita F (2009) Effect of cellulose fibers addition on the mechanical properties and water vapor barrier of starch-based films. Food Hydrocoll 23(5):1328–1333. https://doi.org/10.1016/j.foodhyd.2008.09.002

Musso YS, Salgado PR, Mauri AN (2017) Smart edible films based on gelatin and curcumin. Food Hydrocoll 66:8–15. https://doi.org/10.1016/j.foodhyd.2016.11.007

Nallan Chakravartula SS, Cevoli C, Balestra F et al (2019a) Evaluation of drying of edible coating on bread using NIR spectroscopy. J Food Eng 240:29–37. https://doi.org/10.1016/j.jfoodeng.2018.07.009

Nallan Chakravartula SS, Soccio M, Lotti N et al (2019b) Characterization of composite edible films based on pectin/alginate/whey protein concentrate. Materials 12(15):1–19. https://doi.org/10.3390/ma12152454

Nallan Chakravartula SS, Cevoli C, Balestra F et al (2019c) Evaluation of the effect of edible coating on mini-buns during storage by using NIR spectroscopy. J Food Eng 263:46–52. https://doi.org/10.1016/j.jfoodeng.2019.05.035

Ncama K, Magwaza LS, Mditshwa A et al (2018) Plant-based edible coatings for managing postharvest quality of fresh horticultural produce: a review. Food Packag Shelf Life 16:157–167. https://doi.org/10.1016/j.fpsl.2018.03.011

Nils-Gerrit Wunsch (2020) Bread and bakery products – statistics & facts. https://www.statista.com/topics/3110/bread-and-bakery-products/#dossierKeyfigures. Accessed 12 Dec 2021

Nisar T, Wang ZC, Yang X et al (2018) Characterization of citrus pectin films integrated with clove bud essential oil: physical, thermal, barrier, antioxidant and antibacterial properties. Int J Biol Macromol 106:670–680. https://doi.org/10.1016/j.ijbiomac.2017.08.068

Noshirvani N, Ghanbarzadeh B, Rezaei Mokarram R et al (2017) Novel active packaging based on carboxymethyl cellulose-chitosan-ZnO NPs nanocomposite for increasing the shelf life of bread. Food Packag Shelf Life 11:106–114. https://doi.org/10.1016/j.fpsl.2017.01.010

Ochoa-Yepes O, Di Giogio L, Goyanes S et al (2019) Influence of process (extrusion/thermo-compression, casting) and lentil protein content on physicochemical properties of starch films. Carbohydr Polym 208:221–231. https://doi.org/10.1016/j.carbpol.2018.12.030

Oriani VB, Molina G, Chiumarelli M et al (2014) Properties of cassava starch-based edible coating containing essential oils. J Food Sci 79(2):E189–E194. https://doi.org/10.1111/1750-3841.12332

Ortega F, Versino F, López OV et al (2021) Biobased composites from agro-industrial wastes and by-products. Emergent Mater:1–49. https://doi.org/10.1007/s42247-021-00319-x

Ortiz DE (2016) Cakes, muffins and bagels. In: Wrigley C, Corke H, Seetharaman K, Faubion J (eds) Encyclopedia of food grains, 2nd edn. Academic, Cambridge, MA, pp 30–36. https://doi.org/10.1016/b978-0-12-394437-5.00118-2

Otoni CG, Pontes SFO, Medeiros EAA et al (2014) Edible films from methylcellulose and nanoemulsions of clove bud *(Syzygium aromaticum)* and oregano *(Origanum vulgare)* essential oils as shelf life extenders for sliced bread. J Agric Food Chem 62(22):5214–5219. https://doi.org/10.1021/jf501055f

Otoni CG, Espitia PJP, Avena-Bustillos RJ et al (2016) Trends in antimicrobial food packaging systems: emitting sachets and absorbent pads. Int Food Res J 83:60–73. https://doi.org/10.1016/j.foodres.2016.02.018

Park S-J, Seo M-K (2011) Chapter 3 – Solid-liquid interface. Interface Sci Technol 18:147–252. https://doi.org/10.1016/B978-0-12-375049-5.00003-7

Pasqualone A (2019) Bread packaging: features and functions. In: Preedy Victor RR, Watson R (eds) Flour and breads and their fortification in health and disease prevention, 2nd edn. Academic, Cambridge, MA, pp 211–222. https://doi.org/10.1016/B978-0-12-814639-2.00017-4

Patil S, Sonawane SK, Arya SS (2019) A fuzzy mathematical approach for selection of surface coating and its effect on staling kinetics in a formulated gluten-free flatbread. Food Bioprocess Technol 12:1955–1965. https://doi.org/10.1007/s11947-019-02348-1

Pelissari FM, Yamashita F, Garcia MA et al (2012) Constrained mixture design applied to the development of cassava starch–chitosan blown films. J Food Eng 108(2):262–267. https://doi.org/10.1016/j.jfoodeng.2011.09.004

Peretto G, Du WX, Avena-Bustillos RJ et al (2017) Electrostatic and conventional spraying of alginate-based edible coating with natural antimicrobials for preserving fresh strawberry quality. Food Bioprocess Technol 10:165–174. https://doi.org/10.1007/s11947-016-1808-9

Pérez CD, Flores SK, Marangoni AG et al (2009) Development of a high methoxyl pectin edible film for retention of L-(+)-ascorbic acid. J Agric Food Chem 57(15):6844–6855. https://doi.org/10.1021/jf804019x

Pérez-Vergara LD, Cifuentes MT, Franco AP et al (2020) Development and characterization of edible films based on native cassava starch, beeswax, and propolis. NFS J 21:39–49. https://doi.org/10.1016/j.nfs.2020.09.002

Pranoto Y, Rakshit SK, Salokhe VM (2005) Enhancing antimicrobial activity of chitosan films by incorporating garlic oil, potassium sorbate and nisin. LWT 38(8):859–865. https://doi.org/10.1016/j.lwt.2004.09.014

Priyadarshi R, Sauraj Kumar B, Deeba F et al (2018) Chitosan films incorporated with apricot *(Prunus armeniaca)* kernel essential oil as active food packaging material. Food Hydrocoll 85:158–166. https://doi.org/10.1016/j.foodhyd.2018.07.003

Qian M, Liu D, Zhang X et al (2021) A review of active packaging in bakery products: applications and future trends. Trends Food Sci Technol 114:459–471. https://doi.org/10.1016/j.tifs.2021.06.009

Ramírez C, Gallegos I, Ihl M et al (2012) Study of contact angle, wettability and water vapor permeability in carboxymethylcellulose (CMC) based film with murta leaves (*Ugni molinae* Turcz) extract. J Food Eng 109(3):424–429. https://doi.org/10.1016/j.jfoodeng.2011.11.005

Remya S, Mohan CO, Venkateshwarlu G et al (2017) Combined effect of O_2 scavenger and antimicrobial film on shelf life of fresh cobia (*Rachycentron canadum*) fish steaks stored at 2°C. Food Control 71:71–78. https://doi.org/10.1016/j.foodcont.2016.05.038

Restrepo AE, Rojas JD, García OR et al (2018) Mechanical, barrier, and color properties of banana starch edible films incorporated with nanoemulsions of lemongrass (*Cymbopogon citratus)* and rosemary (*Rosmarinus officinalis*) essential oils. Food Sci Technol Int 24(8):705–712. https://doi.org/10.1177/1082013218792133

Rivero S, Garcia MA, Pinotti A (2010) Correlations between structural, barrier, thermal and mechanical properties of plasticized gelatin films. Innov Food Sci Emerg Technol 11(2):369–375. https://doi.org/10.1016/j.ifset.2009.07.005

Rivero S, Giannuzzi L, García MA et al (2013) Controlled delivery of propionic acid from chitosan films for pastry dough conservation. J Food Eng 116(2):524–531. https://doi.org/10.1016/j.jfoodeng.2012.12.025

Roman L, Eva DLC, Gomez M et al (2018) Specific ratio of A-to B-type wheat starch granules improves the quality of gluten-free breads: optimizing dough viscosity and pickering stabilization. Food Hydrocoll 82:510–518. https://doi.org/10.1016/j.foodhyd.2018.04.034

Rossi D, Rossi D, Pittia P, Realdon N (2019) Contact angle measurements and applications in pharmaceuticals and foods: a critical review. In: Mittal K (ed) Progress in adhesion and adhesives IV. Wiley-Scrivener Publishing LLC, Beverly, pp 193–240. https://doi.org/10.1002/9781119625322.ch5

Rowat SJ, Legge RL, Moresoli C (2021) Plant protein in material extrusion 3D printing: formation, plasticization, prospects, and challenges. J Food Eng 308(March):110623. https://doi.org/10.1016/j.jfoodeng.2021.110623

Roy S, Rhim JW (2020) Anthocyanin food colorant and its application in pH- responsive color change indicator films. Crit Rev Food Sci Nutr:1–29. https://doi.org/10.1080/10408398.2020.17762

Sadygova MK, Kozlov OI (2015) Edible film-forming coating composition for bread and bakery products. RU Patent 2539800, 27 Jan 2015

Sahraiyan B, Sheikholeslami Z, Karimi M (2020) Development of a novel edible surface coating made by *Lepidium sativum Seed Gum and comparison of its effect with traditional glazes of Sorghum Gluten-Free Bread. Res Innov Food Sci Technol 8(4):405–414.* https://doi.org/10.22101/jrifst.2020.214128.1140

Sánchez-Tamayo MI, Vélez Pasos C, Ochoa-Martínez CI (2020) Methods for gas permeability measurement in edible films for fruits and vegetables: a review. Food Sci Technol 41(4):807–815. https://doi.org/10.1590/fst.07520

Scaffaro R, Maio A, Gulino EF et al (2020) PLA-based functionally graded laminates for tunable controlled release of carvacrol obtained by combining electrospinning with solvent casting. React Funct Polym 148:104490. https://doi.org/10.1016/j.reactfunctpolym.2020.104490

Senanayake CM, Nayanakanthi T, Siranjiv P (2021) Development of an edible coating from okra mucilage to preserve the crispiness in soft dough biscuits upon storage. Adv Technol 1(2):307–320. https://doi.org/10.31357/ait.v1i2.4881

Senturk Parreidt T, Müller K, Schmid M (2018a) Alginate-based edible films and coatings for food packaging applications. Foods 7(10):170. https://doi.org/10.3390/foods7100170

Senturk Parreidt T, Schmid M, Müller K (2018b) Effect of dipping and vacuum impregnation coating techniques with alginate based coating on physical quality parameters of cantaloupe melon. J Food Sci 83(4):929–936. https://doi.org/10.1111/1750-3841.14091

Seung YC, Rhee C (2004) Mechanical properties and water vapor permeability of edible films made from fractionated soy proteins with ultrafiltration. LWT 37(8):833–839. https://doi.org/10.1016/j.lwt.2004.03.009

Seydim AC, Sarikus-Tutal G, Sogut E (2020) Effect of whey protein edible films containing plant essential oils on microbial inactivation of sliced Kasar cheese. Food Packag Shelf Life 26:100567. https://doi.org/10.1016/j.fpsl.2020.100567

Sharifi KA, Pirsa S (2021) Biodegradable film of black mulberry pulp pectin/chlorophyll of black mulberry leaf encapsulated with carboxymethylcellulose/silica nanoparticles: investigation of physicochemical and antimicrobial properties. Mater Chem Phys 267:124580. https://doi.org/10.1016/j.matchemphys.2021.124580

Shih YT, Zhao Y (2021) Development, characterization and validation of starch based biocomposite films reinforced by cellulose nanofiber as edible muffin liner. Food Packag Shelf Life 28:100655. https://doi.org/10.1016/j.fpsl.2021.100655

Shih FF, Daigle K, Champagne ET (2011) Effect of rice wax on water vapour permeability and sorption properties of edible pullulan films. Food Chem 127:118–121. https://doi.org/10.1016/j.foodchem.2010.12.096

Silva MA, Gonçalves Albuquerque T, Carneiro Alves R et al (2021) Fruit byproducts as alternative ingredients for bakery products. In: Rajeev Bhat R (ed) Valorization of agri-food wastes and by-products. Academic, Amsterdam, pp 111–131

Smith JP, Simpson BK (1995) Modified atmosphere packaging of bakery and pasta products. In: Farber JM, Dodds KL (eds) Principles of modified atmosphere and sous vide product packaging, 1st edn. Technomic Publishing Company, Lancaster, pp 207–242

Smith JP, Daifas DP, El-Khoury W et al (2004) Shelf life and safety concerns of bakery products – a review. Crit Rev Food Sci Nutr 44(1):19–55. https://doi.org/10.1080/10408690490263774

Soukoulis C, Yonekura L, Gan HH et al (2014) Probiotic edible films as a new strategy for developing functional bakery products: the case of pan bread. Food Hydrocoll 39:231–242. https://doi.org/10.1016/j.foodhyd.2014.01.023

Sucheta Rai SK, Chaturvedi K, Yadav SK (2019) Evaluation of structural integrity and functionality of commercial pectin based edible films incorporated with corn flour, beetroot, orange peel, muesli and rice flour. Food Hydrocoll 91:127–135. https://doi.org/10.1016/j.foodhyd.2019.01.022

Suhag R, Kumar N, Trajkovska Petkoska A et al (2020) Film formation and deposition methods of edible coating on food products: a review. Food Res Int 136:109582. https://doi.org/10.1016/j.foodres.2020.109582

Sun Q, Sun C, Xiong L (2013) Mechanical, barrier and morphological properties of pea starch and peanut protein isolate blend films. Carbohydr Polym 98(1):630–637. https://doi.org/10.1016/j.carbpol.2013.06.040

Tan W, Zhang J, Zhao X et al (2020) Preparation and physicochemical properties of antioxidant chitosan ascorbate/methylcellulose composite films. Int J Biol Macromol 146:53–61. https://doi.org/10.1016/j.ijbiomac.2019.12.044

Tapia-Blácido DR, da Silva Ferreira ME, Aguilar GJ et al (2020) Biodegradable packaging antimicrobial activity. In: Zhang Y (ed) Processing and development of polysaccharide-based biopolymers for packaging applications. Elsevier, Amsterdam, pp 207–238

Tavassoli-Kafrani E, Shekarchizadeh H, Masoudpour-Behabadi M (2016) Development of edible films and coatings from alginates and carrageenans. Carbohydr Polym 137:360–374. https://doi.org/10.1016/j.carbpol.2015.10.074

Tiefenbacher KF (2017) Chapter five: adjuncts – filling creams, inclusions, cacao and chocolate. In: Tiefenbacher KF (ed) Wafer and waffle. Academic, Cambridge, MA, pp 313–404. https://doi.org/10.1016/b978-0-12-809438-9.00005-3

Tiseo I (2021) Global plastic waste production breakdown 2018, by sector. https://www.statista.com/statistics/1166582/global-plastic-waste-generation-by-sector/#statisticContainer. Accessed 12 Dec 2021

Truong T, Kobayashi T (2020) Pectin bioplastic films regenerated from dragon fruit peels. Vietnam J Sci Technol 62(4):18–22. https://doi.org/10.31276/VJSTE.62(4).18-22

Ustunol Z (2009) Edible films and coatings for meat and poultry. In: Huber K, Embuscado M (eds) Edible films and coatings for food applications. Springer, New York, pp 245–268. https://doi.org/10.1007/978-0-387-92824-1_8

Utama-ang N, Sida S, Wanachantararak P et al (2021) Development of edible Thai rice film fortified with ginger extract using microwave-assisted extraction for oral antimicrobial properties. Sci Rep 11(1):14870. https://doi.org/10.1038/s41598-021-94430-y

Valdés A, Ramos M, Beltrán A et al (2017) State of the art of antimicrobial edible coatings for food packaging applications. Coatings 7(4):56. https://doi.org/10.3390/coatings7040056

Varghese SA, Siengchin S, Parameswaranpillai J (2020) Essential oils as antimicrobial agents in biopolymer-based food packaging – a comprehensive review. Food Biosci 38:100785. https://doi.org/10.1016/j.fbio.2020.100785

Versino F, García MA (2014) Cassava (*Manihot esculenta*) starch films reinforced with natural fibrous filler. Ind Crop Prod 58:305–314. https://doi.org/10.1016/j.indcrop.2014.04.040

Versino F, Lopez OV, Garcia MA et al (2016) Starch-based films and food coatings: an overview. Starch – Stärke 68(11–12):1026–1037. https://doi.org/10.1002/star.201600095

Vidaurre-Ruiz J, Matheus-Diaz S, Salas-Valerio F et al (2019) Influence of tara gum and xanthan gum on rheological and textural properties of starch-based gluten-free dough and bread. Eur Food Res Technol 245(7):1347–1355. https://doi.org/10.1007/s00217-019-03253-9

Vilpoux OF, Brito VH, Cereda MP (2019) Starch extracted from corms, roots, rhizomes, and tubers for food application. In: Pedrosa Silva Clerici MT, Schmiele M (eds) Starches for food application. Academic, Cambridge, MA, pp 103–165. https://doi.org/10.1016/B978-0-12-809440-2.00004-6

Wang H, Ding F, Ma L et al (2021) Edible films from chitosan-gelatin: physical properties and food packaging application. Food Biosci 40:100871. https://doi.org/10.1016/j.fbio.2020.100871

Xu J, Zhang Y, Wang W et al (2020) Advanced properties of gluten-free cookies, cakes, and crackers: a review. Trends Food Sci Technol 103:200–213. https://doi.org/10.1016/j.tifs.2020.07.017

Yerramathi BB, Kola M, Annem Muniraj B et al (2021) Structural studies and bioactivity of sodium alginate edible films fabricated through ferulic acid crosslinking mechanism. J Food Eng 301:110566. https://doi.org/10.1016/j.jfoodeng.2021.110566

Zhang M, Biesold GM, Choi W et al (2022) Recent advances in polymers and polymer composites for food packaging. Mater Today (in press). https://doi.org/10.1016/j.mattod.2022.01.022

Zhong Y, Godwin P, Jin Y et al (2019) Biodegradable polymers and green-based antimicrobial packaging materials: a mini-review. Adv Ind Eng Polym Res 3(1):27–35. https://doi.org/10.1016/j.aiepr.2019.11.002

Zoghi A, Khosravi-Darani K, Mohammadi R (2020) Application of edible films containing probiotics in food products. Consum Prot Food Saf 15:307–320. https://doi.org/10.1007/s00003-020-01286-x

Zoumpopoulou G, Tsakalidou E (2019) Gluten-free products. In: Galanakis CM (ed) The role of alternative and innovative food ingredients and products in consumer wellness. Academic, Cambridge, MA, pp 213–237. https://doi.org/10.1016/B978-0-12-816453-2.00008-5

Chapter 8
Gluten Free Pasta Production and Formulation Design

Luciana Carla González, María Ana Loubes, and Marcela Patricia Tolaba

Abbreviations

β_i	coefficient for effect of each component in the MD model
β_{ij}, β_{ijk}	coefficients for double and triple interaction between components *i*, *j* and *k* in the MD model
ΔE*	colour difference
ε_b	strain at break
σ_b	stress at break
a_0, a_i and a_{ii}	coefficients for constant, linear and quadratic effects in RSM model
a_{ij} coefficient	the interaction effect between X_i and X_j factors in RSM model
AF	Amaranth flour
ABTS	antioxidant activity by radical caption (ABTS·+) scavenging activity
B	pasta brightness
BD	bulk density of the pasta
c_1, c_2, c_3	concentration percentages of the mixture components
CIELAB parameter L*	lightness
CIELAB parameter a*	redness
CIELAB parameter b*	yellowness
CL	cooking loss
Ct	cooking time of the pasta
D50	particle size (median)

L. C. González · M. A. Loubes · M. P. Tolaba (✉)
Facultad de Ciencias Exactas y Naturales, Departamento de Industrias, Universidad de Buenos Aires, Ciudad Autónoma de Buenos Aires, Argentina

CONICET – Universidad de Buenos Aires, Instituto de Tecnología de Alimentos y Procesos Químicos (ITAPROQ), Buenos Aires, Argentina
e-mail: mtolaba@di.fcen.uba.ar

M. F. de Escalada Pla, C. E. Genevois (eds.), *Designing Gluten Free Bakery and Pasta Products*, https://doi.org/10.1007/978-3-031-28344-4_8

DPP	dried potato pulp
DPPH	antiradical capacity
EPP	extruded potato pulp
EQ	extruded quinoa flour
F	firmness of the pasta
FR	feed rate
G′	storage modulus
G″	loss modulus
GAE	gallic acid equivalent
GCS	gelatinized corn starch
GF	gluten free
GG	guar gum
HPMC	Hydroxypropyl Methyl Cellulose
LVR	linear viscoelastic region
MC	moisture content
MD	mixture design
NEQ	non-extruded quinoa flour
RSM	response surface method
S	stickiness of the pasta
SS	screw speed
T	extrusion temperature
TPA	texture profile analysis
WA	water absorption
x_i	composition of each of the q components in the mixture
X_i, X_j, … X_n	coded factors
XG	xanthan gum
Y	response (RSM) or dependent variable (MD)

8.1 Introduction

Traditional western pasta is wheat-based pasta and therefore contains gluten, an ingredient that gives the dough the suitable viscoelasticity to make the product. Obtaining gluten free pasta (GF pasta) involves the use of gluten substitutes and the replacement of wheat flour with flours that do not contain gluten (Marti and Pagani 2013). The addition of hydrocolloids, modified starches, gums, egg white, emulsifiers or enzymes as gluten substitutes yields a viscoelastic dough to obtain good quality GF pasta (Schoenlechner et al. 2010; Marti et al. 2014; Linares-García et al. 2019; Loubes et al. 2016).

The development of GF pasta with good acceptance by western consumers was a true challenge back in the 2000s. At that time, the main effort was focused on finding appropriate and inexpensive gluten substitutes to meet the needs of people with celiac disease. A disease that is becoming visible thanks to the development of diagnostic methods for early detection (Gómez and Sciarini 2015).

Rice-based noodle is a staple food in Asia, for its production a flour slurry obtained by wet milling is subjected to steam heating, transforming after cooling into a gelatinized sheet, similar to the production of edible rice paper (Lu and Collado 2019; Ahmed et al. 2016; Yeh 2004; Cham and Suwannaporn 2010). However, this chapter is focused on GF noodles that emulate those obtained by laminating or extrusion processes of wheat flour, according to the preference of Western consumers (Molina-Rosell 2013). Rice, corn and sorghum flours have been widely used alone or in combinations to develop these GF pastas (Yalcin and Basman 2008; Jeong et al. 2017; Ferreira et al. 2016).

Knowledge about celiac disease initially prompted the research and development of GF products. Then, the research was also driven by non-celiac gluten sensitivity incidence and changes in consumer habits, which gradually shifted towards healthier foods with a minor consumption of refined wheat flour, saturated or trans fatty acids, sugar and salt, among others. Consumers are increasingly informed. They demand from the food industry products with high protein and fibre contents, as well as the addition of bioactive food components (i.e., antioxidant, antimicrobial, immunomodulatory, hypocholesterolaemic) for health care (Linares-García et al. 2019; Perez-Gregorio and Simal-Gandara 2017). This is why the current challenge is significant, since the researchers have to work on finding new and better ingredients for formulations development and determining their suitability for making GF pasta. In addition, traditional pasta production methods will have to be adapted to meet the demands of new consumers and the requirements of new products (Padalino et al. 2016).

Recently, it has been proposed to supplement the noodle formulation by adding quinoa, amaranth or buckwheat flours (Fu et al. 2020; Martínez-Villaluenga et al. 2020) as well as legume flours to fortify GF noodles (Bouasla et al. 2017; Sofi et al. 2020a, b). These non-traditional flours can provide high quality proteins composed of essential amino acids, fibre, ω-3 and ω-6 fatty acids, vitamins (E and C) and phenolics compounds, that improve the nutritional value of the final products (Lorenzo et al. 2018).

The circular economy model is being incorporated into the design of formulations with the addition of bioactive fractions extracted from different industrial food waste.

The adoption of the circular economy model is affecting the design of formulations with the incorporation of bioactive fractions extracted from different industrial food wastes. Fradinho et al. (2020) proposed the addition of potato peel autohydrolysis extract to rice noodles, while Bastos et al. (2016) produced GF noodles based on amaranth flour and potato pulp from potato chips industry. Waste recycling is an open challenge to be addressed in future research.

To determine pasta quality, the cooking properties (water absorption index and cooking losses) and texture characteristics (extensibility tests, TPA analysis) of cooked pasta are usually evaluated (Larrosa et al. 2016). However, other tests are also recommended, such as colour evaluation and sensory analysis of cooked pasta or the evaluation of the technological suitability of the dough.

Pasta quality will depend on both the ingredients present in the formulation and the method selected for pasta production. Consumer preference, nutritional needs or health requirements come into play in the selection of ingredients, while different procedures such as lamination, extrusion or extrusion-cooking processes may be adopted to noodle production according to available resources.

Figure 8.1 summarizes the steps for noodles production. Starting with the selection of the flour or flour blends and functional ingredients and their subsequent mixing with water. Then, two ways can be selected: the kneading step followed by dough resting, laminating and cutting stages if the laminating process is chosen; or the production of extruded noodles by extrusion or extrusion-cooking processes. Finally, the drying of the pasta and the evaluation of its quality is performed.

Preliminary trials are required for a first approximation to the formulation. Further optimization of the formula can be performed by using the mixture design method.

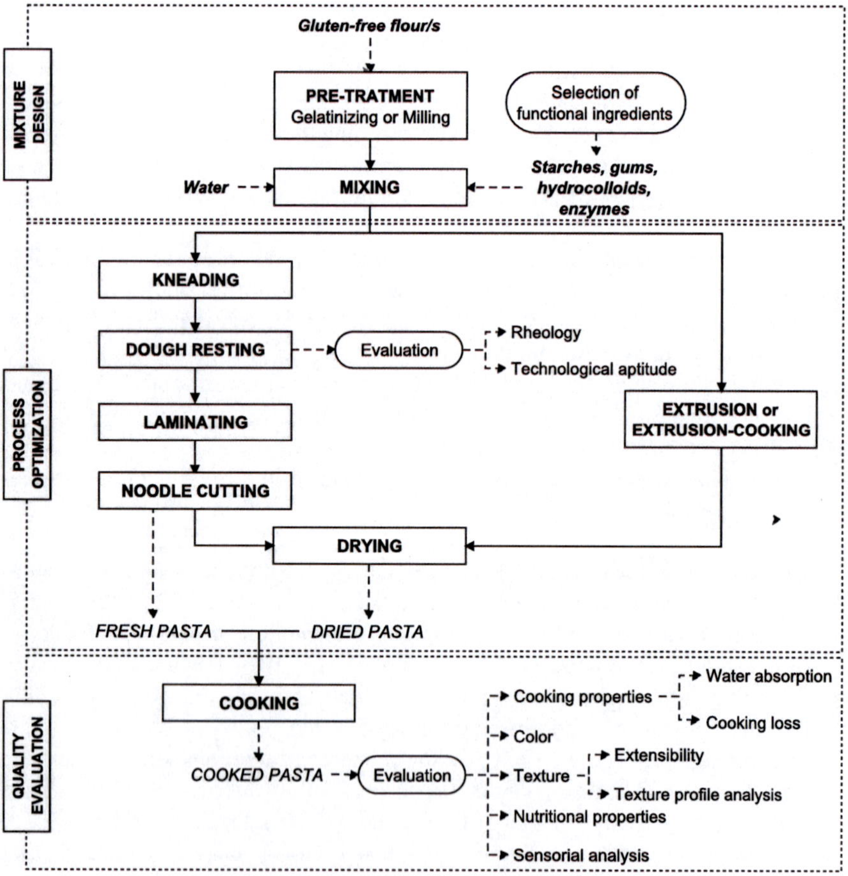

Fig. 8.1 Steps for GF noodles production

Figure 8.1 also shows the topics addressed in this chapter. As the ingredients suitable for the development of GF products, are detailed in a previous chapter, the focus of this chapter is on the methods to produce GF pastas and strategies to address the development of formulations. It is previously described (a) how to evaluate the pasta quality, which is the main criterion for the optimization of both, the formulations and the pasta manufacturing processes; (b) how to model the effects of process variables and formulation on pasta properties. The chapter concludes with a description of techniques to extend the shelf life of noodles and an evaluation of commercial aspects and a cost analysis.

8.2 Evaluation of Dough Characteristics and Pasta Quality

The evaluation of pasta quality is related to consumer acceptance while the evaluation of the dough is associated with its aptitude for lamination step. Dough rheology and technological aptitude of dough are usually evaluated. Pasta quality involves the determination of cooking and texture performance of pasta, as well as others pasta properties such as colour, nutritional aspects and sensorial analysis.

8.2.1 Technological Aptitude of Dough

A qualitative analysis of the homogeneity, elasticity and cohesiveness of the dough is usually performed during kneading to determine if it is acceptable. The ease or difficulty, with which the dough can form a thin sheet without breaking or sticking when passing between the rollers, as well as its behaviour during the noodle cutting operation, must be qualified. This qualitative evaluation makes it possible to determine the technological aptitude of dough. Therefore, this analysis is a useful tool to discard mixtures during preliminary tests (González et al. 2022).

8.2.2 Rheological Characterization of Dough

The viscoelastic properties of dough disks (i.e., 30 mm diameter, 2 mm height) can be measured under isothermal conditions using a rheometer (Fu et al. 2020; Fradinho et al. 2020). A serrated parallel plate geometry, recommended to avoid the slip effect, with a properly gap (i.e. 2 mm) can be adopted. Stress sweep tests are first performed at 1 Hz from 0.1 to 100 Pa to assess the linear viscoelastic region (LVR). Then, the rheological parameters: storage modulus (G'), loss modulus (G'') and loss tangent ($\tan\delta = G''/G'$) are obtained through the frequency sweep test (from 0.1 to 10–20 Hz at fixed strain value within the LVR). These tests are used to determine whether the elastic character predominates over the viscous character and to quantify changes in viscoelastic behaviour due to pasta cooking or formulation variations.

8.2.3 Cooking Quality of Noodles

First, the raw noodles are placed in boiling water at 100 °C by using a noodle to water mass ratio of 1:10. The optimum cooking time is obtained by measuring the time required for disappearance of the white central core when pasta is squeezed between two glass plates (standard procedure AACC 1999a).

Two cooking properties can be determined: cooking loss (CL) by method 16–50 (AACC 1999a) and water absorption (WA) according to Tudorica et al. (2002). Raw noodles are cooked in boiling distilled water (i.e., water to noodles mass ratio of 40) until its optimum cooking time. For CL, cooking water is dried to constant weight at 100 °C and the solid residue is reported as percentage (dry basis) of uncooked pasta. WA is the weight increase of pasta after cooking and draining steps, expressed as percentage (dry basis) of uncooked pasta. A good quality pasta presents low CL values and suitable values of WA. Wheat pasta (WA: 110%, CL: 7.4%) can be consider as a reference (Loubes et al. 2016).

8.2.4 Extensibility Test for Cooked Pasta

The texture behaviour of cooked pasta discs (i.e., 6 cm diameter and 2 mm thickness) can be studied using a universal texture machine, and a spherical measuring tip (diameter of 2 cm), which is moved at a fixed speed (0.1 mm/s). The pasta disc should be appropriately supported by a ring frame (3–4 cm diameter of central free area) to prevent displacement or breakage of the disc (González et al. 2022). The stress and the strain are recorded and the corresponding average values at break are obtained from at least ten replicates. Values of strength and strain at break greater than 0.8 N and 5.4 mm, respectively, indicate good quality GF noodles (Loubes et al. 2016; Heo et al. 2013).

8.2.5 Texture Profile Analysis (TPA) and Cutting Force

TPA of raw and cooked pasta can be performed in a texturometer that emulates chewing or biting action. Raw pasta is moulded in acrylic discs (i.e., 6 cm diameter and 2 cm height) and rest for 15 min before the cylindrical acrylic probe (1 cm diameter) penetrates 8 mm at 1 mm/s into the dough. The hardness (N), adhesiveness (N.s) and cohesiveness are obtained from the force vs. time curve (Fradinho et al. 2020).

The texture profile of cooked pasta (discs samples are dipped in cool water soon after cooking in order to stop the cooking) can be obtained by two compression cycles test using a 25 mm diameter flat-ended cylindrical probe (P/25) with a speed of 0.5 mm/s and a compression distance of 30% of the original size. Hardness, cohesiveness, adhesiveness (negative force of the first compression cycle), springiness, chewiness, and resilience can be estimated from force–time curve (Larrosa et al. 2016).

The AACC method 66 -50.01 (AACC 1999a) is recommended to determine the cutting force, i.e. the maximum force (N) needed to cut the cooked pasta (100% compression). The test simulates the bite action of incisive teeth (speed = 0.5 mm/s).

8.2.6 Colour Measurements

Total colour difference (ΔE*) between pasta samples and control, between pasta samples before and after cooking or colour changes due to drying process can be calculate from the CIELAB parameters L* (lightness), a* (redness) and b* (yellowness), which are obtained by using a colorimeter. The standard illuminant D65, a visual angle of 2° and a white standard (L* = 94.61, a* = −0.53, b* = 3.62) are usually adopted (Fradinho et al. 2020).

8.2.7 Nutritional Composition

The centesimal composition of raw and cooked pasta samples involves the determinations of: moisture content, ash, lipid content, protein content (using nitrogen conversion factor 5.95 for pseudocereals or 6.25 for cereals) and, dietary fibre content, according to the standard AACC (1999b) or AOAC (1998) methods. The carbohydrate content is usually estimated by difference.

8.2.8 Degradation of Bioactive Compounds

Methods to determine bioactive compounds degradation are applied to evaluate, at the end of the pasta production, the conservation of the bioactive components that were incorporated into the mixture. Lyophilized samples of raw and cooked pasta are extracted by using a solution ethanol/water (50:50) at 60 °C/1 h, under magnetic stirring, and filtered. The liquid extract is recovered for the measurements based on spectrophotometric methods. To determine total phenolic content, the liquid extract is incubated in darkness at 20 °C for 1 h together with distilled water (water/liquid extract: 60:1). The Folin-Ciocalteu's phenol reagent and sodium carbonate are added. The absorbance is measured at 765 nm. The result is reported as milligram GAE (gallic acid equivalent) per gram of dry basis sample (Singleton and Rossi 1965).

The antioxidant activity can be determined by ABTS radical caption (ABTS·+) scavenging activity according to Re et al. (1999). ABTS·+solution is added to the liquid extract, the mix is incubated at 30 °C for 6 min, and the absorbance is measured at 734 nm against phosphate buffered saline.

The antiradical capacity can be measured by using DPPH radical following the method proposed by Brand-Williams et al. (1995). Liquid extracts are mixed with the DPPH radical working solution. After few minutes, the decrease in absorbance (515 nm) is recorded and the inhibition percentage is calculated respect to the initial absorbance value. For the last two methods the results are expressed as mmol TEAC (Trolox Equivalent Antioxidant Capacity) per gram of sample (dry basis).

8.2.9 Sensory Evaluation

The evaluation by a trained panel, a semi-trained panel or volunteer judges can be adopted. A panel of 15 semi-trained members (who are regular consumers of pasta) may be adequate for the test. The different samples of cooked pasta could be present in a random order to be assessed for appearance, taste, flavour, colour, hardness, and stickiness among other attributes using at least a 5-point scale while a 9-point hedonic scale is recommended to qualify/quantify the overall acceptability of each pasta sample (Bouasla et al. 2017). Above 5, in a 9-point scale, can be considered as acceptable (Bustos et al. 2011).

8.3 Statistical Tools for Optimization

The response surface method (RSM) commonly used for process optimization is described as well as the mixture design method (MD) to optimize the ingredient proportions of pasta formulations.

8.3.1 RSM Method

The response surface methodology (RSM) introduced by Box and Wilson (1951) is a widely used mathematical and statistical method for empirical model building from experimental data. RSM can be used to relate each response (*Y*), i.e. quality attribute of the product, with the process variables or "factors" in order to find the optimal process conditions to maximize the product quality. A second-degree polynomial expression (Eq. 8.1) has been proposed to estimate the studied responses (*Y*) as a function of coded factors (X_i, X_j, … X_n), which are usually related to process variables by means of linear relationships (Khuri and Cornell 1987).

$$Y = a_0 + \sum_{i=1}^{n} a_i X_i + \sum_{i=1}^{n} a_{ii} X_i^2 + \sum_{i=1}^{n-1} \sum_{\substack{j=2 \\ i<j}}^{n} a_{ij} X_i X_j \tag{8.1}$$

Where a_0, a_i and a_{ii} represent the coefficients corresponding to the constant, linear and quadratic terms, respectively, while the coefficient a_{ij} represents the interaction effect between the studied factors (X_i and X_j).

The different combinations of coded factors (dimensionless) to be evaluated, in order to study their effect on studied responses, can be set by selecting a properly experimental design. RSM is a common analysis tool within the commercial statistical programs: Statgraphics (Statistical graphics Corporation, USA), Systat (Systat Software Inc.), Design – Expert (Stat-Ease Inc.), IBM SPSS (IBM Company), R Studio software (RStudio, PBC, Boston), and R free software (https://www.r-project.org/). These programs offer different options for selecting the most convenient experimental design. There are factorial designs, central composite designs, Doehlert matrix, Box-Behnken design, among others. For each experimental design, the number of factors and the number of levels for each "factor" are well defined. For three levels, it is common to use the coded values −1, 0, 1. At least three levels are required to detect nonlinear effects associated to quadratic coefficients or interaction coefficients between factors in the polynomial model.

8.3.2 *Mixture Design*

In products made from mixtures of two or more ingredients, as in the case of pasta, the quality characteristics of the final product depend on the proportions of the components in the formulation. It is therefore important to identify the optimal mixture, and a region around it, that maximizes product quality (López-Torres et al. 2002).

Since the proportions must add up to a fixed amount, usually 100%, the factors cannot be varied independently (Scheffé 1958). In an experiment with mixtures, the composition x_i of each of the q components must satisfy the following constraints:

$$x_i \geq 0(i = 1,2,\ldots q), \sum_{i=1}^{q} x_i = x_i + x_2 + \ldots + x_q = 1 \tag{8.2}$$

These constraints define the geometry of the experimental region as a simplex design of dimension (q–1). For example, for q = 2 components the experimental region is a line ($x_i + x_2 = 1$) while for $q = 3$ components, an equilateral triangle in the cartesian plane ($x_i + x_2 + x_3 = 1$) represents the experimental region. The objective in MD analysis is to find a mathematical model that allows predicting the value of the dependent variable (Y) as a function of mixture components (x_i, x_j, x_k), fitting the experimental data by mixture models proposed by Scheffé (1958):

Linear Model

$$Y = \sum_{i=1}^{q} \beta_i x_i \tag{8.3}$$

Quadratic Model

$$Y = \sum_{i=1}^{q} \beta_i x_i + \Sigma \sum_{i<j}^{q} \beta_{ij} x_i x_j \tag{8.4}$$

Cubic Model

$$Y = \sum_{i=1}^{q} \beta_i x_i + \Sigma \sum_{i<j}^{q} \beta_{ij} x_i x_j + \Sigma\Sigma \sum_{i<j<k}^{q} \beta_{ijk} x_i x_j x_k \tag{8.5}$$

Where the parameter β_i represents the effect of the pure component *i*, β_{ij} the effect of the interaction between components *i* and *j*, and β_{ijk} the effect of the triple interaction between components *i, j* and *k*.

Model coefficients can be obtained by regression analysis and a stepwise method can be followed to determine the significant terms ($p < 0.05$) in Eqs. 8.3, 8.4 and 8.5.

The experimental designs associated with these models can be of three types: simplex latice, simplex centroid and axial (López-Torres et al. 2002). One of the most commonly used designs is the simplex centroid design. For combinations of three ingredients, seven experimental points are required (Fig. 8.2a). For each component, the coded composition varies between the base of the triangle (level 0) and the vertex of the triangle (level 1). The optimization is carried out considering the constraint imposed on the sum of the ingredients in the ternary mixture. The sum could be 100% if the mixture has only three ingredients (i.e. water, flour and hydrocolloid). However, the sum could also be a fixed percentage less than 100% if there are other components in the mix that are kept constant and therefore, they are not taken into account for the MD analysis (Vandeginste and Rutan 1998). Frequently, the restrictions adopted to limit the experimental region are based on preliminary tests in order to the better use of MD analysis and to enhance the predictions from MD models (Eqs. 8.3, 8.4 and 8.5).

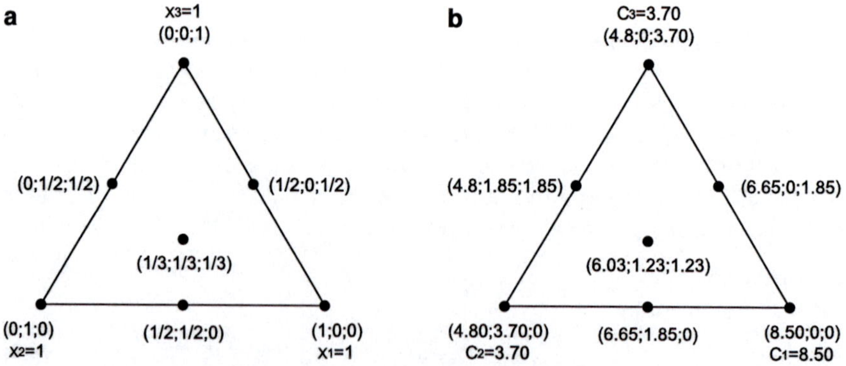

Fig. 8.2 Centroid simplex mixture design for three components. (**a**) coded variables; (**b**) ingredient concentration (%)

8.4 Gluten Free Pasta Production

Pasta production process consists of some consecutive steps: mixing, kneading, shaping, drying and packaging (Giannetti et al. 2021). Mixing step aims to uniformly distribute liquids into the solids and to allow the hydration of the flour particles, since the dispersion and interactions of the ingredients are fundamental to the final product (Alamprese 2017; Gulia et al. 2014). During kneading, starch granules absorb water slowly but starch swelling, and gelatinization are limited due to the low temperature of the process (<50 °C) (De Noni and Pagani 2010). Mixing and kneading are usually followed by dough resting to let further hydration of flour particles and redistribution of water in the dough system (Gulia et al. 2014). Once the ingredients have been properly mixed, kneaded and rested, they undergo a shaping process that is done either by lamination, extrusion, or extrusion-cooking. The extrusion processes are commonly used for dry pasta production, whereas lamination is more suited for fresh, sheeted, and possibly filled pasta products (Alamprese 2017). During shaping stage, the ingredients are chemically and physically transformed as function of the treatment conditions. Finally, the product is dried to extend its shelf-life, trying to keep its technological and nutritional characteristics (Palavecino et al. 2020).

8.4.1 *Extrusion and Extrusion-Cooking Processes*

In GF foods starch plays a key role due to the absence of a gluten matrix. The most common method to improve GF pasta quality is to modify starch structure and functionality (Padalino et al. 2016). As starch assumes a structuring role related to the tendency of amylose and amylopectin molecules to re-associate and interact after gelatinization, heat-treated flours are usually used in GF pasta. Through heating and cooling stages, it is possible to form a rigid network of retrograded starch (Larrosa et al. 2016). Hot-plate and microwave methods for pre-gelatinizing GF flours have been tested and the results showed firmer noodles with less dry matter loss by microwave pre-gelatinization, whereas the hot-plate method showed greater starch gelatinization and retrogradation (Suhendro et al. 2000). Although starch retrogradation is commonly considered a negative phenomenon in food production, it could positively affect the quality of extruded pasta products as starch retrogradation is often associated with an increase in firmness and springiness after cooking. In fact, the production of traditional rice noodles involves cooling cycles in order to decrease stickiness and prevent the dissolution of solid matter into the boiling water (Marti et al. 2011). On the other hand, there is a second technological approach to improve GF pasta called extrusion-cooking process, in which native flour is treated with steam and extruded for a short time at high temperatures (above 100 °C) in order to promote starch gelatinization directly inside the extruder-cooker (Marti and Pagani 2013). During extrusion-cooking food components undergo significant physical and chemical changes. By properly selecting the process parameters (temperature, water content and processing time), the starch present in the mass becomes entirely gelatinized and cooked (Moscicki 2011). In this way, the crystalline starch macromolecules are converted into an amorphous material able to produce a malleable product (Padalino et al. 2016). Depending on the nature and content of starch in the formulation, extrusion-cooking parameters are varied. In the case of a mixture with cereal starch, the working temperature in the gel unit of the extruder is set between the range 90–150 °C, and in the forming unit (where pasta is cooled and shaped) between 65 and 90 °C. Furthermore, it is important to stablish the moisture content of the mixture from 25% to 40% since it determines dough viscosity. High moisture would produce a very sticky dough and result in noodles with low firmness, and low dough moisture may produce cracked surface in the noodles (Moscicki 2011; Palavecino et al. 2020). When extrusion-cooking process is used to obtain expanded products, the range of temperatures and moistures used are different (temperature above 150 °C and moisture lower than 18%) because a high degree of cooking is desired, while in the case of GF pasta, expansion should be avoided, and a low degree of cooking have to be used (lower temperatures and moisture content high enough to avoid too much friction) (Merayo et al. 2011). Wang et al. 2016 showed that the extrusion conditions such as extrusion temperature and screw speed influence the quality of the extruded GF brown rice pasta and the extrusion system parameters, such as die pressure and motor torque, which could also influence the final product quality. Cooking loss decrease sharply with increasing temperature and screw speed. The faster screw, the higher temperature, which strengthens the stability of the retrograded starch network, decreasing the cooking loss. Additionally, water absorption decreases significantly with increasing temperature, but remains constant as the screw speed increases. This was attributed to the formation of new retrograded amylose structures and amylose-lipid complexes which favour the structural stability of pasta, restricting the dissolution of starch and GF pasta hydration. Regarding to textural characteristics, hardness and adhesiveness increase with increasing temperature and screw speed. On the other hand, Bouasla et al. 2016 showed that the screw speed and moisture content-screw speed interaction had a high significant effect on water absorption content and acceptability of rice-yellow pea cooked pasta. Also, a significant effect was observed for screw speed on hardness and adhesiveness. Finally, the selection of suitable dies has a huge impact not only on the shape but also on the functional characteristics and quality of the finished product (Moscicki 2011). Therefore, it is important to test the processing parameters depending on the type of raw material used for the pasta since they have an influence on the quality of the finished product. Extrusion-cooking has been successfully applied for production of pasta based on different GF cereal sources such as corn flour (Giménez et al. 2013; Merayo et al. 2011), pea flour (Wang et al. 1999), rice flour (Marti et al. 2011), brown rice flour (Wang et al. 2016), or flour combinations such as rice-yellow pea (Bouasla et al. 2016), rice-buckweat (Bouasla and Wójtowicz 2019), rice-amaranth (Cabrera-Chávez et al. 2012), maize-rice-sorghum (Toledo et al. 2019).

Marti and Pagani (2013) applied both pre-heated flour and extrusion-cooking processes to native rice flour, without additives or structuring ingredients, to make GF pasta. Pasta prepared from pre-gelatinized flour showed higher firmness compared to that of pasta from single-screw extrusion-cooking of native flour. In fact, the ultrastructure images highlighted differences in starch arrangement inside the two products. At the beginning of cooking, pasta from pre-gelatinized flour showed a compact and homogeneous matrix while the immersion of extruded-cooked pasta from native rice flour in hot water brought a great disruption of surface structure, a higher water absorption and the lower firmness. In addition, some starch aggregates were still recognizable in those pasta made by extrusion-cooking of native rice.

Although the benefits of using pre-gelatinized flours or extrusion-cooking methods are strongly documented and proved, research on GF products is also advancing with the goal of reducing steps, ingredients or temperature, using alternative materials, and lowering processing costs. Shukla et al. (2021) performed rice pasta enriched with pulse and fava protein isolates without a pre-gelatinization step and by a cold extrusion process. From a technical perspective these authors could create cold-extruded GF pasta, nevertheless, further optimization is necessary to reach similar physicochemical and sensory characteristics to the regular glutenous pasta. Chillo et al. (2010) investigated the effect of repeated cold extrusion steps (<46 °C) on the sensory characteristics of GF amaranth, oat and quinoa dried spaghetti. The doughs were obtained by pre-gelatinizing a portion of the flours because the manufacture of pasta based solely on native flours presented difficulties during the spaghetti extrusion step. The repeated extrusion processing method promoted the formation of a more strength structure in the dried spaghettis. Nevertheless, the application of shear stress without the combination of high temperature was not enough to promote further starch gelatinization and, consequently, there was no improvement in the sensory quality of the cooked pasta.

The use of proteins in the formulation of GF pasta is being studied in order not only to improve the nutritional value of the product but also to improve the technological aptitude of the formulation and the quality of the final product. Detchewa et al. (2022) made GF rice spaghetti by extrusion-cooking process in absence of gums or additives but with the substitution of a part of rice flour with rice protein. With the addition of rice proteins, rice flour gel became softer because proteins embedded between the starch granules reduced the reassociation of starch macromolecules in starch gel. The consequence was the production of more porous noodles with better cooking quality and better overall acceptability than those made only with rice flour.

8.4.2 *Laminating Process*

The technological process adopted in GF pasta production as well as the raw materials used have a significant influence on the quality of the final product. The most traditional way to produce wheat pasta is through laminating, a process in which the sheeting provides energy that promotes the formation of the gluten network, which imparts its particular rheological properties and encloses starch granules. However, in GF formulations, it is necessary to replace o re-create the elastic and malleable properties of the wheat dough with other ingredients, additives, or technologies since the lack of gluten leads to fragile and crumbly dough with poor performance (Palavecino et al. 2020). As previously mentioned, one of the most common techniques to produce GF pasta is to use pre-gelatinized starch in which a rigid network created by retrograded starch is formed (Larrosa et al. 2016). In laminated pasta, there is no possibility of a starch gelatinization process during the pasta shaping, so pre-treated flour is usually used. An alternative procedure to the pre-gelatinization of starch involves the addition of other ingredients, such as proteins (Sofi et al. 2020a, b) and hydrocolloids (Chauhan et al. 2017; Loubes et al. 2016; Milde et al. 2020) or the combination of both (Larrosa et al. 2012), to mimic the viscoelastic properties of gluten proteins and achieve the desirable quality attributes through their ability to bind water, forms gels, and control the viscosity (Lorenzo et al. 2018).

In the laminating process, after mixing the ingredients, the dough is compressed between rolls to form a continuous dough sheet. The sheeting process is intended to achieve a smooth dough sheet with desired thickness. The thickness of dough sheet is reduced gradually to avoid damage of the surface. With each successive pass, the roll diameter should decrease gradually so that compression distance and pressure are also reduced (Gulia et al. 2014). As reported by Guillermic et al. 2017, the lamination process is a source of bubble entrapment. These authors studied the difference in the bubble entrapment when the number of lamination steps varied since the presence of bubbles will affect the quality of the manufactured noodles, the drying performance and the texture of the cooked product. The number of lamination steps during manufacturing had a marked effect on the number of bubbles and the bubble size distribution in noodle dough sheets. Besides, bubbles were distributed non-uniformly inside the noodle dough sheets. In general, their number was higher in the middle of the dough sheet, mainly in those which were laminated multiple times. Once the dough is sheeted, it is cut into noodle strands of the desired width with a slitter (Gulia et al. 2014).

Some researchers (Carini et al. 2009; Salimi Khorshidi et al. 2018; Zardetto and Dalla Rosa 2009) have studied the effect of different shaping modes (lamination and extrusion) on the physical-chemical, sensory, mechanical and textural characteristics of fresh semolina or wheat flour pasta, but there is still a luck of this type of comparative information on GF pasta.

8.4.3 Pasta Drying

Dry pasta is one of the most important staple foods consumed in the world. Pasta drying involves heat transfer to reduce the moisture content from around 30% to an approximate range of 12–14% (Alamprese 2017). Drying is the last unit operation in pasta production before packaging and is a technological strategy to ensure microbiological stability, to facilitate its transportation, commercialization, stock management and consumer handling. During drying process several modifications of main constituents can take place, which results in drying being a crucial operation for the pasta quality. Fresh pasta typically has a water activity (aw) of 0.92–0.97 and a moisture content of 26–34% (Manthey et al. 2008; Schebor and Chirife 2000). The higher water activity predisposes the fresh pasta to chemical and microbiological degradation; therefore, it can be stored only for 2–3 days (refrigerated) or 2–3 months (frozen), depending on the temperature of storage. If fresh pasta is pasteurized and packaged in a modified atmosphere its shelf life can be extended up to around 40 days of refrigerated storage (Sanguinetti et al. 2016), or it can be irradiated and kept at room temperature for 90 days (Cassares et al. 2020), but it is still less than the shelf life of dry pasta.

In regard to the pasta production method, the extrusion process is rather used for dry pasta production, whereas lamination is more convenient for fresh sheeted pasta products. Drying technological parameters such as temperature, humidity, and air velocity depend on product shape, dimension, and initial humidity (Alamprese 2017). The drying process generally involves a pre-drying stage to rapidly reduce moisture from 30% to 17–18%, this step favours the creation of a solid film on the surface of pasta, thus preventing structural collapses and sticking phenomena. During drying a protocol of alternate steps of hot air drying and tempering time is usually applied to obtain a stable product. During tempering, water molecules diffuse from the core to the surface of the pasta, minimizing moisture gradients and internal structural tensions that could result in cracking of the dried pasta (Alamprese 2017). There are different types of drying processes: low temperature (below 60 °C) – long time (24–60 h) drying processes, preferred in low scale or traditional production, and high temperature (>60 °C) or very high temperature (≥100 °C) – short time (3–10 h) drying conditions, suitable for larger industrial productions (Alamprese 2017). Since the higher the temperature, the lower the drying time, higher temperature processes have a positive impact on productivity (De Noni and Pagani 2010).

The application of high temperature during the drying process has been shown to perform the cooking quality of wheat pasta (Cubadda et al. 2007). By applying low temperatures drying, cooking quality is related to the protein (gluten) quality rather than its content, while in the case of high temperature drying, only the amount of protein is responsible for pasta quality. The results are analogous in GF pasta. At higher drying temperature (80–100 °C) and longer duration of pre-drying (2–4 h, 40 °C) certain parameters such as cooking loss and protein solubility decrease, indicating greater structural integrity of the pasta. The greater energy input, provided by the high drying temperature and the long pre-drying time, improves all texture properties and allows the firmness to be increased to values comparable to wheat pasta, however, it is still a challenge to reach the elasticity values of wheat pasta (D'Amico et al. 2015). When the traditional drying process at low temperature (<60 °C) is applied, a less organized protein network is produced and no modifications of the inner structure of starch granules is detected. Nevertheless, structural changes do not depend exclusively on the maximum temperature reached during the drying cycle, but also on its length (De Noni and Pagani 2010). Since high protein contents improve cooking quality, egg albumen was shown to enhance texture and cooking properties of GF pasta (GF pasta), because egg proteins form a network which can produce a cohesive mass with a good consistency even in the absence of gluten (Alamprese et al. 2007; Schoenlechner et al. 2010). On the other hand, high temperature drying could also contribute to modify the macromolecular structure and functionality of the starch improving the GF pasta quality.

Another feature to be considered after the drying process is the cooling step. It is important for pasta to remain in the drier until it is cooled near to room temperature in order to prevent cracking of the pasta. The cooling period from the maximum temperature of drying to room temperature can last several hours (2–5 h), depending on the drying temperature (D'Amico et al. 2015).

It should be mentioned that some publications reported the use of microwaves for the pasta drying process. Physical, textural and cooking properties of pasta dried with combined hot air/microwave drying processes were found to be equal to or better than those dried with hot air. Also, hot air/microwave combination shortened the drying time (Altan and Maskan 2004). Compared with conventional drying methods whereby heat is transported from the surface to the centre, heating on a microwave field is 10–20 times faster. The shorter drying time is due to the additional energy input and rapid heat penetration of microwaves. However, at present no industrial plants are reported to use this drying method (Sicignano et al. 2014).

Although drying process carries benefits related to manipulation, storage time and microbiological stability, the high temperature-short time system generally can strongly affect not only the sensorial properties but also the nutritional value of the finished product (De Noni and Pagani 2010). The high temperature process promotes heat damage, mostly related to changes in the colour of the pasta (Acquistucci 2000), the loss of bioavailability of some essential amino acids such as lysine, and the formation of volatile compounds responsible for the occurrence of off-flavour (Giannetti et al. 2021). During drying process pasta reaches aw values of 0.70–0.80, optimal for occurring Maillard reaction and the release of melanoidins end products (De Noni and Pagani 2010). The heat damage can be monitored and evaluated by furosine or maltulose determinations which arises from the early stage of Maillard reaction (García-Baños et al. 2004; Gasparre et al. 2019), ε-pyrrole-lysine and glucosylisomaltol both produced during the advanced stage (De Noni and Pagani 2010). Stuknyte et al. 2014, found more heat damage resulting from high temperature than from low temperature pasta drying process by means of furosine amount. Acquistucci 2000 showed that more furosine is formed when high temperature is applied at the beginning of the process when pasta still has a moisture content around 18% than if the highest temperature is applied at the final drying cycles when the moisture has already reached 13%. As mentioned above these results are related to the water activity of samples that affects the reaction rate and the products formed.

Table 8.1 shows examples of some methods used in GF pasta making and drying.

Table 8.1 Formulations of fresh rice noodles for the selection of functional ingredients

Ingredients	Formulations							
(g/100 g dough)	F1	F2	F3	F4	F5	F6	F7	F8
Rice flour	47.37	46.45	50.00	46.45	50.00	46.45	46.45	–
Gelatinized rice flour	5.26	5.16	–	5.16	–	5.16	5.16	–
Xanthan gum	–	1.94	–	–	–	–	–	–
Gelatinized cassava starch	–	–	5.00	–	–	–	–	–
HPMC[a]	–	–	–	1.94	–	–	–	–
Gelatinized corn starch	–	–	–	–	5.00	–	–	–
Guar gum	–	–	–	–	–	1.94	–	–
Espina corona gum	–	–	–	–	–	–	1.94	–
Reference[b]	–	–	–	–	–	–	–	60.24
Water	47.37	46.45	45.00	46.45	45.00	46.45	46.45	39.76
Total	100	100	100	100	100	100	100	100

Source: Loubes et al. (2016)
[a]hydroxy propyl methyl cellulose (E464)
[b]Durum wheat semolina

8.4.4 *Process Optimization by RSM*

Wang et al. (1999) investigated the effects of four extrusion variables on properties of pea-based pasta, by means of RSM method. A high temperature extrusion was performed in a twin-screw co-rotating extruder. A low temperature extrusion (room temperature) in a single screw extruder was adopted as control. Pasta was dried at room temperature to reach 10% of moisture content. A fractional factorial design 2^3 was employed to study the effects of moisture content of dough (MC: 24.3, 28.2, 32%), extrusion temperature (T: 90, 100, 110 °C), screw speed (SS: 100, 125, 150 rpm), and feed rate of pea flour (FR: 22.7, 27.3, 31.8 kg/h), on brightness (B), bulk density (BD), cooking loss (CL), stickiness (S), cooking time (Ct) and firmness (F) of the pasta. The mathematical model (Eq. 8.1) included the linear effect of process variables and the interactions of MC with T, SS and FR. The model provided a satisfactory fit of the different studied responses ($R^2 > 0.97$). Increasing MC and T decreased B, BD and CL but increased Ct and F. In other hand, S increased with increasing T but decreased with MC growing. A positive effect of SS was observed on CL, S, Ct and F, however for B and BD a negative influence of SS was found. In contrast, the influence of FR on the responses was significantly lower. To obtain pasta with good textural and cooking attributes, the optimal conditions were MC = 30%, T = 110 °C, and SS = 125 rpm. In comparison with wheat spaghetti, the optimal pea-pasta was more red and more yellow, its cooking weight was similar to control; it had shorter cooking times, was firmer and less sticky, but its CL value was higher (20.5% vs. 7.8% for wheat control). Quality of pasta obtained by low temperature extrusion was lower (inferior integrity, flavour and texture) in comparison with high temperature extruded pasta.

D'Amico et al. (2015) investigated the effect of high drying temperature (60, 80 and 100 °C) and pre-drying time (0, 2 and 4 h) at 40 °C (low temperature drying) on pasta attributes (cooking behaviour, texture properties, protein solubility) adopting wheat pasta as control. These authors adopted a factorial design (9 experimental points) and they applied the RSM methodology to quantify the mentioned effects. The drying time was set for each temperature to have a similar overall energy input; 5 h at 60 °C, 1.6 h at 80 °C, and 1 h at 100 °C). The same criterion was adopted for cooling stage at 30 °C (2 h from 60 °C, 4.5 h from 80 °C, and 5 h from 100 °C), which was performed after drying to avoid pasta cracking. Two GF pasta formulations were evaluated. The formula 8.1 (F1) involved flours of amaranth (20%), quinoa (20%) and buckwheat (60%) while the formula 8.2 (F2) was a blend of millet flour (70%) and white bean flour (30%). Both formulation and control also included egg (6%), emulsifier (1%) and water (water to flour mass ratio: 31–33.3).

By RSM a significant and positive effect (p-value <0.05) of drying temperature on tensile strength (F1) and firmness (F1, F2) were determined. The effects were more marked in formula 8.1. Pre-drying time affected the values of tensile strength (F2) and firmness (F2). Formula 8.2 showed higher firmness than formula 8.1, probably due to its higher protein content; the observed differences were also attributed to the differences in the amino acid profile of both recipes. At higher drying temperature, cooking loss and protein solubility decreased. Good quality pasta was obtained, however in all cases the elasticity was inferior to the wheat reference. As a resume, higher drying temperature is recommended to enhance product texture lowering cooking loss and reducing process costs.

8.5 Strategies to Address the Development of Formulations

A common strategy is to search for a GF pasta recipe and try to adapt it. However, it is not as simple as it seems because each flour and functional ingredient has its own effect in the formula and a small modification can affect the product characteristics. It is therefore advisable to consider this strategy only as a starting point for formulation developing. There are two stages for the formulation progress: (1) selection of ingredient by preliminary tests; (2) optimization of the formulation by mixture design.

8.5.1 Selection of Ingredients

At this stage, the basic requirements for product development must be considered. Is a rice-based noodle required? Is a noodle based on mixtures of rice and corn needed? Is it intended to substitute part of the rice flour with flours from other grains (quinoa, amaranth, buckwheat, millet or canary seed, among others), legume flours (beans, lentils) or protein or bran fractions from different sources? The availability of raw material and resources should also be taken into account in this step. Preliminary tests can be planned to select flours and functional ingredients based on their performance in producing quality pastas. These tests will allow limiting the experimental region, i.e. limiting the ingredients and their proportions to the most promising combinations. This proposal will facilitate the later implementation of the mixture design (second step) to optimize the formulation.

Loubes et al. (2016) evaluated the effect of several gluten substitutes based on tensile strength tests of cooked noodles in order to select the best ones for the development of a rice-based GF pasta. Wheat-based pasta was adopted as reference (control). Each rice noodle formulation including rice flour obtained by planetary ball-milling, water and each functional ingredient are shown in Table 8.2. The authors recommended adding the amount of water to obtain an easily laminated dough for each mixture. Due to its pregelatinized character (starch gelatinization degree of 62.1%) and particle size (D50: 131.1 ± 1.6 μm between 100 and 150 μm), the ball- milled rice flour resulted very suitable to obtain a firm microstructure and therefore good quality noodles (Yeh 2004).

Gelatinized corn and cassava starches, gelatinized rice flour and binary blends of gelatinized rice flour and one of the following hydrocolloids: HPMC, xanthan gum, guar gum and espina corona (*Gleditsia amorphoides*) gum were tested as gluten substitutes. The values of σ_b (stress at break) and ε_b (strain at break) are shown for the tested formulations and control in Fig. 8.3a, b respectively. In comparison with the reference (ε_b: 27 ± 4%), a significant decrease ($p < 0.05$) in strain at break was observed for cassava starch (55%), corn starch (59%), HPMC (55%) and espina corona gum (73%). In relation to formulation F1 (only rice flour, gelatinized rice flour and water); the addition of gums or gelatinized corn starch caused an increase of mechanical parameters in accordance with literature reports (Larrosa et al. 2013; Huang et al. 2001; Marti et al. 2012; Sozer 2009). Based on the results shown in Fig. 8.3, the formulations F2, F5 and F6 resulted the most promising formulations. Therefore, gelatinized corn starch, xanthan gum and guar gum can be chosen as appropriate functional ingredients to be added in a blend based on ball-milled rice flour and gelatinized rice flour.

Other objective in preliminary test is to select the more suitable proportion or range of a given ingredient. In this case, essays with different amounts of target ingredient are planned to study its effect on product properties. Some cases found in the literature are discussed below.

Bouasla et al. (2017) evaluated different levels (10, 20, 30 g/100 g) of legumes flours (yellow pea, chickpea and lentil) as ingredient of rice-based spaghetti obtained by extrusion-cooking method. These authors found that addition of legumes flours up to 30 g/100 g led to good quality pasta with low cooking loss (<6%) without change in cooking time (8–9 min). The expansion ratio, hardness and lightness decreased as legume flours content increased while firmness and adhesiveness increased.

Effects of partial replacement (0, 15, 30, 45, 60%) of rice flour by buckwheat flour on quality attributes of GF noodles were investigated by Fu et al. (2020). At replacement of 30% the formation of more integrated starch network was observed

Table 8.2 Technological options used in GF pasta making and drying

Author	Flour/starch	Type of pasta	Forming method	Drying method
Detchewa et al. (2022)	Rice flour and rice protein concentrate powder	Spaghettis	Extrusion. Single-screw extruder (50 °C, 90 °C, 90 °C and 90 °C)	Hot air oven at 50 °C until a final moisture of 12%
Shukla et al. (2021)	Rice flour and pulse protein isolates	Lasagna	Extrusion. Single-screw extruder	Food dehydrator for 6 h at 74 °C. Final moisture: 7.4–8.7%
D'Amico et al. (2015)	Amaranth, quinoa and buckwheat flour	Noodle and lasagna sheets	Extrusion	Pre-drying and drying at different conditions. Pre-drying at 40 °C for 0, 2 and 4 h. Drying at 60 (5 h), 80 (1.6 h) or 100 °C (1 h). After drying pasta was to 30 °C before removing them from the oven
Wang et al. (1999)	Pea flour	Spaghetti	Extrusion-cooking. Twin-screw extruder (30-90-90-100-95-95 °C). Moisture: 18–23%	Ambient temperature. Final moisture: 10%
Giménez et al. (2013)	Corn and broad bean flour	Spaghetti	Extrusion-cooking. Single-screw extruder (80, 90 or 100 °C). Moisture: 28, 31 or 34%	40 °C and 40% relative humidity for 16 h
Merayo et al. (2011)	Corn flour	Spaghetti	Extrusion-cooking. Single-screw extruder (80, 90 or 100 °C). Moisture: 27, 31 or 35%	40 °C and 60% relative humidity for 16 h
Wang et al. (2016)	Brown rice flour	Macaroni	Extrusion-cooking. Twin-screw extruder (70-70-(100, 110 or 120)-70-50). Moisture: 28%	Fluidized bed dryer at 45 °C for 65–80 min. Final moisture: <15%
Bouasla et al. (2016)	Rice and yellow pea flours	Spaghetti	Extrusion-cooking. Single screw extruder (90-100-70 °C)	Air oven at 40 °C for 4 h. final moisture: 12%
Chillo et al. (2010)	Amaranth, quinoa and oat flours	Spaghetti	Four repeated steps of cold extrusion (<46 °C)	Step I: 50 °C for 30 min Step II: 85 °C for 400 min Step I: 50 °C for 30 min

(continued)

Table 8.2 (continued)

Author	Flour/starch	Type of pasta	Forming method	Drying method
Marti et al. (2011)	Parboiled rice flour	–	Extrusion (<55 °C) Extrusion cooking (115 °C for pre-treatment) Water content: 40%	Drying cell using low-temperature drying cycle (50 °C for 14 h)
Larrosa et al. (2016)	Corn flour and corn starch	Tagliatelle and lasagna	Lamination	(Fresh pasta)
Loubes et al. (2016)	Rice flour	Noodles	Lamination	(Fresh pasta)
Oupathumpanont and Wisansakkul (2021)	Banana flour and modified starch	Noodles	Lamination	Hot air oven at 60 °C until a final moisture of 10%
Choobthaisong and Oupathumpanont (2021)	Brown rice powder, modified starch *cladophora* spp. powder	Macarroni	Lamination	Hot air oven at 60 °C until a final moisture of 10%
Milde et al. (2020)	Cassava starch and corn flour	Spaghetti	Lamination	(Fresh pasta)

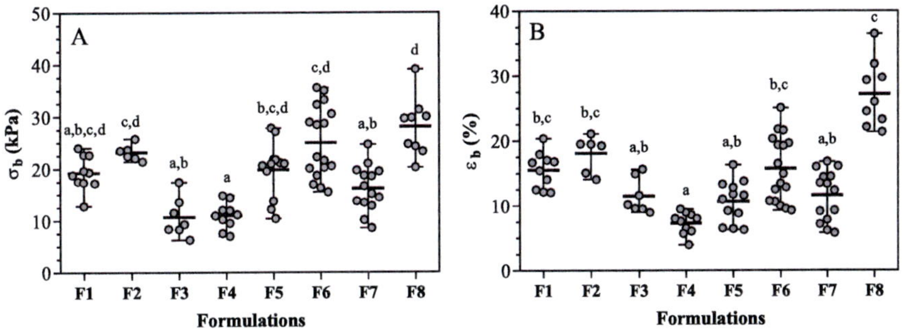

Fig. 8.3 Mechanical properties of cooked rice noodle as function of pasta composition (F1: gelatinized rice flour, F2: gelatinized rice flour and xanthan gum, F3: gelatinized cassava starch, F4: gelatinized rice flour and HPMC, F5: gelatineze corn starch, F6: gelatinized rice flour and guar gum, F7: gelatinized rice flour and espina corona gum, F8: control). a) stress at break (σ_b), b) strain at break (ε_b). (Source: Loubes et al. 2016)

by SEM analysis, together with beneficial effects on product quality. Among others good attributes, the optimal product presented a low glycaemic index; besides it was observed the lowest values of cooking loss and broken rate of extruded noodles and, the higher retention rate of polyphenols and flavonoids after extrusion cooking for 30% substitution level.

Jeong et al. (2017) tested three rice flours with different amylose contents (12, 19, and 26%) to be blended with zein (corn protein) as gluten substitute, in order to select the mixture that rendered the best quality rice noodles obtained by lamination-cutting processes. These authors observed a significant effect of amylose content on mixing properties of rice-zein dough. High amylose rice-zein mixture (26%) had, in comparison with the other samples, higher values of pasting parameters and storage modulus, indicating greater elastic properties, as well as higher water absorption. As regards the noodles quality, high amylose noodles showed a firm texture (greater breaking stress and resistance to extension) that contributed to their reduced cooking loss.

When the combination of many ingredients is required, different series of experiments are usually planned to perform a stepwise screening. It is laborious task, but necessary in these cases. The most promising combinations are selected in each series and the worst ones are discarded.

This strategy was developed by Linares-García et al. (2019), who evaluated the combination of extruded (EQ) and non-extruded (NEQ) quinoa flour (red and white) with potato starch, tara gum (*Caesalpinia spinose*), egg white and vegetable protein from different sources (potato, pea and rice protein isolates). Three series of experiments were performed. In the first series, the use of EQ and NEQ was contrasted, as well as the need to add or not to add tara gum. As a result, NEQ was eliminated. In the second series of experiments, the effect of replacing egg white with lupine flour was studied. It was found that lupine flour (6–12%) was insufficient to replace egg white. In addition, it was decided to discard the tara gum because it reduced the firmness of the pasta. In the third series of experiments, the content of lupine four was increased to 30% because its protein is complementary to the quinoa protein. The effects of adding vegetable proteins (potato, pea or rice protein) and the oxidizing enzyme-Pox to quinoa flour-lupine flour mixture (70/30) were investigated. Since the firmness of the quinoa pasta decreased when potato or rice proteins were added, these protein sources were discarded. Addition of the enzyme-Pox could even further improve pasta firmness. The optimal mixture containing quinoa (70%) and lupine (30%) flours, pea protein (12%) and enzyme-Pox (1%) lead to noodles with good nutritional quality (GF and egg-free), high protein (27.9%) and dietary fibre (15.2%) contents.

8.5.2 *Optimization of Formulation by Mixture Design*

This analysis is applied to optimize the formulation. It is based on the selection of an appropriate mixture design to study the effect of the blend ingredients on product attributes as well as to notice interactions between ingredients that may be or not beneficial to product quality.

Simplex centroid design (Fig. 8.2) based on seven combinations was adopted by Loubes et al. (2016) to optimize rice noodle formulation. The effect of concentrations (expressed as percentages in dry basis) of three functional ingredients:

gelatinized corn starch (GCS as c_1), guar gum (GG as c_2) and xanthan gum (XG as c_3) on texture and cooking properties were analysed. Experimental points are shown as function of coded values (Fig. 8.2a) and, in terms of dry basis ingredient percentages (Fig. 8.2b). The sum of the functional ingredients was constrained at 8.5%, while ball-milled rice flour (86.7%) and gelatinized rice flour (4.8%) were constant. Water was added to have 0.9 g water/g (dry basis) in all combinations tested. Higher water contents produced a sticky dough, and lower water amount results in defective lamination process. These authors, based on preliminary trials, defined the experimental region by adopting 0% and 3.7% as lower and upper bound for both, XG and GG. Experimental range for GCS was 4.8–8.5% as it was obtained from the mass balance taking into account the adopted constrain ($c_1 + c_2 + c_3 = 8.5\%$ or $x_1 + x_2 + x_3 = 1$).

Effects of ingredient concentrations on texture and cooking parameters were satisfactorily modelled (R^2: 0.94–0.97) by means of cubic model (Eq. 8.5); the results are shown in Fig. 8.4. Although several values of stress at break were similar to wheat control ($\sigma_b = 28 \pm 4$ kPa), all values of strain at break and the values of cooking loss resulted worse in comparison to wheat control ($\varepsilon_b = 27 \pm 4\%$; CL = $7.4 \pm 1.4\%$).

Mathematical expressions for stress at break (Eq. 8.6), strain at break (Eq. 8.7) and cooking loss (Eq. 8.8) are presented as function of concentration considering that: $c_1 = 3.7\,x_1 + 4.8$, $c_2 = 3.7\,x_2$, and $c_3 = 3.7\,x_3$. As concentration percentages (c_i,

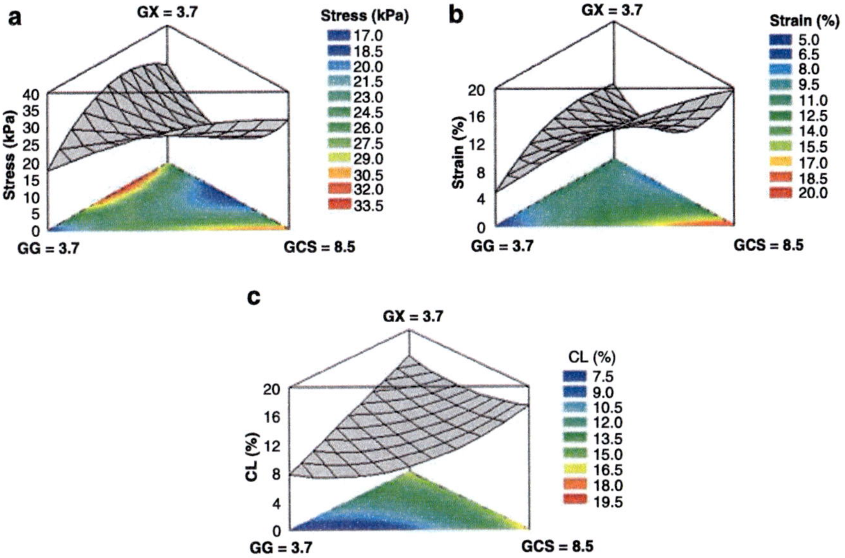

Fig. 8.4 Surface plots of selected mechanical and cooking properties of cooked rice noodle as function of pasta composition. Gelatinized corn starch (GCS: 4.8–8.5%), guar gum (GG: 0–3.7%), xanthan gum (XG: 0–3.7%). a) stress at break, b) strain at break, c) cooking loss (CL). (Source: Loubes et al. 2016)

c_j, c_k) are adopted instead of coded variables (x_i, x_j, x_k), the equations show a constant term in contrast with Eq. (8.5):

$$\sigma_{b(kPa)=} -41.2 + 8.6c_1 - 1.1c_2 + 24.9c_3 + 1.2c_1c_2 - 3.6c_1c_3 + 13.3c_2c_3 - 2.2c_1c_2c_3 \quad (8.6)$$

$$\varepsilon_{b(\%)=} -25.5 + 5.3c_1 - 1.6c_2 + 12.2c_3 + 0.61c_1c_2 - 1.9c_1c_3 + 0.8c_2c_3 \quad (8.7)$$

$$CL_{(\%)=} -22.7 + 4.8c_1 + 8.5c_2 + 7.3c_3 - 1.3c_1c_2 - 0.6c_1c_3 - 6.1c_2c_3 + 1.3c_1c_2c_3 \quad (8.8)$$

The significant interaction coefficients (p-value <0.05, in bold) reflect the synergistic effects between gums (Fig. 8.4a) and antagonist effects among GCS and gums (Fig. 8.4a–c).

By maximizing strain at break (ε_b = 17.9%) and at the same time minimizing cooking losses (CL = 13%), the optimum combination (7.8% GCS, 0.7% GG) was obtained. This mixture also showed satisfactory values of water absorption (58.7%) and stress at break (σ_b = 31.5 kPa). The capacity of gelatinised rice flour and GCS to induce starch network formation was enhanced by the pregelatinised character of ball-milled rice flour. The use of gums in pasta formulated with ball-milled rice flour could be significantly reduced by substituting them partially with GCS, without reduction of noodle quality.

Bastos et al. (2016) adopted a simplex design with constrains to optimize the amounts of three selected ingredients in mixtures for fresh spaghetti production as an approach to recycle the wastes of potato chips industry. Amaranth flour (AF: 10–25%, [0–0.83]), dried potato pulp (DPP: 65–80%, [0–0.83]) and extruded potato pulp (EPP: 7–17%, [0–0.56]) were selected (coded compositions are shown in brackets). Spaghetti formula also included water 18.8 mL water and 56 g of fresh egg per 100 g mixture. The optimization criteria were short optimum cooking time, low loss of solids, intermediate mass increase due to water absorption after cooking, and low b* chromaticity coordinate for pasta before cooking. Considering that the sum of the three selected ingredients as 100%, the combination of 65% DPP, 10% EPP and 25% AF yielded fresh spaghetti with good colour and cooking characteristics. In comparison with wheat spaghetti (WS) a more yellowish colour was obtained, as well as a cooking time (2 min) 13% lower than WS, cooking loss (3.8%) 70% lower than WS, and water absorption (96.2%) 73% higher than WS. The authors concluded that the use of the wastes from potato chip production, proved to be highly successful for spaghetti making.

Larrosa et al. (2013) optimized, by using a mixture design, the formulation of laminated fresh corn-based noodles. The effect of formulation on extensibility and rheological properties of dough was investigated. Based on preliminary experiments, these authors selected combinations of gums (0.5–2.5%), proteins (0.7–6.7%), and water (35.5–39.5%), maintaining the sum of gums and proteins between 3.2 and 7.2%. The other ingredients: corn starch (42.8%), corn flour (10.7%), NaCl (1%), and sunflower oil (2.8%) remained constant. As gums, a mix of xanthan gum and locust bean gum (2:1) was adopted while as proteins, a blend of dry egg and dry egg-white (10:1) was selected.

When water, which plays a plasticizing role in the mix, is included as a component in the MD analysis, some points of the design may present difficulties in mixing or rolling steps. Therefore, the experimental region should be limited to the domain suitable for pasta production. In this case, a mixture design with constrains is appropriate and each component will be restricted by upper and lower bounds.

Larrosa et al. (2013) evaluated 12 formulations within a quadrangular region circumscribed into the triangular domain (Fig. 8.2). These authors found the desirable textural properties (the highest values of storage modulus (G′), breaking force, and extensibility) by using a formulation containing 35.5% water, 2.5% gums, and 4.7% proteins.

Choobthaisong and Oupathumpanont (2021) developed a GF pasta supplemented with *Cladophora* spp., a green alga which has high contents of protein (19.90%) and fibre (21.50%). The effects of brown rice flour (50–70%), modified starch (15–25%), and *Cladophora* spp. powder (10–20%) on physicochemical properties and consumer acceptance of pasta were analysed by MD method. Formulations evaluated (16) also included guar gum (0.05%), NaCl (0.05%), egg (2%), olive oil (2%), and water (20%). The highest levels of cutting and shearing force were found within a sub-region of the experimental range: 68–70% brown rice flour, 15–22% modified starch and 10–15% *Cladophora* spp. The higher amount of modified starch in these mixtures favoured dough cohesiveness and elasticity. The optimal mixture involved 68% of brown rice flour, 22% of modified starch, and 10% of *Cladophora* spp. This formulation provided 379 kcal/100 g of total energy, 7.09% of protein, 1.91% of dietary fibre, and antioxidant activity of 48.50 mg eq Trolox. Overall consumer preference was at moderate level (about 5) from sensory evaluation based on 9-point hedonic scale. A significant percentage (>85%) of the participants consider that the algae-supplemented pasta is a healthy product and expressed their interest in acquiring it.

8.6 Techniques to Extend the Shelf Life of Noodles

A wide variety of GF pasta, characterized by shape, composition, and moisture content, is produced around the world (Mariotti et al. 2011). The water content greatly determines the shelf life and storage conditions of products (Herawati and Kamsiati 2021). Dry pasta (maximum moisture content 12–14%) can be stored at room temperature and has a shelf life of over one year (Alamprese 2017; Schettino et al. 2020). The water activity should be below 0.65 to avoid any microbiological growth. However, some hydrophilic moulds can survive down to this a_w (Lorenzo et al. 2018). Conversely, fresh pasta (moisture between 26% and 34%) requires storage under refrigerated conditions and is easily perishable (Manthey et al. 2008). Fresh pasta spoilage is mainly due to the metabolic activity of bacteria, yeasts, and especially moulds, which negatively alter the sensorial characteristics of this food, limiting considerably the shelf life. In addition, the risk of these microorganisms being pathogenic could also product safety (Sanguinetti et al. 2015; Schettino et al.

2020). Common filamentous fungi, for example, *Alternaria*, *Aureobasidium*, *Cladosporium*, *Epicoccum*, *Fusarium*, *Helminthosporium*, *Claviceps*, *Aspergillus*, *Penicillium*, are derived from the field, post-harvest, or processing contamination (Oliveira et al. 2014).

In general, the industrial production of fresh pasta includes heat treatments after packaging to preserve the hygiene and quality of the product (Schettino et al. 2020). Pasteurization is among the most widely used methods in the food industry. Heating kills microorganisms, which considerably reduces the number of these in the food, improving its quality and prolonging its shelf life (Li et al. 2021). The operation is done with a specified time-temperature combination to achieve sufficient microbial inactivation (Sanguinetti et al. 2015). Pasteurization is generally carried out under normal pressure because high pressure will make fresh noodles stick together into a mass and modify the organoleptic characteristics (Li et al. 2021). After pasteurization immediately, the product must be cooled to 4 °C (Verma et al. 2020). Nevertheless, the thermal stress generally compromises the sensory characteristics of fresh pasta (Schettino et al. 2020). Unlike traditional heat treatments, the microwave does not require a heat-conducting medium and heats the product inside and outside simultaneously, reducing the undesirable effects of heat on food (Li et al. 2021). Thus, the use of microwaves to sterilize or pasteurize food has received increasing attention, and microwave technology has enjoyed a wider application. Microwaves with frequencies of 915 MHz and 2450 MHz are most used to kill pathogenic bacteria and the organisms responsible for food spoilage (Li et al. 2021; Verma et al. 2020). An increase in frequency leads to a decrease in the penetration depth, so 915 MHz microwaves have a deeper penetration depth than the 2450 MHz microwaves, therefore may provide more uniform heating (Verma et al. 2020). The mechanism for the inactivation of microorganisms by microwaves at sublethal temperatures includes both thermal and non-thermal effects, as penetrating microwaves cause deleterious biological effects in organisms after they have been subjected to a certain degree of radiation (Li et al. 2021; Chandrasekaran et al. 2013). Microwaves prolong the shelf life of food products while preserving nutritive qualities and maximizing flavour. Therefore, microwave sterilization can be successfully used with heat-sensitive GF pasta (Li et al. 2021).

However, other techniques can be applied, such as antimicrobial compounds addition in the dough and modified headspace conditions during packaging. Among chemical preservatives commonly used for improving microbial stability and extending the shelf life of fresh pasta include: potassium sorbate, calcium propionate, glyceryl monocaprylate, sodium diacetate and sodium dehydroacetate (Schettino et al. 2020; Li et al. 2021; Yang et al. 2021). Nevertheless, there are several human pathogenic fungi and spoilage moulds able to adapt to food preservatives due to their frequent use in industry (Oliveira et al. 2014). Nowadays, consumers increasingly request for more natural food (Del Nobile et al. 2009). For this reason, natural preservatives, such as chitosan, lemon extract, grapefruit seed extract, thymol, and lactic acid, have been investigated as GF pasta additives (Klinmalait et al. 2017; Del Nobile et al. 2009; Lu and Collado 2019). Moreover, transglutaminase, an enzyme often used in GF products to improve texture, has been evaluated, demonstrating its potential to extend the shelf life of fresh pasta (Kiyat et al. 2020). However, the use of latter additive is being questioned due to its undesirable effect on human health, especially in celiac patients (Lerner and Matthias 2020).

On the other hand, ozone treatments of pasta or raw materials have been reported as a green method to modify quality characteristics, suppress microbial growth, and extend the shelf life of fresh pasta (Zhu 2018). Varying packaging technologies are widely used in the food industry to extend the shelf life of products. Vacuum packaging is not suitable for fresh pasta due to the surface adhesion and deformation of noodles caused by the squeeze (Wang et al. 2018). Modified atmosphere packaging (MAP) is a well-tested and simple technology helpful for extending the shelf life of fresh pasta. MAP is achieved by using very low O_2 concentrations, high CO_2 concentrations (20% or higher) for its bacteriostatic and fungistatic activities, and N_2 as an inert filler and anti-packaging collapse gas (Sanguinetti et al. 2016).

Frozen storage can be used for the long-term preservation of pasta, maximizing its shelf life by reducing enzymatic and microbial activity. However, the ice crystal size within the food, which varies with freezing temperature, can result in a loss of textural properties throughout the storage period (Vieira et al. 2021).

Those strategies, alone or in combination, provide extensive and efficient preservation, thus assuring shelf-life periods ranging from 14 days to 6 months (Vieira et al. 2021; Sanguinetti et al. 2015, 2016; Yang et al. 2021; Kiyat et al. 2020).

At present, few studies have been executed to extend the shelf life of GF fresh pasta. Future research is needed to develop more effective and safer preservatives and explore the synergistic interactions among preservatives, temperature, physical treatment, and packaging technologies for the long-term storage of GF pasta.

8.7 Gluten Free Pasta Market

In recent years, the demand for GF products has increased considerably, either for health or lifestyle reasons, which has driven the growth of the GF pasta market. The global GF pasta market is estimated to reach a value of US$1.29 billion by the year 2025, registering a Compound Annual Growth Rate (CAGR) of 4.5% from 2018 to 2025 (Deshmukh and Thomas 2019).

The price of GF foods is one of the most considered factors for the selection of products, in addition to sensory characteristics (Hopkins and Soon 2019; Demirkesen and Ozkaya 2020).

Although the market for GF food is growing, it has not led to the expected transformation into lower product prices (Demirkesen and Ozkaya 2020), including pasta.

Data from around the world (Table 8.3) indicates that GF pasta is approximately two to six times more expensive than comparable gluten-containing products. Price differences between GF and gluten-containing products could be attributable to the higher cost of raw materials replacing the wheat used in GF production. The need

Table 8.3 Relative price of gluten-free (GF) and gluten-containing (GC) pasta by store and country

Authors	Country	Types of stores	Product	Monetary units	Gluten-containing (price/100 g)	GF (price/100 g)	GF/GC
Own source (2021)[a]	Argentina	Websites of supermarkets	Fusilli – Spaghetti	Argentine peso	13.68–14.69	45.33–38.13	3.31–2.60
da Silva et al. (2021)	Brazil	Online	Pasta and cereals	Euro	0.38	0.8	2.11
Jegede et al. (2021)	Canada	Grocery stores (national chain)	Pasta	Canadian dollar	0.47	0.88	1.87
Jegede et al. (2021)	Canada	Grocery stores (local chain)	Pasta	Canadian dollar	0.77	1.17	1.52
Panagiotou and Kontogianni (2017)	Greece	Supermarkets	Pasta	Euro	0.21	0.63	3.00
Panagiotou and Kontogianni (2017)	Greece	Pharmacies	Pasta	Euro	0.21	1.21	5.76
Mohd Fauad et al. (2020)	Malaysia	Grocery stores	Lasagna sheet – Spaghetti	Malaysia Ringgit	2.22–1.38	6.17–5.71	2.78–4.14
Arias-Gastelum et al. (2018)	Mexico	Supermarkets and health food stores	Lasagna sheet – Noodle	Mexican peso	9.20–11.80	35.20–31.50	3.83–2.67
Myhrstad et al. (2021)	Norway	Online and grocery stores	Pasta	Norwegian kroner	4.90	10.60	2.16
FACE (2021)	Spain	Hypermarket	Lasagna sheet – Noodle	Euro	0.4–0.09	1.06–0.34	2.67–3.78
Abdulla and Garemo (2018)	United Arab Emirates	Supermarkets	Pasta	Dirham	1.50	6.30	4.20
Hopkins and Soon (2019)	United Kingdom	Regular stores, health food shops and online	Pasta	Pound sterling	0.29	0.70	2.41
Lee et al. (2019)	United States	Mass-market	Pasta	United States dollar	0.46	0.99	2.15

[a]Data were collected in the month of October 2021

for more stringent quality controls to ensure the food safety of the final product, I + D to improve the nutritional quality and organoleptic properties of GF products, changes in the facilities and equipment used in the production line, among other additional costs that cannot be ignored (FACE 2021; Hopkins and Soon 2019).

Nowadays, GF manufacturers are yet smaller than their main market competitors (Demirkesen and Ozkaya 2020). It may be another relevant factor significantly affecting GF pasta costs. The need for different production lines to avoid the risk of cross-contamination (Demirkesen and Ozkaya 2020) may also influence the high prices of different types of GF pasta.

On the other hand, several studies have shown that price of GF pasta was affected by store class. Comparing the price of GF pasta available at supermarkets with the price of similar products available at pharmacies, this last was 92% higher in Greece (Table 8.3) (Panagiotou and Kontogianni 2017). Similarly, Hanci and Jeanes (2019) observed a significant difference in the price of GF pasta sold by different types of shopping venues in the United Kingdom. It was 47% higher in premium supermarkets compared with regular supermarkets. In the same way, GF pasta was 33% more costly at local stores than at chain stores in Canada (Table 8.3). Nevertheless, gluten-containing pasta was also concerned by this trend (Jegede et al. 2021). The price of GF products continues to be an economic burden for people who need to follow a GF diet, even though many countries provide some form of financial assistance to cover these expenses (Panagiotou and Kontogianni 2017; Myhrstad et al. 2021; Abdulla and Garemo 2018; Demirkesen and Ozkaya 2020). Hence, it is a challenge for food producers and technologists to reduce the production costs of GF pasta without detriment of sensory characteristics and improvement of nutritional quality.

8.8 Conclusions

The pasta production process includes extrusion or lamination shaping methods. The selection of ingredients and formulation will depend on the selected method. Extrusion is one of the most broadly used technologies; its main advantages are the ease of producing pasta through a continuous process with a minimal transformation of the ingredients and the versatility to produce a wide of different shapes. Obtaining good quality GF pasta by cool extrusion requires the use of structuring ingredients such as pre-gelatinized starch or flour, whereas the extrusion-cooking methods develop the retrograded starch three-dimensional network directly inside the extruder and it is possible to use native starch. Moisture content of the dough and extrusion conditions influence the quality of the GF pasta.

On the other hand, lamination is the most traditional method to produce pasta. As in cold extrusion, for the production of laminated GF pasta, it is very common to use pre-gelatinized ingredients that recreate the elastic properties of the gluten. In the sheeting method, lower variety of shapes can be obtained than in extrusion, nevertheless, it is a simple and inexpensive method.

Drying process turns pasta into a more stable product, with a longer shelf life. For the production of dry pasta, pasta made by extrusion is commonly used. The drying process at high temperature and short time is preferred in large industrial productions; however, it is important to control the heat damage, which can be monitored by Maillard reaction markers. Dry pasta can be stored at room temperature and has a shelf life of over one year. Conversely, fresh pasta requires storage under refrigerated conditions and is easily perishable. In general, the industrial production of fresh pasta includes heat treatments after packaging to preserve the safety and quality of the products. Other techniques can also be applied, such as antimicrobial compounds addition in the dough, modified headspace conditions during packaging, and frozen storage. These strategies, alone or in combination, can provide a shelf life of up to approximately 6 months.

The RSM method has proven to be useful to simulate the effect of process conditions on the pasta attributes. This methodology allows the optimization of the process in order to find the best conditions for obtaining good quality pasta. On the other hand, for the development of a suitable ingredient formulation, the mixture design analysis is an effective tool that takes into account the mass balance between the components of the mixture. Optimization is an iterative process that starts with preliminary screening tests to obtain an initial recipe, whose optimization will also affect the adjustment of the process variables.

Despite the growth of the GF pasta market, price differences between gluten-containing and GF products (associated with higher production costs of the latter) are still very significant, leading to an excessive economic burden for people suffering from gluten intolerance. Thus, it is a challenge for food manufacturers to reduce the production costs of GF pasta without detriment of organoleptic properties and improving nutritional quality.

Acknowledgments This work was supported by the Agencia Nacional de Promoción Científica y Tecnológica, ANPCyT, (PICT 2018–01619), CONICET, and the Universidad de Buenos Aires (UBACYT 20020170100367BA).

References

AACC (1999a) Method 66-50.01 pasta and noodle cooking quality-firmness approved methods of analysis, 11th edn. AACC International, St Paul. https://doi.org/10.1094/AACCIntMethod-66-50.01

AACC (1999b) Method 44-15.02 moisture: air-oven methods. Approved methods of analysis, 11th edn. AACC International, St Paul. https://doi.org/10.1094/AACCIntMethod-44-15.02

Abdulla A, Garemo M (2018) High cost of gluten-free products might be challenging for people with celiac disease in The United Arab Emirates. Int J Celiac Dis 6(2):37–41. https://doi.org/10.12691/ijcd-6-2-2

Acquistucci R (2000) Infuence of maillard reaction on protein modification and color development in pasta. Comparison of different drying conditions. LWT Food Sci Technol 33:48–52. https://doi.org/10.1006/fstl.1999.0606

Ahmed I, Mabood Qazi I, Li Z et al (2016) Rice noodles: materials, processing and quality evaluation. Proc Pak Acad Sci B Life Environ Sci 53(3):215–238

Alamprese C (2017) The use of egg and egg products in pasta production. In: Hester P (ed) Egg innovations and strategies for improvements. Academic, San Diego, pp 251–259

Alamprese C, Casiraghi E, Pagani M (2007) Development of gluten-free fresh egg pasta analogues containing buckwheat. Eur Food Res Technol 225:205–213. https://doi.org/10.1007/s00217-006-0405-y

Altan A, Maskan M (2004) Microwave assisted drying of short-cut (ditalini) macaroni: cooking process and textural properties. Food Sci Tech Int 10(3):0187–0110. https://doi.org/10.1177/1082013204044903

AOAC (1998) Method 991.43. Total, soluble, and insoluble dietary fibre in foods. AOAC official methods of analysis, 16th edn. AOAC international, Gaithersburg

Arias-Gastelum M, Cabrera-Chávez F, de Jesús M (2018) The gluten-free diet: access and economic aspects and impact on lifestyle. Nutr Diet Suppl 10:27–34. https://doi.org/10.2147/NDS.S143404

Bastos G, Soares Júnior M, Caliari M et al (2016) Physical and sensory quality of gluten-free spaghetti processed from amaranth flour and potato pulp. LWT Food Sci Technol 65:128–136. https://doi.org/10.1016/j.lwt.2015.07.067

Bouasla A, Wójtowicz A (2019) Rice-buckwheat gluten-free pasta: effect of processing parameters on quality characteristics and optimization of extrusion cooking process. Foods 8(10):496. https://doi.org/10.3390/foods8100496

Bouasla A, Wójtowicz A, Zidoune M et al (2016) Gluten-free precooked rice-yellow pea pasta: effect of extrusion-cooking conditions on phenolic acids composition, selected properties and microstructure. J Food Sci 81(5):C1070–C1079. https://doi.org/10.1111/1750-3841.13287

Bouasla A, Wójtowicz A, Zidoune M (2017) Gluten-free precooked rice pasta enriched with legumes flours: physical properties, texture, sensory attributes and microstructure. LWT Food Sci Technol 75:569–577. https://doi.org/10.1016/j.lwt.2016.10.005

Box G, Wilson K (1951) On the experimental attainment of optimum conditions. J R Stat Soc B 13:1–38. https://doi.org/10.1111/j.2517-6161.1951.tb00067.x

Brand-Williams W, Cuvelier M, Berset C (1995) Use of a free radical method to evaluate antioxidant activity. Lebensmittel-Wissenschaft Tech 28(1):25–30. https://doi.org/10.1016/S0023-6438(95)80008-5

Bustos M, Perez G, León A (2011) Sensory and nutritional attributes of fibre enriched pasta. LWT Food Sci Technol 44(6):1429–1434. https://doi.org/10.1016/j.lwt.2011.02.002

Cabrera-Chávez F, de la Barca A, Islas-Rubio A et al (2012) Molecular rearrangements in extrusion processes for the production of amaranth-enriched, gluten-free rice pasta. LWT Food Sci Technol 47(2):421–426. https://doi.org/10.1016/j.lwt.2012.01.040

Carini E, Vittadini E, Curti E et al (2009) Effects of different shaping modes on physico-chemical properties and water status of fresh pasta. J Food Eng 93:400–406. https://doi.org/10.1016/j.jfoodeng.2009.02.002

Cassares M, Sakotani N, Kunigk L et al (2020) Effect of gamma irradiation on shelf-life extension of fresh pasta. Radiat Phys Chem 174:108940. https://doi.org/10.1016/j.radphyschem.2020.108940

Cham S, Suwannaporn P (2010) Effect of hydrothermal treatment of rice flour noodles quality. J Cereal Sci 51(3):284–291

Chandrasekaran S, Ramanathan S, Basak T (2013) Microwave food processing – a review. Food Res Int 52(1):243–261. https://doi.org/10.1016/j.foodres.2013.02.033

Chauhan A, Saxena D, Singh S (2017) Effect of hydrocolloids on microstructure, texture and quality characteristics of gluten-free pasta. Food Measure 11:1188–1195. https://doi.org/10.1007/s11694-017-9495-4

Chillo S, Civica V, Iannetti M et al (2010) Influence of repeated extrusions on some properties of non-conventional spaghetti. J of Food Eng 100(2):329–335. https://doi.org/10.1016/j.jfoodeng.2010.04.01

Choobthaisong P, Oupathumpanont O (2021) The nutritional quality improvement of dried gluten-free pasta supplemented with *Cladophora* spp. Em J Food Agric 33(5):395–399. https://doi.org/10.9755/ejfa.2021.v33.i5.2703

Cubadda R, Carcea M, Marconi E et al (2007) Influence of gluten proteins and drying temperature on the cooking quality of durum wheat pasta. Cereal Chem 84(1):48–55. https://doi.org/10.1094/CCHEM-84-1-0048

D'Amico S, Mäschle J, Jekle et al (2015) Effect of high temperature drying on gluten-free pasta properties. LWT Food Sci Technol 63:391–399. https://doi.org/10.1016/j.lwt.2015.03.080

da Silva LA, de Carvalho Tavares IM, de Oliveira CP et al (2021) Nutritional quality and price of regular food versus gluten-free on E-commerce platforms. Res Soc Dev 10(10). https://doi.org/10.33448/rsd-v10i10.18751

De Noni I, Pagani M (2010) Cooking properties and heat damage of dried pasta as influenced by raw material characteristics and processing conditions. Crit Rev Food Sci Nutr 50(5):465–472. https://doi.org/10.1080/10408390802437154

Del Nobile MA, Di Benedetto N, Suriano N et al (2009) Use of natural compounds to improve the microbial stability of amaranth-based homemade fresh pasta. Food Microbiol 26(2):151–156. https://doi.org/10.1016/j.fm.2008.10.003

Demirkesen I, Ozkaya B (2020) Recent strategies for tackling the problems in gluten-free diet and products. Crit Rev Food Sci Nutr 62(3):571–597. https://doi.org/10.1080/10408398.2020.1823814

Deshmukh R, Thomas A (2019) Report: gluten-free pasta market by product type (brown rice pasta, quinoa pasta, chickpea pasta, and multigrain pasta) and distribution channel (retail shops, supermarkets/hypermarkets, and E-commerce): global opportunity analysis and industry forecast, 2018–2025. In: Gluten-free Pasta Market. Allied Market Research. https://www.alliedmarketresearch.com/GF-pasta-market. Accessed 11 Oct 2021

Detchewa P, Prasajak P, Phungamngoen C et al (2022) Substitution of rice flour with rice protein improved quality of gluten-free rice spaghetti processed using single screw extrusion. LWT Food Sci Technol 153:112512. https://doi.org/10.1016/j.lwt.2021.112512

FACE (2021) Informe de precios sobre productos sin gluten 2021. In: Informe de precios 2021. Federación de Asociaciones de Celiacos de España. https://celiacos.org/tratamiento/informe-de-precios/. Accessed 25 Jan 2022

Ferreira S, de Mello A, dos Anjos M et al (2016) Utilization of sorghum, rice, corn flours with potato starch for the preparation of gluten-free pasta. Food Chem 191:147–151. https://doi.org/10.1016/j.foodchem.2015.04.085

Fradinho P, Oliveira A, Domínguez H et al (2020) Improving the nutritional performance of gluten-free pasta with potato peel autohydrolysis extract. Innov Food Sci Emerg Technol 63:102374. https://doi.org/10.1016/j.ifset.2020.102374

Fu M, Sun X, Wu D et al (2020) Effect of partial substitution of buckwheat on cooking characteristics, nutritional composition, and in vitro starch digestibility of extruded gluten-free rice noodles. LWT Food Sci Technol 126:109332. https://doi.org/10.1016/j.lwt.2020.109332

García-Baños J, Corzo N, Sanz M et al (2004) Maltulose and furosine as indicators of quality of pasta products. Food Chem 88:35–38. https://doi.org/10.1016/j.foodchem.2004.01.018

Gasparre N, Betoret E, Rosell C (2019) Quality indicators and heat damage of dried and cooked gluten-free spaghetti. Plant Foods Hum Nutr 74:481–488. https://doi.org/10.1007/s11130-019-00765-3

Giannetti V, Boccacci Mariani M, Colicchia S (2021) Furosine as marker of quality in dried durum wheat pasta: impact of heat treatment on food quality and security – a review. Food Control 125:108036. https://doi.org/10.1016/j.foodcont.2021.108036

Giménez M, González R, Wagner J et al (2013) Effect of extrusion conditions on physicochemical and sensorial properties of corn-broad beans (*Vicia faba*) spaghetti type pasta. Food Chem 136:538–545. https://doi.org/10.1016/j.foodchem.2012.08.068

Gómez M, Sciarini L (2015) Gluten-free bakery products and pasta. In: Arranz E, Fernández-Bañares F, Rosell C, Rodrigo L, Peña A (eds) Advances in the understanding of gluten related pathology and the evolution of gluten-free foods. OmniaScience Monographs, Barcelona, pp 565–604

González L, Loubes M, Tolaba M (2022) Effect of ball-milled rice starch and other functional ingredients on quality attributes of rice-based dough and noodles. Starch-Stärke:2100241. https://doi.org/10.1002/star.202100241

Guillermic R, Koksel F, Sun X et al (2017) Bubbles in noodle dough: characterization by X-ray microtomography. Food Res Int 105:548–555. https://doi.org/10.1016/j.foodres.2017.11.050

Gulia N, Dhaka V, Khatkar B (2014) Instant noodles: processing, quality, and nutritional aspects. Crit Rev Food Sci Nutr 54(10):1386–1399. https://doi.org/10.1080/10408398.2011.638227

Hanci O, Jeanes YM (2019) Are gluten-free food staples accessible to all patients with coeliac disease? Frontline Gastroenterol 10(3):222–228. https://doi.org/10.1136/flgastro-2018-101088

Heo S, Lee S, Shim J-H et al (2013) Effect of dry- and wet-milled rice flours on the quality attributes of gluten-free dough and noodles. J Food Eng 116(1):213–217. https://doi.org/10.1016/j.jfoodeng.2012.11.01

Herawati H, Kamsiati E (2021) Characteristics of various flour and gluten free noodles from Indonesian local food. IOP Conf Ser Earth Environ Sci 803:012036. https://doi.org/10.1088/1755-1315/803/1/012036

Hopkins S, Soon JM (2019) Nutritional quality, cost and availability of gluten-free food in England. Br Food J 121(11):2867–2882. https://doi.org/10.1108/BFJ-09-2018-0607

Huang JC, Knight S, Goad C (2001) Model prediction for sensory attributes of nongluten pasta. J Food Qual 24(6):495–511

Jegede O, Enns A, Kantounia M et al (2021) Cost, nutritional content and number of gluten-free staple foods available in Winnipeg, Manitoba, Canada. Plant Foods Hum Nutr 76(2):196–202. https://doi.org/10.1007/s11130-021-00889-5

Jeong S, Kim M, Yoon M-R et al (2017) Preparation and characterization of gluten-free sheeted doughs and noodles with zein and rice flour containing different amylose contents. J Cereal Sci 75:138–142. https://doi.org/10.1016/j.jcs.2017.03.022

Khuri A, Cornell J (1987) Response surfaces, designs and analyses. Marcel Dekker, New York

Kiyat W, Christopher A, Rianti A et al (2020) Application of transglutaminase in developing cassava-based wet noodle for quality and shelf-life improvement: a review. Recent Pat Food Nutr Agric 11(3):229–234. https://doi.org/10.2174/2212798411666200124105614

Klinmalait P, Hagiwara T, Sakiyama T et al (2017) Chitosan effects on physical properties, texture, and microstructure of flat rice noodles. LWT Food Sci Technol 7(Part A):117–123. https://doi.org/10.1016/j.lwt.2016.10.052

Larrosa V, Lorenzo G, Zaritzky N et al (2012) Effect of the addition of proteins and hydrocolloids on the water mobility in gluten-free pasta formulations. Water 4:1–17. https://doi.org/10.14294/WATER.2012.2

Larrosa V, Lorenzo G, Zaritzky N et al (2013) Optimization of rheological properties of gluten-free pasta dough using mixture design. J Cereal Sci 57(3):520–526. https://doi.org/10.1016/j.jcs.2013.03.003

Larrosa V, Lorenzo G, Zaritzky N et al (2016) Improvement of the texture and quality of cooked gluten-free pasta. LWT Food Sci Technol 70:96–103. https://doi.org/10.1016/j.lwt.2016.02.039

Lee A, Wolf R, Lebwohl B et al (2019) Persistent economic burden of the gluten-free diet. Nutrients 11(2):399. https://doi.org/10.3390/nu11020399

Lerner A, Matthias T (2020) Processed food additive microbial transglutaminase and its cross-linked gliadin complexes are potential public health concerns in celiac disease. Int J Mol Sci 21(3):1127. https://doi.org/10.3390/ijms21031127

Li C, You Y, Chen D et al (2021) A systematic review of rice noodles: raw material, processing method and quality improvement. Trends Food Sci Technol 107:389–400. https://doi.org/10.1016/j.tifs.2020.11.009

Linares-García L, Repo-Carrasco-Valencia R, Glorio Paulet P et al (2019) Development of gluten-free and egg-free pasta based on quinoa (*Chenopdium quinoa* Willd) with addition of lupine four, vegetable proteins and the oxidizing enzyme POx. Eur Food Res and Technol 245(10):2147–2156. https://doi.org/10.1007/s00217-019-03320-1

López-Torres R, Ramírez-Guzmán M, González-Cossio F et al (2002) A confidence region for the explanatory variables in experiments with mixtures using calibration. Agrociencia 36:579–592

Lorenzo G, Sosa M, Califano A (2018) Alternative proteins and pseudocereals in the development of gluten-free pasta. In: Holban A, Grumezescu A (eds) Handbook of food bioengineering. Academic, pp 433–458

Loubes M, Flores S, Tolaba M (2016) Effect of formulation on rice noodle quality: selection of functional ingredients and optimization by mixture design. LWT Food Sci Technol 69:280–286. https://doi.org/10.1016/j.lwt.2016.01.055

Lu Z-H, Collado L (2019) Rice noodles. In: Jinsong B (ed) Rice, 4th edn. AACC International Press, pp 557–588

Manthey F, Sinha S, Wolf-Hall C et al (2008) Effect of flaxseed flour and packaging on shelf life of refrigerated pasta. J Food Process Preserv 32:75–87. https://doi.org/10.1111/j.1745-4549.2007.00166.x

Mariotti M, Iametti S, Cappa C et al (2011) Characterization of gluten-free pasta through conventional and innovative methods: evaluation of the uncooked products. J Cereal Sci 53(3):319–327. https://doi.org/10.1016/j.jcs.2011.02.001

Marti A, Pagani A (2013) What can play the role of gluten in gluten-free pasta? Trends Food Sci Technol 31:63–71. https://doi.org/10.1016/j.tifs.2013.03.001

Marti A, Pagani M, Seetharaman K (2011) Understanding starch organization in gluten-free pasta from rice flour. Carbohydr Polym 84(3):1069–1074. https://doi.org/10.1016/j.carbpol.2010.12.070

Marti A, Caramanico R, Bottega G et al (2012) Effect of thermal treatments on rice flour and cooking behavior of rice pasta. Cereal Foods World 57:4A

Marti A, Barbiroli A, Marengo M et al (2014) Structuring and texturing gluten-free pasta: egg albumen or whey proteins? Eur Food Res Technol 238(2):217–224. https://doi.org/10.1007/s00217-013-2097-4

Martínez-Villaluenga C, Peñas E, Hernández-Ledesma B (2020) Pseudocereal grains: nutritional value, health benefits and current applications for the development of gluten-free foods. Food Chem Toxicol 137:111178. https://doi.org/10.1016/j.fct.2020.111178

Merayo Y, González R, Drago S et al (2011) Extrusion conditions and zea mays endosperm hardness affecting gluten-free spaghetti quality. Int J Food Sci Technol 46:2321–2328. https://doi.org/10.1111/j.1365-2621.2011.02752.x

Milde L, Chigal P, Olivera J et al (2020) Incorporation of xanthan gum to gluten-free pasta with cassava starch. Physical, textural and sensory attributes. LWT Food Sci Technol 131:109674. https://doi.org/10.1016/j.lwt.2020.109674

Mohd Fauad SNA, Kaur S, Shafie SR (2020) Nutritional composition and cost differences between gluten-free and gluten-containing food products in Kuala Lumpur, Malaysia. Mal J Med Health Sci 16:178–183

Molina-Rosell C (2013) Alimentos sin gluten derivados de cereales. In: Rodrigo L, Peña A (eds) Enfermedad celíaca y sensibilidad al gluten no celíaca. Omnia Publisher, Barcelona, pp 447–461

Moscicki L (2011) Extrusion-cooking techniques: applications, theory and sustainability. Wiley, Hoboken

Myhrstad MCW, Slydahl M, Hellmann M et al (2021) Nutritional quality and costs of gluten-free products: a case-control study of food products on the Norwegian marked. Food Nutr Res 65. https://doi.org/10.29219/fnr.v65.6121

Oliveira PM, Zannini E, Arendt E (2014) Cereal fungal infection, mycotoxins, and lactic acid bacteria mediated bioprotection: from crop farming to cereal products. Food Microbiol 37:78–95. https://doi.org/10.1016/j.fm.2013.06.003

Oupathumpanont O, Wisansakkul S (2021) Gluten-free pasta products with improved nutritional profile by using banana flour. J Food Nut Res 9(6):313–320. https://doi.org/10.12691/jfnr-9-6-7

Padalino L, Conte A, Del Nobile M (2016) Overview on the general approaches to improve gluten-free pasta and bread. Foods 5(4):87. https://doi.org/10.3390/foods5040087

Palavecino P, Curti M, Bustos M et al (2020) Sorghum pasta and noodles: technological and nutritional aspects. Plant Foods Hum Nutr 75:326–336. https://doi.org/10.1007/s11130-020-00829-9

Panagiotou S, Kontogianni M (2017) The economic burden of gluten-free products and gluten-free diet: a cost estimation analysis in Greece. J Hum Nutr Diet 30:746–752. https://doi.org/10.1111/jhn.12477

Perez-Gregorio R, Simal-Gandara J (2017) Critical review of bioactive food components, and of their functional mechanisms, biological effects and health outcomes. Curr Pharm Des 23(19):2731–2741. https://doi.org/10.2174/1381612823666170317122913

Re R, Pellegrini N, Proteggente A et al (1999) Antioxidant activity pplying an improved ABTS radical cation decolorization assay. Free Radic Biol Med 26(9–10):1231–1237. https://doi.org/10.1016/S0891-5849(98)00315-3

Salimi Khorshidi A, Hatcher D, Page J et al (2018) A novel method to assess the mechanical behavior of Asian noodles during the sheeting process I. The effect of repeated lamination. Food Bioprod Process 112:131–136. https://doi.org/10.1016/j.fbp.2018.10.001

Sanguinetti A, Secchi N, Del Caro A et al (2015) Gluten-free fresh filled pasta: the effects of xanthan and guar gum on changes in quality parameters after pasteurization and during storage. LWT Food Sci Technol 64(2):678–684. https://doi.org/10.1016/j.lwt.2015.06.046

Sanguinetti A, Del Caro A, Scanu A et al (2016) Extending the shelf life of gluten-free fresh filled pasta by modified atmosphere packaging. Food Sci Technol 71:96–101. https://doi.org/10.1016/j.lwt.2016.03.010

Schebor C, Chirife J (2000) A survey of water activity and pH values in fresh pasta packed under modified atmosphere manufactured in Argentina and Uruguay. J Food Prot 63(7):965–696. https://doi.org/10.4315/0362-028X-63.7.965

Scheffé H (1958) Experiments with mixtures. J R Stat Soc B 20:344–360. https://doi.org/10.1111/j.2517-6161.1958.tb00299.x

Schettino R, Pontonio E, Gobbetti M et al (2020) Extension of the shelf-life of fresh pasta using chickpea flour fermented with selected lactic acid bacteria. Microorganisms 8(9):1322. https://doi.org/10.3390/microorganisms8091322

Schoenlechner R, Drausinger J, Ottenschalaeger V, Jurackova K, Berghofer E (2010) Functional properties of gluten-free pasta produced from amaranth, quinoa and buckwheat. Plants Foods Hum Nutr 65(4):339–349. https://doi.org/10.1007/s11130-010-0194-0

Shukla V, Martínez A, Li Y et al (2021) Optimization of gluten-free pasta formulation enriched with pulse protein isolates. J Culin Sci Technol 21:99–117. https://doi.org/10.1080/15428052.2021.1888836

Sicignano A, Di Monaco R, Masi P et al (2014) From raw material to dish: pasta quality step by step. J Sci Food Agric 95:2579–2587. https://doi.org/10.1002/jsfa.7176

Singleton V, Rossi J (1965) Colorimetry of total phenolics with phosphomolybdic-phosphotungstic acid reagents. Am J Enol Vitic 16(3):144–158

Sofi S, Singh J, Chhikara N et al (2020a) Quality characterization of gluten-free noodles enriched with chickpea protein isolate. Food Biosci 36:100626. https://doi.org/10.1016/j.fbio.2020.100626

Sofi S, Singh J, Mir S et al (2020b) In vitro starch digestibility, cooking quality, rheology and sensory properties of gluten-free pregelatinized rice noodle enriched with germinated chickpea flour. LWT Food Sci Technol 133:110090. https://doi.org/10.1016/j.lwt.2020.110090

Sozer N (2009) Rheological properties of rice pasta dough supplemented with proteins and gums. Food Hydrocoll 23:849–855

Stuknyte M, Cattaneo S, Pagani M et al (2014) Spaghetti from durum wheat: effect of drying conditions on heat damage, ultrastructure and in vitro digestibility. Food Chem 149:40–46. https://doi.org/10.1016/j.foodchem.2013.10.071

Suhendro E, Kunetz C, McDonough CM et al (2000) Cooking characteristics and quality of noodles from food sorghum. Cereal Chem J 77:96–100. https://doi.org/10.1094/CCHEM.2000.77.2.96

Toledo V, Carvalho C, Vargas-Solórzano J (2019) Extrusion cooking of gluten-free whole grain flour blends. J Food Process Eng 43(2):e13303. https://doi.org/10.1111/jfpe.13303

Tudorica C, Kuri V, Brennan C (2002) Nutritional and physicochemical characteristics of dietary fiber enriched pasta. J Agric Food Chem 50(2):347–356. https://doi.org/10.1021/jf0106953

Vandeginste B, Rutan S (1998) Mixture designs. In: Massart D, Vandeginste B, Buydens L, De Jong S, Lewi P, Smeyers-Verbeke J (eds) Handbook of chemometrics and qualimetrics: Part A, vol 20. Elsevier, Amsterdam, pp 739–769. https://doi.org/10.1016/s0922-3487(97)80055-x

Verma D, Naveen M, Mamta T et al (2020) Microwave heating: alternative thermal process technology for food application. In: Srivastav P, Verma D, Patel A (eds) Emerging thermal and non-thermal technologies in food processing. Apple Academic Press, New York, pp 25–67. https://doi.org/10.1201/9780429297335-2

Vieira A, Silva A, Albuquerque A et al (2021) Effects of long-term frozen storage on the quality and acceptance of gluten-free cassava pasta. Heliyon 7(8):e07844. https://doi.org/10.1016/j.heliyon.2021.e07844

Wang N, Bhirud P, Sosulski F et al (1999) Pasta-like product from pea flour by twin-screw extrusion. J Food Sci 64(4):671–678. https://doi.org/10.1111/j.1365-2621.1999.tb15108.x

Wang L, Duan W, Zhou S et al (2016) Effects of extrusion conditions on the extrusion responses and the quality of brown rice pasta. Food Chem 204:320–325. https://doi.org/10.1016/j.foodchem.2016.02.053

Wang X, Ma Z, Li X et al (2018) Food additives and technologies used in Chinese traditional staple foods. Chem Biol Technol Agric 5(1). https://doi.org/10.1186/s40538-017-0113-9

Yalcin S, Basman A (2008) Effects of gelatinization level, gum and transglutaminase on the quality characteristics of rice noodle. Int J Food Sci Technol 43(9):1637–1644. https://doi.org/10.1111/j.1365-2621.2007.01674.x

Yang S, Shan C-S, Xu Y-Q et al (2021) Dissimilarity in sensory attributes, shelf life and spoilage bacterial and fungal microbiota of industrial-scale wet starch noodles induced by different preservatives and temperature. Food Res Int 140:109980. https://doi.org/10.1016/j.foodres.2020.109980

Yeh A (2004) Preparation and applications of rice flour. In: Champagne E (ed) Rice: chemistry and technology. American Association of Cereal Chemists, St Paul, pp 495–539

Zardetto S, Dalla Rosa M (2009) Effect of extrusion process on properties of cooked, fresh egg pasta. J Food Eng 92:70–77. https://doi.org/10.1016/j.jfoodeng.2008.10.027

Zhu F (2018) Effect of ozone treatment on the quality of grain products. Food Chem 264:358–366. https://doi.org/10.1016/j.foodchem.2018.05.047

Chapter 9
Sensory Analysis Tools in Developing Gluten-Free Bakery and Pasta Products and Their Quality Control

Vanessa Dias Capriles, Etiene Valéria de Aguiar, Fernanda Garcia Santos, Marión Elizabeth Aguilar Fernández, Bruna Guedes de Melo, Bruna Lago Tagliapietra, Michele Scarton, Maria Teresa Pedrosa Silva Clerici, and Ana Carolina Conti

Abbreviations

BF	bean flour
CATA	Check-all-that-apply
CD	celiac disease
CF	chickpea flour
fwb	flour weight basis
GCC	gluten-containing counterparts
GF	gluten free
GFB	gluten-free bread
GI	glycaemic index
GL	glycaemic load
GRD	gluten related diseases

V. D. Capriles (✉) · E. V. de Aguiar · F. G. Santos · M. E. A. Fernández
Department of Biosciences, Federal University of São Paulo (UNIFESP), Institute of Health and Society (Campus Baixada Santista), Santos, SP, Brazil
e-mail: vanessa.capriles@unifesp.br; etiene.aguiar@unifesp.br; fg.santos@unifesp.br; marion.aguilar@unifesp.br

B. G. de Melo · B. L. Tagliapietra · M. Scarton · M. T. P. S. Clerici
School of Food Engineering, Department of Food Science and Nutrition, University of Campinas (UNICAMP), Campinas, SP, Brazil
e-mail: mclerici@unicamp.br

A. C. Conti
Department of Food Engineering and Technology, São Paulo State University (UNESP), Institute of Biosciences, Humanities and Exact Sciences (IBILCE), Campus São José do Rio Preto, São José do Rio Preto, SP, Brazil
e-mail: ac.conti@unesp.br

M. F. de Escalada Pla, C. E. Genevois (eds.), *Designing Gluten Free Bakery and Pasta Products*, https://doi.org/10.1007/978-3-031-28344-4_9

JAR	Just-about-right
P	psyllium
PS	potato starch
QDA	quantitative descriptive analysis
RF	rice flour
W	water
WB	wheat bread

9.1 Introduction

As pointed out in the previous chapters of this book, the rising interest in a gluten-free (GF) diet has led to increased research into the development of GF foodstuffs, aiming to obtain products that resemble their gluten containing counterpart (GCC). However, wheat gluten has unique properties that confer high quality and palatability to bakery and pasta products. As a result, obtaining high-quality GF bakery and pasta products continues to be a huge task for food scientists and producers, especially with an increasing need due to the growing number of individuals following a GF diet.

Even though there has been an impressive research effort with the growth of the GF food market in recent years, important issues remain to be addressed for GF bakery and pasta products, such as improvements in the sensory and nutritional quality, shelf life, cost reduction, and increased availability of GF products. People with gluten-related disorders (GRD) rely on an increasing range of healthier, tastier GF foodstuffs to implement a more satisfying diet and to improve aspects related to their nutrition, health, and quality of life (Capriles et al. 2021).

The previous chapters presented information regarding the unique properties of gluten that confer high quality and acceptability to bakery and pasta products, as well as approaches used to design and improve GF product quality. Food researchers and industry face the task of producing high-quality GF products and making them more like their GCC to meet consumer demands. There has been an increasing interest in the application of sensory analysis over the last decade, as shown in Fig. 9.1, which highlights the importance of sensory and consumer research for developing GF bakery and pasta products and their quality control.

Data from Fig. 9.1 were obtained in the Elsevier Scopus database which was explored using the following research string in topic and title: 1 - "gluten-free" and "cakes" or "brownies" or "muffins", 2 - "gluten-free" and "cookies" or "biscuits" or "crackers", 3 - "gluten-free" and "pasta" or "noodles", 4 - "gluten-free" and "pizza" and 5 "gluten-free" and "bread" to selected original articles published between 2011 and 2021. There were no restrictions regarding language. The papers were screened by reading the title and abstract and duplicated articles and papers that were not pertinent to GF bakery and pasta products were excluded. The search resulted in a total of 1631 articles found, 1244 of which met the inclusion criteria. The figure shows the increase in the number of studies with sensory analysis in them

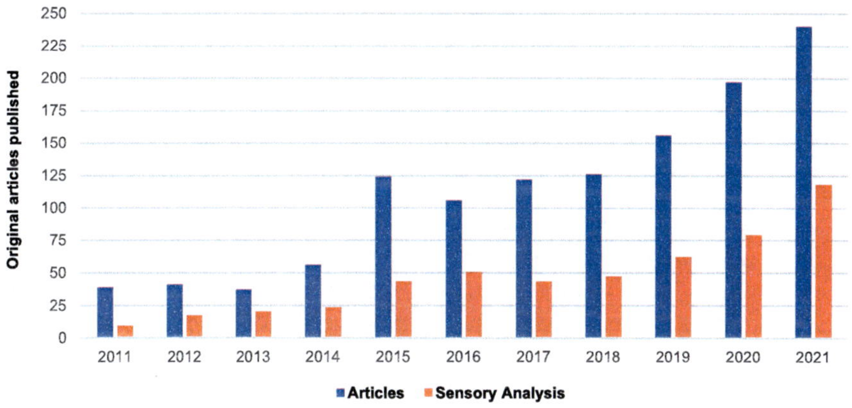

Fig. 9.1 Annual scientific production of original articles about gluten-free bakery and pasta products (in blue) and those that include sensory analysis (in orange) registered by Scopus (2011 until 2021)

since, in 2011, it represented 23% of the articles and, in 2021, it grew representing 49% of the total articles published.

This chapter presents theoretical information regarding sensory tests, as well as consumer opinion and expectations about commercially available GF food products. Then, it concentrates on research application of sensorial analyses to overcome technological, nutritional, sensory, and shelf-life issues currently related to GF foods and explores both analytical and affective sensory tests. Some examples of recently published papers (within the last 10 years) are presented.

9.2 Sensory Analysis and Consumer Research

> "Sensory evaluation has been defined as a scientific method used to evoke, measure, analyse, and interpret those responses to products as perceived through the senses of sight, smell, touch, taste, and hearing". (Stone and Sidel 2004, cited by Lawless and Heymann 2010)

Therefore, sensory analysis investigates attributes that are perceived through human senses, i.e., appearance, odour/aroma, specific texture, and taste/flavour.

Traditional sensory methods, which are still widely used today, and novel methodologies, with their advantages and disadvantages, are very useful in the development of food products and quality control. Moreover, all these techniques may be applied with the support of software specially designed to assist the planning, execution, data collection and statistical analysis of sensory analyses.

However, other factors besides sensory properties, such as social aspects, nutrition facts, specific diets, emotions, health, and packaging, also have a very important influence on drivers of purchase and consumption of a food product. Currently, sensory analysis is applied together with consumer research for new product development, reformulation, and quality control and for companies to achieve a better market position.

Nowadays, sensory and consumer scientists intend to collect a variety of consumer information to obtain insight and a better knowledge of experiences with products. According to Kock and Magano (2020), focusing on conceptual views of consumers, e.g., adequacy of a product for certain uses, willingness to consume or purchase a product, willingness to compromise on sensory quality in view of a health or other perceived or real benefit, and evaluation of post-ingestive measures, can be useful for development and reformulation of GF products.

Traditionally, sensory evaluation has been divided into *analytical tests* to objectively evaluate the sensory characteristics of products and *affective tests* to measure product acceptance/preference with regular consumers of the target products. The sensory tests are divided into three classes: *Discriminative, Descriptive and Affective*, each with a different goal and using participants selected using different criteria. Moreover, both analytical and affective tests can be applied in a sensory laboratory or a real-world setting, such as Central Location Tests (CLTs), In-Home Use Tests (IHUTs), internet testing, etc.

- *Discriminative tests* are applied to determine whether panellists will notice or not a difference between two or more products.
- *Descriptive tests* describe and quantify the perceived intensities of the sensory properties of the product. These are traditionally performed by specifically screened and trained panellists. However, in the last couple of decades, a variety of new methods for descriptive sensory characterization using regular consumers or semi trained panellists for describing products have been proposed and recognised (Ares and Varela 2017). Varela and Ares (2012) present detailed information about theory and implementation, data analysis, applications, advances, and limitations of each of these novel techniques.
- *Affective tests* quantify and/or qualify the affective opinions of consumers towards product options.

Trained panellists should not execute hedonic tests, as they are trained to give out their own preferences and to assess products using objectively criteria. In addition, a small, trained panel (usually close to 10) does not represent consumer perception and cannot be considered as a measure of the potential product performance in the marketplace (Ares and Varela 2017). This misconception still occurs in sensory evaluation of GF products as seen in the current literature.

Nowadays, a very interesting trend is the evaluation of the drivers of liking/disliking by relating descriptive characteristics of products to consumer opinions using statistical techniques. Moreover, results from sensory analyses can be related to instrumental measures. Sections 9.4, 9.5, 9.6, and 9.7 presents some examples applied to GF bakery and pasta product development and quality control, drivers of liking, and the relationship between different sensory parameters, as well as with instrumental analyses for fresh products and during and/or after a given storage period.

9.3 Panorama of Sensory Evaluation of GF Bakery and Pasta Products

Regarding sensory analysis, detailed information about important factors to be considered during GF product sensory evaluation, such as sample preparation and presentation, and the test environment are presented in the article by Kock and Magano (2020). These authors also propose a reflection about who are the most suitable panellists for evaluating GF products; celiac or non-celiac consumers and/or trained panels and point out that GF products are targeted at celiac and consumers with GRD. However, regular consumers also eat GF foods. In addition, all difficulties recruiting consumers with CD and additional care to ensure GF food safety should be taken into consideration. Current issues occurring in sensory analysis of GF products include trained panellists performing hedonic tests, which is not is not recommended as was point out in Sect. 9.2; few consumers participating in affective studies; and the discussion about studies with celiac and non-celiac consumers. These and other factors need attention and would be improved if researchers and the food industry followed good sensory practices and included a Sensory and Consumer Research Specialist in their team.

Studies have shown that the main attribute considered by individuals with CD in the purchase of GF products is the sensory aspect, especially taste and texture (do Nascimento et al. 2014, 2017; Potter et al. 2014; Alencar et al. 2021) and the same was noticed for non-celiac consumers (unpublished results). This strengthens the importance of sensory analyses for GF products. Moreover, sensory techniques are useful for product development, quality control, product improvement, monitoring shelf-life changes, and evaluating effects of ingredients and manufacturing processes on food product characteristics and/or consumer opinions. They are also useful in gaining insight on consumer views on products, which are essential to better understand GF food systems and improve GF food quality. These techniques are illustrated by the examples in the following sections of this chapter.

There has been a pronounced increase in the number of original and review articles about GF food over the last decade, while there are few publications regarding commercial GF food. This clearly shows the problem of insufficient knowledge of the characteristics of GF foods on the market. So, some research groups, recently studied the nutritional and sensory quality of commercially available GF products (Roman et al. 2019; Aguiar et al. 2021a; Alencar et al. 2021). Such information is essential to understand the range of currently available products, the potential of experimental products, possible future investigations, and the needs of consumers suffering from GRD, as well those of the gluten-tolerant consumers that choose to follow a GF diet or eat GF foods.

9.4 GF Bread

GF bread (GFB) is the most sought after and consumed GF product among celiac and non-celiac consumers (Alencar et al. 2021; Capriles et al. 2021). GFB is commonly identified as a product with an unsatisfactory appearance, texture, mouthfeel, and taste. It is also known for its lack of nutritional content and short shelf life, with limited availability and a significant price tag compared to GCC (do Nascimento et al. 2014, 2017; Fry et al. 2018; Hanci and Jeanes 2019; Alencar et al. 2021).

As a result, numerous studies have centered on the development and quality improvement of GFBs, as discussed in the previous chapters. There is a huge variation in the formulation, process, and storage conditions, which consequently affect the GFB final quality (Matos and Rosell 2015; El Khoury et al. 2018). The research on GFB is very divergent, with tremendous variability in formulation and processing conditions, as well as methods used for analyzing batter/dough and bread (Masure et al. 2016). Consequently, any comparison between the reported results is difficult.

Table 9.1 presents some examples of sensory tests as applied, showing diverse ways to guide GFB development, to evaluate the effect of ingredients on consumer perceptions, and to investigate staling effects on consumer liking and drivers of liking.

Sensory and nutrition aspects are crucial issues to be addressed in improving GFB quality. To this end, nutrient-dense alternative raw materials and functional dietary fibers have been explored for simultaneous improvement of GFB physical-chemical, nutritional, and sensory properties. Another key aspect in recent studies is the shelf life of the bread contribute to fill the gap related to reliable predictors that can correlate GF dough parameters and GFB physical properties with the sensory parameters of fresh and stored GFB. Some results are described in the next sections.

9.4.1 Approaches to Improve Sensory and Nutritional Quality of GFB

Flours derived from alternative raw materials, such as non-gluten cereals, pseudocereals, legumes, seeds and nuts, and fruit and vegetable-based materials, have been applied to increase the levels of nutrients and bioactive compounds and to diversify GFB formulations (Capriles et al. 2016; Conte et al. 2019; Bender and Schönlechner, 2020; Cappelli et al., 2020). Regardless of the nutritional benefits, the use of these alternative raw materials usually changes GFB sensory attributes (i.e., appearance, colour, odour, texture, aroma, and flavour), which might impact consumer liking. Thus, assessment of the sensory characteristics and consumer perception during GF research is critical (Capriles and Arêas 2014).

Various literature reviews (e.g., Capriles and Arêas 2014; Capriles et al. 2016; Conte et al. 2019; Bender and Schönlechner 2020) condensed some of the studies

Table 9.1 Summary of reviewed articles regarding sensory analysis of gluten-free bread

Country and sensory focus	Gluten-free bread formulation(s)	Participants	Sensory methodology	Main sensory conclusions	References
United States Consumer liking	20% amaranth or Montina flour (fwb) added compared to a control formulation of white bread	222 untrained volunteers recruited from faculty staff and students, and celiac support groups Divided in GF consumers (n = 93), who eating GF products at least 2–3 times per week, and non-GF consumers (n = 129)	9-point hedonic scale to assess appearance, texture, flavour, tenderness, and overall acceptability	The mean acceptance scores for the GF/ non-restricted groups were 5.8/5.9 for amaranth and 6.5/6.2 for Montina, with no significant differences regarding the sensory attributes between consumer groups The commercial GFB was preferred over either developed bread and the Montina-based bread was preferred over the amaranth-based bread	Breshears and Crowe (2013)
Poland Consumer Liking	Enriched with 10% albumin, collagen, ppea or soy proteins (fwb) compared to a control with no added ingredients	14 non celiac experts with established sensory sensitivity and trained	7-point hedonic scale to assess overall appearance, structure and porosity, crumb colour, smell, and taste acceptability	An increase over the control in the acceptability gluten-free bread with added pea protein, followed by gluten-free bread with added collagen, and the lowest acceptability was recorded for a gluten-free bread with added soy protein	Ziobro et al. (2013)

(continued)

Table 9.1 (continued)

Country and sensory focus	Gluten-free bread formulation(s)	Participants	Sensory methodology	Main sensory conclusions	References
Brazil Consumer liking	Enriched with inulin-type fructans at 8.6%, 17.9%, 22.7% and 28% (fwb), compared to a control with no inulin-type fructans	60 regular consumers	9-point hedonic scale to evaluate the appearance, colour, texture, flavour, and overall acceptability	All levels of added inulin-type fructans increased the appearance, colour, texture, and overall acceptability All enriched formulations were acceptable, with scores ranging from 6.2 to 7.4	Capriles and Arêas (2013)
Brazil Sensory profiling and drivers of liking	Prepared with 0.16% sucralose, 0.75% fructose, 0.25% stevia, 0.75% fructooligosaccharides (FOS) or 0.75% inulin compared to control (prepared with sugar)	65 celiac consumers – Affective test 15 trained assessor – Sensory profiling	9-cm linear hedonic scale (not structured, with anchors of "dislike extremely" and "like extremely"), to evaluate appearance, crumb colour, aroma, flavour, softness, and overall liking Quantitative descriptive analysis (QDA)	Products that presented the Highest acceptability by celiac consumers were the ones developed with raw sugar and FOS The drivers of liking are crumb Colour, sweetness, traditional bread aroma, and apparent softness, whereas hardness, chewiness, and yeast aroma were drivers of disliking	Morais et al. (2014)
Iran consumer liking	Prepared with 5, 10 and 15% soy flour (fwb) compared to control with no soy flour.	30 tasting panel judges comprising of workers with more than 10 years of experience in baking and teachers, scientific officers, and students	5-point hedonic scale to access taste, texture, colour, and overall acceptability	The highest total score of sensory evaluation was for the bread sample containing 15% soybean flour The evaluation of crust and crumb showed that bread samples with 15% soy flour were significantly darker than the other bread samples	Taghdir et al. (2016)

Spain Sensory profiling and drivers of liking Consumer preference	Prepared with teff flour (5, 10 and 20%) and different dried (buckwheat or rice) or fresh (with *Lactobacillus helveticus*) sourdoughs	15 selected and trained assessors (non-celiac) 30 celiac consumers (above 14 years old and diagnosed for at least 1 year In a screening questionnaire, 82% stated they consumed bread daily, while the other 18% consumed bread at least 2 or 3 times per week	Descriptive test (20 samples) Ranking test: Consumers rank 4 samples from "least liked" (left) to "most liked" according to visual appearance and overall taste. They were also asked to provide a few terms that described the tasted products	The combination of teff (10%) with cereal sourdough (rice or buckwheat) enhanced bread aroma, increasing the fruity, cereal, and toasty notes The visual appearance of breads with 20% teff was highly appreciated by consumers, while bread combining 10% teff and rice sourdough was preferred in terms of flavour The bitter taste of buckwheat sourdough was considered as a negative attribute. However, a group of consumers liked bitter bread as they associated it to a traditional, artisan, "malty-like" product	Campo et al. (2016)

(continued)

Table 9.1 (continued)

Country and sensory focus	Gluten-free bread formulation(s)	Participants	Sensory methodology	Main sensory conclusions	References
Brazil Consumer Liking	Optimized and enriched with psyllium fibre. Psyllium level ranges from 0 to 17.14% (fwb) and water levels range from 82.14 to 117.96 (fwb), totalizing 7 formulas and a control of 0% psyllium and 100% water fwb	53 non-celiac bread consumers	10-cm hybrid hedonic scale (unstructured, with anchors of "dislike extremely" on the left and "like extremely" on the right), to evaluate the appearance, colour, odour, texture, flavour, and overall acceptability of the formulations	Significant predicted model equations for all sensory attributes (R^2_{adj} 95.7–99.8% $p < 0.01$) The psyllium and water interactions enhanced the sensory acceptability scores for appearance, texture, and overall liking. The optimum formulation (desirability of 0.89) was prepared with 2.86% P and 82.14% W and overall liking of 8.8, like wheat bread. It is possible to add 17.14% psyllium and 117.86% water (fwb) to obtain an acceptable product with score 7 for all attributes, enriched with 3 g psyllium/ portion	Fratelli et al. (2018)

Brazil consumer liking	Prepared with chia seed and chia flour at 2, 4, 6, 8 and 10% (fwb), compared with control with no added chia	100 non-celiac bread consumers	9-point hedonic scale to evaluate the global acceptance, appearance, colour, odour, flavour, and texture	Only the formulations with 4% chia flour and 6% chia seeds were sensorially evaluated because they had the best technological characteristics These products showed no significant difference in evaluated parameters, with average scores between 6 and 7	Borges et al. (2021)
Brazil Consumer liking	Prepared with psyllium levels ranges from 0 to 17.14% (fwb) and water levels range from 82.14 to 117.96 (fwb) compared to wheat bread (WB) during 3 days of storage	54 consumers (non-celiac)	10-cm hybrid hedonic scale (unstructured, with anchors of "dislike extremely" on the left and "like extremely" on the right), to evaluate the aroma, texture, and flavour of the formulations fresh and stored	The longest delay in GFB staling was observed with the addition of 17.14% psyllium, maintaining Acceptability during storage comparable to that of the wheat bread counterparts GFB17.14P was well accepted During the 72 h of storage, with acceptable scores for aroma, texture, and flavour ranging From 6.8 to 8.3, which were comparable to the scores of WB1 and WB2. Control formulation was rejected after 24 h of storage.	Fratelli et al. (2021)

(continued)

Table 9.1 (continued)

Country and sensory focus	Gluten-free bread formulation(s)	Participants	Sensory methodology	Main sensory conclusions	References
Brazil Sensory profiling and drivers of liking	Prepared with 75% (fwb) chickpea or rice flour combined with 0 or 5.5% (fwb) psyllium during 7 days at storage room	65 consumers without gluten-related disorders participated in four sessions, organized for the evaluation of samples after 0, 1, 4, and 7 days of storage 10 gluten-related disorder consumers participated in a single session carried out to evaluate the products after 7 days of storage	9-point structured hedonic scale to evaluate appearance, aroma, flavour, texture, and overall acceptability Softness intensity using the 5-point Just-About-Right scale Check-All-That-Apply question using 18 terms comprising descriptive and hedonic attributes. Test conducted only with consumers without gluten-related disorders	During all storage, the combination of chickpea flour and psyllium maintained acceptability (scores for all attributes ranging from 6.3 to 8.2). Also, the softness was considered ideal by approximately 70% of all consumers In addition, this formulation was described as 'soft', with 'uniform alveoli' and 'rounded slice top' by consumers without gluten-related disorder	Santos et al. (2021b)

Brazil Consumer Liking	Prepared with 0 to 100% (fwb) amaranth, buckwheat or quinoa flour combined with rice flour and/or potato starch	54 consumers (non-celiac)	10-cm hybrid hedonic scale (unstructured, with anchors of "dislike extremely" on the left and "like extremely" on the right), to evaluate the appearance, colour, odour, texture, flavour, and overall acceptability of the formulations	The interaction effects between pseudocereal flours and rice flour increase the degree of liking Blends of 50% pseudocereals flour with 50% rice flour result in GFB with high degree of liking (overall of 8) like the control bread The maximum pseudocereal proportions to obtain acceptable GFB (liking scores ≥7 for all evaluated attributes were 60%, 85% and 82% of amaranth, buckwheat, and quinoa flour respectively	Aguiar et al. (2021b)
Brazil sensory profiling and drivers of liking	Prepared with 0, 50 or 100% (fwb) beans or rice flour combined with 2.86% (fwb) psyllium	64 consumers (non-celiac)	9-point structured hedonic scale to evaluate appearance, aroma, flavour, texture, and overall liking Softness intensity using the 5-point Just-About-Right scale Food-related emotion questionnaire (33 emojis)	The combination of beans and rice flour increase the liking of appearance, texture, flavour and overall, as well as the degree of softness, which is correlated with a positive food-related emotion	Aguiar et al. (2022)

fwb flour weight basis

concerning raw materials and ingredients used to increase the nutrient and bioactive compound content of GFB, together with improving the physical and sensory properties of the bread, as well as its potential health benefits. Many investigations focused on developing GFB formulas by testing different alternative raw material ratios and assessing dough and bread quality parameters (e.g., Genevois et al. 2021; Genevois and de Escalada 2021; Locke et al. 2019; Milde et al. 2012). Nevertheless, few studies have been made using statistical approaches to define and optimize the levels of these alternative raw material.

Recent studies have been applying mixture design experiments, factorial design experiments and response surface methodology to optimize GFB formulations based on alternative nutrient-dense raw materials, blended with traditional GF raw materials, that yield GFB with improved nutritional quality and sensory profiles. Principal component analysis and multiple factor analysis have also been used to identify new formulations with physical properties and sensory acceptability like those of conventional white GFB formulations.

Aguiar et al. (2021b) showed that it is possible to produce new GFB formulations based on pseudocereals. However, combining those alternative flours with traditional GF raw materials (rice flour – RF and potato starch – PS) improves product quality and acceptance. GFBs prepared with up to 60% amaranth, 85% buckwheat and 82% quinoa flours, on a flour weight basis (fwb), present good physical properties (loaf volume and crumb texture) and degrees of liking (i.e., appearance, colour, odour, texture, taste, and overall) higher than 7.0 on a 10-cm hybrid hedonic scale, evaluated by 54 regular consumers.

The GFB made from chickpea flour alone was accepted by consumers. Nevertheless, blends of 75% chickpea flour with cassava or PS improved bread acceptability. Detailed information about the mixture design approach to optimize chickpea-based GFB was provided by Santos et al. (2018), considering physical properties (loaf volume, crumb firmness, and moisture), degree of liking by 50 regular consumers (appearance, colour, aroma, texture, taste, and overall), and proximate composition.

Centeno et al. (2021) applied a 2^2 factorial design to study sorghum flour and water level effects on GFB physical properties and acceptability. Experimental bread was prepared based on a single formulation made with sorghum flour and composite formulations prepared with 50% and 75% sorghum flour combined with PS. The water levels ranged from 100% to 140% on a fwb. All GFB formulations containing red sorghum flour had a high degree of liking (scores ranging from 7.4 to 8.5 a 10-cm hybrid hedonic scale, evaluated by 54 regular consumers), with no significant effect of sorghum flour or water on GFB acceptability. A similar approach was used to study the effects of millet flour (50–75%), and composite formulations blended with maize starch and water levels ranging from 100% to 130% fwb. Results show that all formulations had high degrees of liking (overall liking ranged from 7 to 8 on a 10-cm hybrid hedonic scale) (Personal Communication).

Table 9.2 shows eleven promising GF whole grain bread formulations, considering both optimized and higher levels - containing alternative whole grain flours to

Table 9.2 Whole grain flour and dietary fibre content and degree of liking of whole-grain gluten-free bread formulations and their comparison with white gluten-free and wheat bread counterparts

Bread formulation (flour/starch base)	Content of Whole grain flour (g/100 g)	Content of dietary fibre (g/100 g)	Degree of liking (mean values of 50–54 regular consumers on a 10-cm hybrid hedonic scale)						References
			Appearance	Colour	Odour	Texture	Flavour	Global	
100% chickpea flour	–	10	8.4	8.2	7.8	7.0	6.9	7.0	Santos et al. (2018)
75% chickpea flour +25% cassava or potato starch	–	8	8.8	8.8	8.0	8.3	8.0	8.2	Santos et al. (2018)
50% quinoa flour +50% rice flour	22	6	8.8	8.3	8.1	7.7	8.2	8.3	Aguiar et al. (2021b)
82% quinoa flour +18% rice flour	36	7	8.1	8.2	7.9	7.4	7.3	7.6	Aguiar et al. (2021b)
50% amaranth flour +50% rice flour	22	5	8.8	8.8	7.9	7.7	7.7	8.0	Aguiar et al. (2021b)
60% amaranth flour +40% rice flour	26	6	8.9	9.0	7.7	7.3	7.3	7.6	Aguiar et al. (2021b)
50% buckwheat flour +50% rice flour	22	6	8.3	7.9	7.6	8.1	8.1	8.1	Aguiar et al. (2021b)
85% buckwheat flour +15% rice flour	36	7	7.8	7.4	7.6	8.0	7.3	7.6	Aguiar et al. (2021b)
50% white sorghum flour +50% potato starch	18	5	8.5	8.6	8.6	8.4	8.7	8.9	Centeno et al. (2021)
100% white sorghum flour	44	8	8.2	3.0	8.0	7.2	7.7	7.6	Centeno et al. (2021)
50% brown sorghum flour +50% potato starch	18	5	7.8	7.6	8.5	8.4	8.6	8.5	Centeno et al. (2021)
100% brown sorghum flour	44	8	8.4	8.3	8.5	8.2	8.1	8.2	Centeno et al. (2021)

Table 9.2 (continued)

Bread formulation (flour/starch base)	Content of Whole grain flour (g/100 g)	Content of dietary fibre (g/100 g)	Degree of liking (mean values of 50–54 regular consumers on a 10-cm hybrid hedonic scale)						References
			Appearance	Colour	Odour	Texture	Flavour	Global	
50% millet flour + 50% maize starch	22	5	6.6	6.5	8.1	7.6	8.1	7.8	Capriles et al. (2021)
50% rice flour + 50% potato starch	0	2	8.5	8.2	8.2	7.8	7.9	8.0	Santos et al. (2018)
100% rice flour	0	2	8.3	8.3	8.0	7.6	7.9	7.9	Capriles et al. (2021)
100% wheat flour (standard formula)	0	4	8.4	8.3	8.0	7.6	8.1	7.9	Santos et al. (2018)
100% wheat flour (lab. formula)	0	4	9.0	9.1	8.5	8.8	8.6	8.9	Santos et al. (2018)

obtain acceptable products and their comparison with two white GFBs and two wheat bread (WB) counterparts.

These new GFBs have a consumer overall acceptability score like or better than that of white GFB and some were even comparable to their WB counterparts. Thus, it is feasible to use a higher proportion of alternative flour (50–100% fwb) to prepare well-accepted and nutritionally superior products than conventional white GFB. Compared to white GFB, these new whole grain GFBs presented a 2.5–5 times increase in total fibre content. The formulations can be considered "high in fibre" since they contain more than 6% dietary fibre, except the GFBs prepared with 50% amaranth or millet flours which can be considered a "fibre source" since they contain more than 3% dietary fibre (Codex Alimentarius Commission 1996). According to Brazilian food legislation, all these new GFBs can be deemed "fibre sources" since they contain over 2.5 g of fibre/50 g bread portion (Brazil 2012).

Considering the criteria established to bear a Whole Grain Stamp (Whole Grains Council 2021), GFB prepared with sorghum flour met the "100% whole grain" criterion, as it provides a 22 g of whole grain/50 g portion. The other alternative grain-based GFBs met the "50% whole grain" criterion since they have a 9–18 g of whole grain/50 g of bread portion. There is a minimum requirement of 16 g and 8 g of whole grain per labelled serving to attend the 100% and 50% whole grain stamp criteria, respectively. According to Brazilian food legislation, all those GFB can be deemed "whole grain" (Brazil 2021). According to Aguiar et al. (2021b), this is the first report on whole grain content in GFB and no product with those characteristics was mentioned in a recent literature review regarding commercially available GFB worldwide.

In a recent preliminary study, Drub et al. (2021) showed the potential of whole grain flours to produce fibre and protein enriched acceptable GF rolls. Figure 9.2 shows these new product appearances. Briefly, the white roll made with RF and cassava starch had a high degree of liking (overall 8.3 on a 10-cm hybrid hedonic scale), as well as the roll made with brown RF (scored 7.5), and the remaining bread roll had a moderate degree of liking (overall of 6.3–6.8) by consumers. Liking scores of the assessed attributes of GF rolls are satisfactory (6.0–8.6). These results are promising, showing the feasibility of preparing a new GFB variety, a non-pan bread roll, as well as the wholegrain versions using grain like millet, sorghum and pseudocereals which are not yet frequently consumed by the population.

In short, all those new healthier GFBs (Table 9.2 and Fig. 9.2) have good consumer appeal and could help to expand the consumption of whole grain, fibre, and bioactive compounds. The sensory studies were done with non-GF consumers and a good liking evaluation by this group suggests a closer similarity to regular WB. This could be judged an especially good aspect of these products. However, further sensory studies with GF consumers, especially those people with CD, will be made to verify whether the developed product meets their expectations.

The use of dietary fibre ingredients, especially soluble fibres, has been suggested to promote better GFB physical properties, sensory acceptance, shelf life, nutritional content and glycaemic response (Capriles and Arêas 2014; Capriles et al.

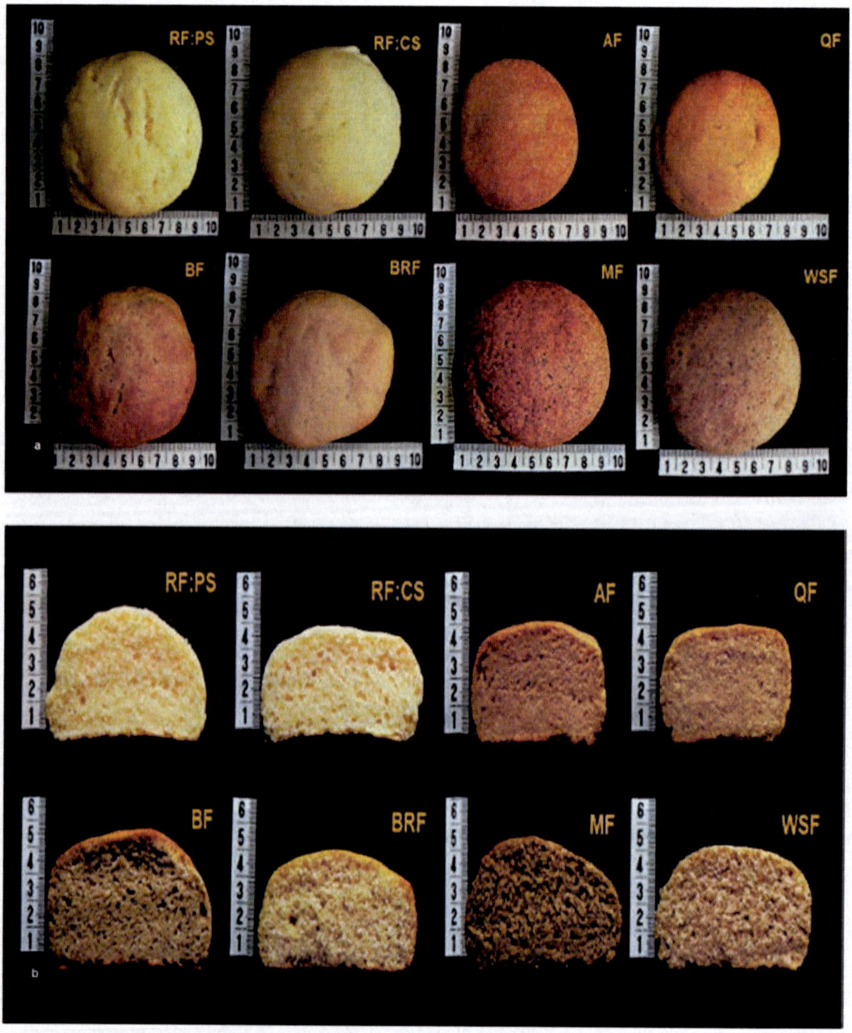

Fig. 9.2 Appearance of gluten-free yeast rolls made with traditional raw materials and with whole grain flour.[a] Bread identification: RF, rice flour; PS, potato starch; CS, cassava starch; AF, amaranth flour; QF, quinoa flour; BF, buckwheat flour; ML, millet flour; BRF, brown rice flour; WSF, white sorghum flour. (Source: Drub et al. (2021), with permission from Elsevier)

2016; Tsatsaragkou et al. 2016). These effects are connected to water-binding, thickening, gelling, and structure-building characteristics.

Design of experiments and response surface methodology were used by Fratelli et al. (2018) to optimize fibre enriched GFB quality. Impressive results were obtained showing that the psyllium (P) and water (W) interactions improve the bread quality by yielding better loaf volume, softer crumbs and enhanced appearance as well as improving the sensory acceptability scores, as summarized in

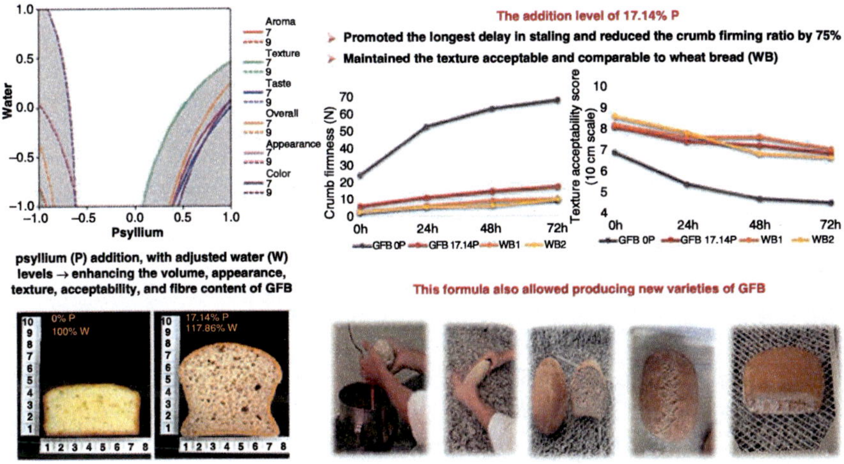

Fig. 9.3 Overlaid contour plots for the acceptability scores for the gluten free bread (GFB) formulations prepared with different combinations of psyllium and water addition levels. The appearance of psyllium enriched gluten-free bread (GFB 17.14P) and its crumb firmness and texture acceptability score at 0–72 h post-production, and its comparison to the control (GFB 0P) and wheat bread (WB1 — standard and WB2 — lab. formulas) counterparts. (Source: Adapted from Fratelli et al. (2018, 2021) and Capriles et al. (2022))

Fig. 9.3. The formulation prepared with 17.14% P and 117.86% W fwb results in acceptable GFB with nearly a four-fold increase in the fibre content and 33% decreased glycaemic response, presenting low-glycaemic index (GI = 50) and low-glycaemic load (GL = 9), while the control GFB presented high GI ≈ 70 and high GL ≈ 14 (Fratelli et al. 2018).

Another advantage is that dough can be worked by hand to produce a variety of non-pan bread buns and rolls (Fig. 9.3). This psyllium-enriched formula and others developed by the researchers had an improved volume, a rounded top, no cracked crust, and an appealing-looking crust and crumbs because of an increase in the dough consistency and gas-holding capacity (Capriles et al. 2022).

9.4.2 Approaches to Delay GFB Staling and Maintain Softness and Texture Liking

Bread staling includes the physical-chemical changes that occur during storage due to the reduction of crust crunchiness, increased firmness, and reduced cohesiveness of the crumb and the sensory changes in the texture, flavor, and aroma of the bread, which together gradually decrease consumer acceptance. Although bread staling mechanism is not well established, the leading causes for these changes are starch retrogradation and the migration of water from the crumb to the crust (Fadda et al. 2014).

GFBs are characterized by a short shelf life due to faster staling and greater susceptibility to microbial deterioration (Axel et al. 2017; Melini and Melini 2018), which imply additional challenges in the development of GFB with a pleasant texture and that maintains freshness during storage Santos et al. (2021b). Thus, researchers focus on the use of ingredients, additives, and technologies as strategy to extend GFB shelf life.

Fratelli et al. (2021) investigated the potential of P in delaying GFB staling, and the main results are shown in Fig. 9.3. Crumb firming was observed during 72 h of storage, especially for the GFB control, which had a crumb firmness eightfold higher than that of the WB. The P-enrichment reduced the crumb firming ratio by 75% and maintained an acceptable texture comparable to that of WB during the storage time. Adding 17.14% P to the GFB formula delayed bread staling, maintaining it compared to the physical and sensory properties more similar than those of WB samples during 72 h of storage. So, this approach is promising in overcoming some of the limitations of GF breadmaking (Fratelli et al. 2021).

Recently, Santos et al. (2021a) obtained an optimum combination of 75% chickpea flour (CF) and 5.5% P fwb that improves GFB quality by yielding a better loaf volume and crumb texture, enhancing the appearance, texture, and overall liking scores. A double increase in protein, dietary fibre and resistant starch contents was obtained, reducing the GI and GL, and increasing the satiety index (Santos et al. 2021a). In a continuation study, Santos et al. (2021b) reported that CF and its combination with P were promising for reducing and delaying GFB staling, thus maintaining texture and overall liking, softness, and freshness after 7 days of storage, according to the perceptions of consumers with and without GRD.

9.4.3 Promising Instrumental Predictors of Sensory Quality of Fresh and Stored GFB

Studies also contribute to fill the gap associated with reliable predictors that can correlate GF dough parameters, as well as GFB physical properties, with the sensory quality of fresh and stored GFB.

In a factorial study, varying P and W effects, Fratelli et al. (2018) reported that increasing the GFB specific volume decreased the crumb firmness ($r = -0.945$, $p = 0.001$), which also improved the degree of liking of appearance ($r = 0.908$, $p = 0.005$), texture ($r = 0.936$, $p = 0.002$) and overall ($r = 0.936$, $p = 0.002$). The authors also observed a strong negative correlation between the crumb firmness and the bread texture liking scores during storage ($r = -0.808$, $p = 0.000$). These data show the importance of these instrumental indicators for bread quality and, indeed, crumb firmness obtained using the AACC Bread Firmness Standard Method may be a predictor of texture acceptability of both fresh and stored WB and GFB (Fratelli et al. 2021).

A statistical technique that has been recently applied in the search to identify relationships between the set of variables studied is Multiple Factor Analysis (MFA). MFA is considered a simple, versatile, and robust statistical technique that can be used to integrate multiple data tables collected in the same dataset. MFA has gained attention in studies regarding GFB characteristics and makes it possible to identify how the key ingredients relate to the properties studied.

To the best of our knowledge, Santos et al. (2021a, b) were one of the pioneers who used MFA to relate thermomechanical dough parameters using the Mixolab2 (Chopin Technologies, France) to the physical and sensorial properties of GFB. Later, they used MFA to relate the dough parameters to the physical, compositional, and sensory properties of fresh GFB (Santos et al. 2021a). In continuation studies, they found a relationship between the physical properties (moisture content and instrumental texture), degree of liking (on 9-point hedonic scale), descriptive profile (by CATA), and softness intensity (by 5-point Just-About-Right scale) to describe the changes observed in GFB during 7 days of storage (Santos et al. 2021b). They also reported the relationship between the Mixolab dough parameters and the changes in both instrumental and sensorial texture parameters of GFB during 7 days of storage (Santos and Capriles 2021). Briefly, all these studies identified a data variation from 77.1 to 96.25% explained by the influence of the ingredients (chickpea flour and psyllium, especially) on the improvement of dough characteristics, dietary fibre composition and increases in expansion and softness, which relates to consumer liking and adequacy of softness intensity of GFB, both fresh and stored for 7 days after production.

In a recent study, Aguiar et al. (2022) investigated relations between instrumental and sensory techniques. They applied a 2^2 factorial design to investigate the effects between RF and BF combined with different W levels. The thermo-mechanical properties of the dough were analyzed using the Chopin +90 protocol in a Mixolab2 dough characterizer (Chopin Technologies, France), some GFB physical properties also being verified such as, specific volume, crumb cell structure, moisture content and instrumental texture (crumb firmness and texture profile analysis) and proximate composition. Sensory analyses assessing degree of liking on a 9-point hedonic scale, softness intensity on a 5-point Just-About-Right scale (JAR), and a facial emoji-based questionnaire (containing 33 facial emojis) to investigate the emotions related to GFB based on RF and bean flour (BF). Assessment of the intensity of a given sensorial attribute using the JAR scale and facial emoji-based questionnaires are some of the methods currently used to acquire information on the liking, softness and emotions response related to food products. However, these techniques are still little used in studies regarding GFB characteristics.

Figure 9.4 shows the relationship between the variables studied in a multiple factor analysis, where the three factors explained 91.51% of the total data variation. Briefly, this research highlights promising predictors able to correlate Mixolab dough parameters, such as the primary parameters (initial consistency – C1, protein network weakening – C2, starch gelatinization – C3, stability – C4, and

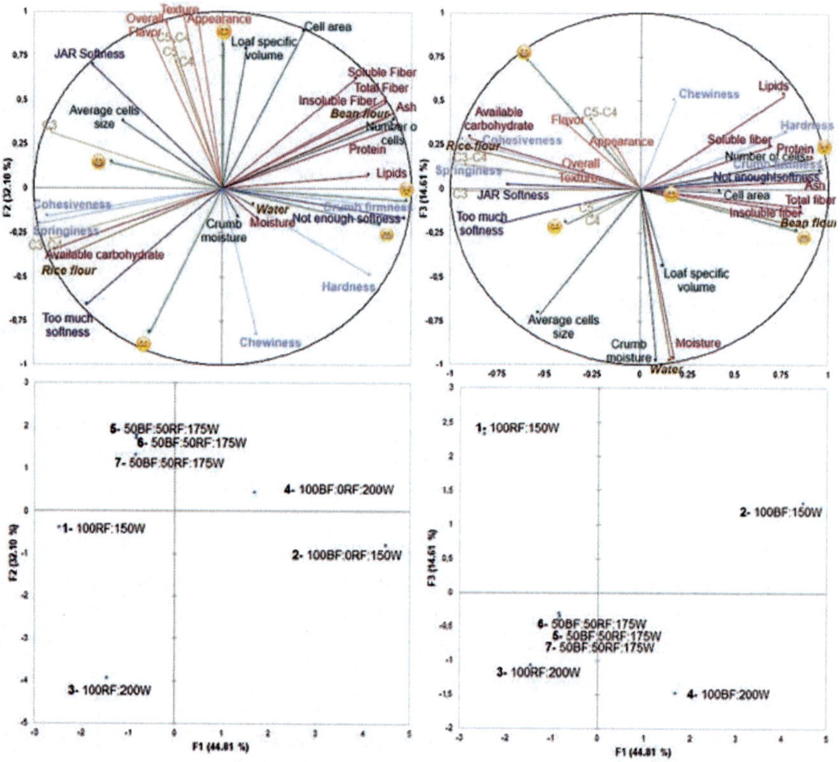

Fig. 9.4 Multiple factor analysis correlating the active variables of the dough and of the evaluated gluten-free breads. (a-b) Mixolab® dough parameters (in beige), physical properties (in green), instrumental texture (indigo), proximate composition (in pink), sensory acceptability (in red), Just-About-Right scale of softness (in blue), and facial emojis of feeling and the ingredients bean flour and water as supplementary variables. (c-d) Map of gluten-free breads coded by different levels of bean flour (BF), rice flour (RF) and water (W). (Source: Aguiar et al. 2022)

retrogradation – C5) and the secondary ones (C4-C3, C5-C4 – which refer to the starch hydrolysis and retrogradation rates respectively) (Rosell et al. 2011), as well as physical properties of bread with the sensory quality of GFB; this could be helpful to food scientists and producers to conduct extensive sensory and consumer research regarding both commercial and experimental GFB to establish whether those products meet consumer expectations. BF has an enormous potential to improve the nutritional quality of GFB, since it can contribute with better dietary fiber and mineral content. The GFB developed with BF alone presented a greater specific volume, but the GFB prepared with the mixture of BF with RF presented a better acceptance, obtaining a product with improved technological, nutritional, and sensory properties, inducing a positive feeling from the consumers.

These studies show that a combination of different sensory and instrumental methods can identify quality parameters of GFB and how these influence liking, softness, descriptive and emotional profiling of new clean label GFB formulations.

9.5 GF Cakes and Muffins

Cakes, muffins, brownies, and cupcakes are bakery products frequently consumed for breakfast or for snacking due to their sensory appeal and easy preparation (Nath et al. 2018), making them the GF products most prepared by celiac and non-celiac consumers (Alencar et al. 2021).

Xu et al. (2020) presented an interesting review regarding chemically leavened GF products such as cookies, biscuits, cakes, muffins, and crackers. Information regarding ingredients, dough properties, technological limitations, nutrient composition, and sensory properties are addressed. The authors reported that few studies described sensory results for those products, especially those with consumers with CD. Some research aimed at optimizing GF cake and muffin formulations was discussed.

Table 9.3 presents the recent studies regarding GF cakes, brownies, muffins, and cupcakes.

Table 9.3 shows the potential of new food matrices that are being used to improve the nutritional composition and diversity of the GF diet. Different ingredients have been used, like non-gluten cereals (Cayres et al. 2020, Haas et al. 2022), pulses (Jeong et al. 2021), pseudocereals (Bhatt et al. 2021), seeds (Brigagão et al. 2021) and fruit, vegetable, and food by-products (Levent et al. 2021; Radünz et al. 2021; Brigagão et al. 2021; Konuk et al. 2021). The performance of the key ingredient on cakes properties is usually evaluated through comparison to a control formulation. Some studies apply a mixture design approach (Brigagão et al. 2021; Nespeca et al. 2021) to investigate a number of single ingredients, and their combined binary and ternary effects on GF cakes and muffins properties to achieve promising and optimum formulas.

As seen for other GF products, affective testing to access consumer liking is the most frequent. All the 12 studies presented in Table 9.3 applied affective tests using a 5, 7 or 9-point hedonic scale to evaluate consumer liking. Some studies including additional sensory methods, like purchase intention (Radünz et al. 2021; Brigagão et al. 2021; Haas et al. 2022), and JAR (Pio Ávila et al. 2019). Three studies also applied the descriptive test of CATA, (Cayres et al. 2020; Gomez and Colina 2019; Pio et al. 2019) allowing access to the drivers of liking and disliking. Only one study included 50 consumers with GRD (Gomez and Colina 2019).

Further studies should consider the effect of different flavours in GF cakes, muffins and cupcakes prepared with traditional and alternative nutrient and bioactive-dense ingredients, as well as including consumers with GRD from different ages in the sensory analysis.

Table 9.3 Summary of reviewed articles regarding sensory analysis of gluten-free cakes, brownies, and cupcakes

Country and sensory focus	Gluten-free cakes, muffins, and brownies formulations	Participants	Sensory methodology	Main sensory conclusions	References
Brazil Consumer Liking and purchase intention	9 muffin formulations prepared with rice and peel/seed flours in the ratio 40:60. Pineapple peel flour, banana peel flour and pumpkin seed flour were blended in different proportions according to a mixture design experiment	47 regular consumers who consume cakes frequently	9-point hedonic scale to access colour, flavour, texture, and overall liking Purchase intention test with 5-point scale	Muffins prepared with pineapple peel flour and the mixture of pineapple peel and pumpkin seed flours showed the highest overall liking and purchase intention	Brigagão et al. (2021)
Brazil Consumer liking	1 muffin based on green banana flour	100 regular consumers	9-point hedonic scale to access the colour, odour, flavour, and overall liking Purchase intention test with 5-point scale Acceptability Index (AI)	Scores ≥7 were attributed by 84% of consumers for odour, 75% for texture, 85% for flavour, and 83% for overall liking of the green banana flour muffin 75% of the evaluators would certainly or probably buy the product GF muffins received 84.5% acceptability index	Radünz et al. (2021)

(continued)

Table 9.3 (continued)

Country and sensory focus	Gluten-free cakes, muffins, and brownies formulations	Participants	Sensory methodology	Main sensory conclusions	References
Korea Consumer liking	6 muffin formulations prepared with pulse flour (mungbean and cowpea) and waxy rice with three different ratios (80:20, 65:35, 50:50), compared to a wheat muffin	24 trained panellists (non-celiacs)	7-point hedonic scale to assesses appearance, odour, flavour, texture and overall linking	The appearance, odour, and flavour pulse - rice muffins had marginally lower scores than the wheat muffin Muffins containing 80:20 mixtures could be associated with a beany flavour and taste The proportion with the highest acceptance was 50:50 pulse flour and rice	Jeong et al. (2021)
India Consumer liking	6 muffins based on black rice flour replaced by amaranth flour at various levels (0%, 10%, 20%, 30%, 40% and 50%)	15 trained panellists	9-point hedonic scale to access colour, taste, texture, appearance, and overall liking	The proportion with the highest degree of liking in terms of texture, taste/flavour and colour was 50% amaranth flour and 50% black rice flour A sharp decrease in bitterness was observed after replacement of black rice flour with amaranth flour	Bhatt et al. (2021)

(continued)

Table 9.3 (continued)

Country and sensory focus	Gluten-free cakes, muffins, and brownies formulations	Participants	Sensory methodology	Main sensory conclusions	References
Turkey Consumer liking	4 cupcakes prepared with rice flour added with fig seed pomace flour in rations of 100/0, 90/10 70/30 and 50/50	10 Semi-trained panellists, who consume cakes frequently	5-point hedonic scale to access colour, taste, texture, and overall liking	GF cupcakes prepared with 30% fig seeds in flour base showed the highest degree of liking for appearance, colour, and overall linking GF cupcakes prepared with 10% fig seeds flour were the most preferred in terms of texture and taste	Konuk et al. (2021)
Brazil Consumer liking	9 chocolate cakes prepared with rice, sorghum, and teff flours and their binary and ternary blends according to a mixture design experiment	100 regular consumers, 61 consumers claimed to eat cake at least once month, while 39% consumed cake at least once every 2 week	9-point hedonic scale to evaluate colour, odour, flavour, texture, and overall liking	The cake samples did not differ significantly for colour, texture, and flavour attributes, but they are different in odour and overall linking The odour score varied from 6.7 to 7.6 and overall liking from 7.3 to 8.0 The higher odour liking was achieved for cake prepared from the blend of sorghum, rice and teff flours (1:1:1)	Nespeca et al. (2021)

(continued)

Table 9.3 (continued)

Country and sensory focus	Gluten-free cakes, muffins, and brownies formulations	Participants	Sensory methodology	Main sensory conclusions	References
Turkey Consumer liking	5 cakes supplemented with 5% of grape seed, pomegranate seed, poppy seed, flaxseed, and turmeric, compared to a GF formula (75% rice flour +15% chickpea flour +10% carrot flour) and to a wheat cake	26 regular consumers	9-point hedonic scale to evaluate appearance, texture, odour, mouthfeel, and overall liking	Cakes prepared with flaxseed and poppy seed obtained degrees of liking equal or higher than control GF cake for all the evaluated attributes The turmeric-enriched sample had the lowest degree of liking	Levent et al. (2021)
Brazil Consumer liking	4 chocolate cakes using Teff (*Eragrostis tef*) in different ratios (100%, 75%, 50%, 25%) complemented with rice flour and cassava starch	60 regular consumers	9-point hedonic scale to access colour, flavour texture, and overall liking 5-point scale for purchase intention	Cakes with 75%, 50% and 25% of teff flour reached 6 or 7 points for all attributes No effect on colour was observed for chocolate cakes containing 25–100% teff No difference in purchase intention between samples	Haas et al. (2022)

(continued)

Table 9.3 (continued)

Country and sensory focus	Gluten-free cakes, muffins, and brownies formulations	Participants	Sensory methodology	Main sensory conclusions	References
Brazil Sensory profiling, Consumer Liking, drivers of liking and purchase intention	5 optimized premix sorghum cakes (i) 20% sorghum +80% polished rice flour, (ii) 3% sorghum +97% pregelatinized blend flour, (iii) 100% pregelatinized blend flour, (iv) 3% sorghum +39% polished rice flour +58% pregelatinized blend flour, (v) 40%polished rice flour +60% pregelatinized blend flour	151 regular consumers	9-point structured hedonic scale to evaluated, appearance, odour, texture, flavour and overall linking CATA: the attributes were grouped into 4 categories (appearance, aroma, flavour, and texture) Purchase intention	The result suggests a greater potential to discriminate appearance, aroma, and flavour Purchase intention was 85% of the evaluation on "Would certainly buy" and "would probably buy" for the formulation prepared with 20% of sorghum flour and 80% of polished rice For CATA, no statistical differences were found between samples in 4 attributes: roast, caramel, sourness, and sweet aftertaste	Cayres et al. (2020)

(continued)

Table 9.3 (continued)

Country and sensory focus	Gluten-free cakes, muffins, and brownies formulations	Participants	Sensory methodology	Main sensory conclusions	References
Brazil Sensory profiling, Consumer Liking, drivers linking and purchase intention	2 brownies prepared with (i) 75% rice flour +25% white bean flour and (ii) 75% rice flour +25% lentil flour, compared to a wheat flour brownie	20 trained panellists 100 regular consumers	9-point structured hedonic scale to evaluated, appearance, colour, odour, and flavour linking CATA: 20 attributes were selected JAR: 3-point scale (above ideal, ideal, and below ideal)	Results from both trained panellists and consumers indicate that colour and texture were the principal attributes that need improvement in gluten – free brownie formulations	Pio Avila et al. (2019)
Venezuela Sensory profiling, Consumer Liking	2 cupcake formulations, one based on rice flour and another on cassava flour	50 consumers with celiac disease or gluten-related disorders	9-point hedonic scale to evaluated overall liking CATA: evaluated 11 attributes	Cupcake prepared with rice flour was preferred to those based on cassava flour The cassava flour cupcake was associated with "more flavour", while the rice flour cupcake was "spongy"	Gomez and Colina (2019)

9.6 GF Cookies, Biscuits, and Crackers

Cookies, biscuits, and crackers represent a large proportion of bakery products, with celiac people consuming more of these than bread (Valitutti et al. 2017). Biscuits have a long shelf life, crispness, convenience, and easy preparation (Manley Duncan 2011). Among bakery products, they have the lowest requirements in terms of gluten providing structure to the products (Di Cairano et al. 2018). However, they still offer many challenges that reflect on the nutritional, technological, and sensory quality of the products.

Recent studies (Table 9.4) show that GF cookies, biscuits and crackers are made mainly with starchy flours such as rice (Torbica et al. 2012; Radočaj et al. 2014; Mancebo et al. 2016; Mir et al. 2017; Giuberti et al. 2018; Sulieman et al. 2019; Hamdani et al. 2020; Silva et al. 2021; Christ-Ribeiro et al. 2021), corn (Paesani

Table 9.4 Summary of reviewed articles regarding sensory analysis of gluten-free cookies, biscuits, and crackers

Country and sensory focus	Gluten-free cookie, biscuit, or cracker formulations	Participants	Sensory methodology	Main sensory conclusions	References
Serbia Sensory profiling	2 cracker formulations based on 100% refined or whole grain buckwheat flour [a]controls: 100% refined or whole grain wheat flour	7 experienced regular panellists were selected from the previously trained academic staff	Generic descriptive analyses of representative properties of crackers: appearance, texture, aroma, taste. Evaluated using a 5-point method (Scores: 1 – unacceptable, 2 – acceptable, 3 – good, 4 – very good, 5 – excellent)	The best cracker quality was obtained for refined buckwheat cracker – excellent quality The scores for all sensory properties were higher for the refined buckwheat cracker than for the refined wheat cracker. No significant differences were observed in the sensory quality of wholegrain buckwheat crackers compared to wholegrain wheat crackers	Sedej et al. (2011)
Serbia Consumer Liking	3 cookie formulations prepared with blends of rice and buckwheat flour in the ratios of 90:10; 80:20 and 70:30 compared with a control cookie made with wheat flour	10 semi-trained regular panellists who were familiar with sensory analysis techniques	5-point hedonic scale to assess the shape, upper surface appearance, bottom surface appearance, rupture, cross-section structure, chewiness, and flavour	Raising the ratio of buckwheat flour from 10% to 20% increases sensory scores for flavour, rupture, and chewiness Cookies prepared with 20% buckwheat flour were better scored by the sensory panel	Torbica et al. (2012)

(continued)

Table 9.4 (continued)

Country and sensory focus	Gluten-free cookie, biscuit, or cracker formulations	Participants	Sensory methodology	Main sensory conclusions	References
Serbia and Canada Sensory profiling	5 cracker formulations: Hemp seed oil press-cake from 0 until 40% blended with brown rice flour and decaffeinated green tea leaves 2 components mixture experimental design	12 expert regular assessors	Quantitative descriptive analysis (QDA): 9-point scale to assess the appearance, colour, flavour, crunchiness, and overall texture	Appearance, colour, and taste were different between samples. The formulation with the addition of 40% hemp flour was darker and received the lowest sensory score Optimum formula, based on nutrient and bioactive composition as well as overall score, contains 20% hemp seed oil press-cake and 4 g decaffeinated green tea leaves that received an overall score of 8.9	Radočaj et al. (2014)
India Consumer liking	2 cookie formulations prepared with 100% raw or germinated amaranth flour [a]control: 100% wheat flour	20 semi-trained regular panellists drawn from within the University community	9-point hedonic scale to assess colour, appearance, aroma, taste, texture, and overall acceptability	Cookies prepared with germinated amaranth flour show the highest score for all sensory attributes compared with cookies prepared with raw amaranth flour or wheat flour	Chauhan et al. (2015)

(continued)

Table 9.4 (continued)

Country and sensory focus	Gluten-free cookie, biscuit, or cracker formulations	Participants	Sensory methodology	Main sensory conclusions	References
Romania Sensory profiling and consumer liking	5 cookie formulations prepared with oat flour replaced by 30%, 50%, 70% e 100% of oat bran, compared to control without oat bran	10 trained regular panellists 73 consumers	Quantitative descriptive analysis (QDA): 5-point method to assess (1 low intensity, 5 high intensity) appearance, surface colour, hardness at the first bite, oat flavour, sweet degree, effort of chewing, after-taste after swallowing 9-point hedonic scale to determine overall liking	With the increase in oat bran, the appearance became more grained. Addition of up to 30% oat grain did not change the colour on the cookie surface The higher the oat bran levels, the higher the colour and oat flavour intensity Oat bran levels did not change the sweet degree and after-taste intensity Cookies prepared with 50% or more oat bran become harder to chew Overall liking ranges from 5.6 to 7. The higher the oat bran levels, the lower the overall liking.	Duta and Culetu (2015)
India Consumer liking	5 cookie formulations: 100% buckwheat flour with no gum, or with acacia, guar, tragacanth, or xanthan gum added [a]control: Wheat flour	10 regular panellists trained with commercial cookies	9-point hedonic scale to assess colour, appearance, flavour, texture, taste, and overall acceptability	The control formulation had the highest scores while buckwheat flour preparations had the lowest scores The incorporation of gums, mainly xanthan gum, improved the sensory scores	Kaur et al. (2015)

(continued)

Table 9.4 (continued)

Country and sensory focus	Gluten-free cookie, biscuit, or cracker formulations	Participants	Sensory methodology	Main sensory conclusions	References
Spain Consumer liking	3 cookie formulation selected from instrumental results obtained in an experimental design Cookies prepared with the blends of (i)- 80% maize starch and 20% pea protein, (ii) – 30% rice flour, 50% maize starch and 20% pea protein, and (iii) – 70% rice flour and 30% maize starch, compared to 100% rice flour, as a [a]control	66 regular volunteers, staff, and students from the university who were habitual cookie consumers	9-point hedonic scale to assess the appearance, odour, texture, taste, and overall appreciation	Consumers attributed the highest overall liking to Cookies 1 and 2 prepared with protein, a score of 5.9 for each, although it was not significantly different from the control cookie. Cookie 3, without protein, got the worst overall liking (5.2) lower than control (5.7)	Mancebo et al. (2016)
India Consumer liking	4 cracker formulations based on brown rice flour and apple pomace powder ratios of 0%, 3%, 6%, and 9%.[a]control: 100% brown rice flour	15 regular panellists	9-point hedonic scale to access appearance, colour, flavour, texture, and overall liking	The liking for appearance was higher for the formulation with 3% pomace and, for flavour, it increased with an increasing pomace level up to 6%	Mir et al. (2017)
Italy Consumer liking	4 cookie formulations prepared with rice flour replaced by 0, 15%, 30%, and 45% of alfalfa seed flour [a]control: rice flour	10 trained regular panellists	9-point hedonic scale to assess colour, texture, flavour, and overall acceptability	The control formulation presented the best sensory scores, however, the supplemented cookies showed moderate acceptability for all parameters tested	Giubert et al. (2018)

(continued)

Table 9.4 (continued)

Country and sensory focus	Gluten-free cookie, biscuit, or cracker formulations	Participants	Sensory methodology	Main sensory conclusions	References
China Consumer liking	6 biscuit formulations made with 3%, 6%, and 10% fermented and non-fermented *Agaricus bisporus* polysaccharide [a]control: Sweet potato flour and rice flour	61 untrained and semi-trained regular panellists comprised mainly of students and staff members of the university	9-point hedonic scale to assess colour, appearance, aroma, taste, crispiness, and overall acceptability	Biscuits with fermented *Agaricus bisporus* polysaccharide flour (3%) were the best in all sensory characteristics due to softer texture, lighter colour, and better flavour	Sulieman et al. (2019)
Brazil Consumer liking	4 cracker formulations produced with 2% mucilage from cactus, or 5, 10, and 15% of cladode flour from cactus, without commercial gum, compared to a [a]control: Prepared with 2% commercial gums ([b]CMC and xanthan gum)	50 regular panellists untrained	9-point hedonic scale to assess the appearance, colour, odour, crunchiness, taste, aftertaste, and overall liking	Sensory analysis did not indicate differences for the appearance, colour, and odour attributes of all cookies Cookies containing cactus mucilage and those supplemented with 5% cladode flour were the ones that had the highest overall liking	Dick et al. (2020)
India Consumer liking	6 cookie formulations: addition of acacia, apricot, and karaya gum at levels of 0.5% and 1.0%. [a]control: Rice-chickpea composite flour (80:20)	15 semi-trained regular members	9-point hedonic scale to assess the texture, appearance, mouthfeel, flavour, and overall liking	The lowest scores were found for the control. The incorporation of gums increased the sensory score of the cookies	Hamdani et al. (2020)

(continued)

Table 9.4 (continued)

Country and sensory focus	Gluten-free cookie, biscuit, or cracker formulations	Participants	Sensory methodology	Main sensory conclusions	References
Spain Consumer liking	4 cookie formulations: (i) whole grain maize flour, (ii) extruded whole grain maize flour and (iii) flour + stabilized bran and germ. (iv)[a]control: maize flour	95 recruited regular volunteers at university	9-point hedonic scale to assess the appearance, odour, texture, taste, and overall acceptability	The most accepted formulation was that prepared with wholemeal flour with stabilized bran and germ	Paesani et al. (2020)
Brazil Consumer liking and intention to consume	4 cookie formulations prepared with cassava flour added with 0%, 3.7%, 5.5% and 7.4% of cooked cassava leaves [a]control: white cassava flour	120 regular untrained volunteers	9-point hedonic scale for accessing appearance, colour, odour, crispness, flavour and overall linking 5-point hedonic scale (1: would not consume, 5: would certainly consume) for assessing the intention to consume	All formulations obtained scores higher than 6 for all evaluated attributes. The addition of cassava leaves did not affect the liking nor the intention to consume the biscuits	Neves et al. (2021)
Brazil Consumer liking and Intention to buy	6 biscuit formulations, produced with blends of rice and beans in the proportion of 3:1, for nutrition/health reasons. Biscuits were prepared using (i) brown rice flour, (ii) polished rice flour, (iii) cooked polished rice, (iv) white bean flour and (v) cooked beans, compared to [a]control: whole wheat biscuit	120 regular participants for all tests	9-point hedonic scale to assess the appearance, odour, taste, texture, and overall impression 5-point hedonic scale (5: would not certainly buy; 1: certainly, would buy)	The use of cooked beans instead of bean flour resulted in higher liking. The formulation with cooked beans and a blend of brown rice flour and polished rice obtained the highest liking in all attributes and in the purchase intention of consumers	Silva et al. (2021)

(continued)

Table 9.4 (continued)

Country and sensory focus	Gluten-free cookie, biscuit, or cracker formulations	Participants	Sensory methodology	Main sensory conclusions	References
Italy Consumer liking	3 biscuit formulations: Commercial gluten-free flour mix with replacement of 15%, 30%, and 45% for sorghum starch (rich in resistant starch). [a]control: commercial gluten-free flour mix	20 regular trained panellists	9-point hedonic to assess appearance, structure, odour, flavour, and overall liking	The overall liking was negatively influenced by the addition of white sorghum starch, but all attributes remained above the acceptability limit of 5	Cervini et al. (2021)
Brazil Consumer liking and intention to consume	4 cookie formulations prepared with rice flour and 0, 7.1%, 14.2%, and 28.3% of rice bran fermented by *Saccharomyces cerevisiae*. [a]control: without the addition of fermented rice bran	101 regular consumers	7-point hedonic scale to assess the colour, crispness, sweetness, and overall liking 7 points (7: would always eat, 1: would never eat) for evaluate the consume intention	The cookies were accepted by the consumer. Cookie prepared with 7.1% fermented rice bran was highlighted for consumer liking and intention to consume	Christ-Ribeiro et al. (2021)
Germany Sensory profiling	6 cookies formulations: 100% of 6 different *Vicia faba* bean varieties [a]there was no control formulation	17regular trained panellists	Flash Profiling, containing 54 descriptors, with approx. 20% being related to smell, and approx. 40% each to taste and texture	The bean variety affected the flavour, but all cookies were acceptable	Schmelter et al. (2021)

Where: [a]control: formulation developed in the study used for comparison. [b]*CMC* carboxymethyl cellulose

et al. 2020), cassava (Neves et al. 2021), buckwheat (Sedej et al. 2011; Torbica et al. 2012; Kaur et al. 2015) and oats (Duta and Culetu 2015) and others that currently stand out, being a source of protein, such as chickpeas (Hamdani et al. 2020), beans (David et al. 2021), amaranth (Chauhan et al. 2015) and fava beans (Schmelter et al. 2021). This demonstrates the tendency to diversify the raw materials used in GF cookies, biscuits, and crackers in an attempt to improve the nutritional value, technological properties, and sensory perception of products.

The sensory analyses in Table 9.4 show that the products are being developed in their entirety for a wide audience, who may or may not be consumers of GF products.

Few studies reported details about participants, i.e. if they are regular consumers of GF products or if they are GCC consumers, which implies they could compare GF to wheat crackers. In addition, there is no information regarding consumer characteristics like age, gender, race, and region which can make a big difference to this comparison. For example, in Asian countries, the consumption of rice crackers belongs to the food habit, in which they present sensory memory for GF products. Another factor that can affect the sensory evaluation and that could be considered in the studies is the production and consumption of wheat products as a local habit. In non-wheat producing countries, where the consumption of biscuits often homemade with regional raw materials such as potatoes, cassava, and corn is stronger, in addition to being local and low-cost products, this consumer public can more readily accept GF cookies produced under laboratory conditions, which facilitates advances in this area of research.

For research and development laboratories for various products with and without wheat, it is difficult to guarantee the safety of GF products, which are free from cross contamination. Due to the specificity of GF cookies, the articles do not present how the panellist selection and training was carried out and how the selection of participants for the sensory analysis took place, including what "semi-trained participant" means (Table 9.4). If this training was carried out with commercial cookies with or without gluten, this causes technological disadvantages for cookies produced on a laboratory scale, since industrial technology allows laminating, cutting, baking, and cooling of the product under mechanized and controlled conditions while, in laboratories, equipment, including ovens, suitable for cakes and bread is often used, with a minority of laboratories having appropriate production lines for cookies.

Regarding the sensorial methods applied, these are conservative and are frequently repeated, there being acceptance tests in 15 of the 18 studies (Table 9.4). Studies with quantitative descriptive analysis (QDA) were found in 3 studies and affective tests using the purchase intent or consumption intent were found in 3 studies.

Of the 18 studies (Table 9.4), five studies compared cookies with a control sample of wheat flour (Sedej et al. 2011; Torbica et al. 2012; Kaur et al. 2015; Silva et al. 2021), in general, the objective of most of these studies was to develop GF cookies with new raw materials and/or to evaluate the technological properties and feasibility of these raw materials, demonstrating that there is a search for standardization and similarity to cookies with gluten.

There is a need for more research efforts and the construction of specific laboratories to further and strengthen the development of GF products and to create a solid identity for the GF cookie. In addition, it is relevant that research expands beyond laboratories and universities, investigating new approaches that include greater variety and diversity of consumers concerning gender, ethnicity, social class, and age group, making the sensory analysis produce more reliable results for a region for which the product is intended. As an example, concerning social class, GF products in developing countries are seen as high-cost products and inaccessible to the lower income classes. Consequently, these products are not present in the basic food basket.

9.7 GF Pasta

For GF pasta production, rice flour or starch (Giménez et al. 2015; Bouasla et al. 2017; Ferreira et al. 2016; Albuja-Vaca et al. 2020; Demir and Bilgiçli 2021; Aínsa et al. 2021; Rungsardthong et al. 2021; Scarton et al. 2021) was frequently used as a basis for the formulation of these products, especially due to its mild flavour. Corn flour and starch have also been used (Padalino et al. 2011; Flores-Silva et al. 2015; Mirhosseini et al. 2015; Demir and Bilgiçli 2021), resulting in GF pasta with characteristic colour and flavour (O'Shea et al. 2014). Despite their lower production costs, these ingredients are rich in carbohydrates and make a strong contribution to the nutritional value and sensory characteristics of GF pastas. Consequently, recent studies have focused on new ingredients for improvement in the nutritional value as well as the flavour, aroma, colour, and texture.

Table 9.5 shows some examples of GF pasta research. There is a preference for natural ingredients, with a tendency to adopt raw materials and co-products of low cost, for example, cassava fibre (Fiorda et al. 2013), mango peel fibre (Rungsardthong et al. 2021), green banana flour (Zandonadi et al. 2012), and fish by-products (Aínsa et al. 2021) aiming to increase the consumption of these ingredients and reduce the monotony of a GF diet.

Studies with long and dry pasta, mainly the spaghetti format, are predominant (Padalino et al. 2011; Fiorda et al. 2013; Flores-Silva et al. 2015; Giménez et al. 2015; Bastos et al. 2016; Rungsardthong et al. 2021). However, this format leads to higher rates of breakage and defects, especially in the stages of drying, packaging, transport, and storage, impairing the cooking quality characteristics of these pastas. In this way, GF pastas produced with other formats, such as *fusilli* (Scarton et al. 2021) or *penne* (Demir and Bilgiçli 2021), can be a technological alternative for a better consumption experience.

Sensory analysis methods (Table 9.5) were mostly affective tests – with a predominance of acceptance tests using a structured hedonic scale in 10 of the 15 studies. Studies with QDA (Ferreira et al. 2016; Aínsa et al. 2021) and CATA (Giménez et al. 2015) were also found but, perhaps, it is necessary to stimulate more descriptive studies to obtain more specific information about GF pastas. The purchase intention was evaluated in a few studies (Fiorda et al. 2013; Giménez et al. 2015; Bastos et al. 2016). However, the purchase of a product is dependent on many aspects besides the sensory attributes, such as price, packing, quantity or how-to-prepare.

Of the 15 studies (Table 9.5), only two (Zandonadi et al. 2012; Giménez et al. 2015) focused on recruitment of celiac or gluten-intolerant individuals for the sensory panel. The use of control pastas was also a point for discussion, since durum wheat semolina (Flores-Silva et al. 2015; Aínsa et al. 2021), or standard commercial

Table 9.5 Summary of reviewed articles regarding sensory analysis of gluten-free pasta

Country and sensory focus	Gluten-free pasta	Participants	Sensory methodology	Main sensory conclusions	References
Italy Sensory profiling	*Spaghetti* Step 1: 6 samples prepared with heat treated maize flour with oat bran added at levels ranging from 5% to 20% [a]control: 100% heat treated maize flour. Step 2: 8 samples produced with heat treated maize flour, oat bran (20%) + 2% of hydrocolloids (xanthan gum, carboxymethylcellulose, hydroxypropyl cellulose, agar, egg protein powder, tapioca starch, guar seed flour, or chitosan) plus a [a]control: 100% heat treated maize flour	10 regular trained panellists	9-point hedonic scale (1: extremely unpleasant; 9: extremely pleasant) to assess the raw fresh and dry samples (colour, homogeneity, resistance to break and overall quality) and cooked (elasticity, firmness, bulkiness, adhesiveness, colour, odour, taste, and overall quality)	Fresh extruded spaghetti samples (non-cooked and cooked) were scored higher for overall quality than dry samples. Increasing the oat bran decreased the overall quality, due to the decrease in elasticity and firmness. The sample prepared with 20% oat bran was at the limit of acceptance (5.4). The structuring agents (hydrocolloids) improved the sensory (firmness and adhesiveness) characteristics of the samples	Padalino et al. (2011)
Brazil Consumer liking	*Fettuccine* 1 sample: green banana flour (47.0%), egg white (31.5%), guar gum (2.5%), and xanthan gum (2.5%) [a]control: wheat pasta	50 regular consumers (tested both products) 25 celiac consumers (tested only GF pasta)	9-point hedonic scale to assess the odour, flavour, texture, and overall liking	Acceptance means of the green banana pasta were higher for celiac tasters	Zandonadi et al. (2012)

(continued)

Table 9.5 (continued)

Country and sensory focus	Gluten-free pasta	Participants	Sensory methodology	Main sensory conclusions	References
Brazil Consumer liking and Buying intention	*Spaghetti* 1 sample: pregelatinized cassava starch and bagasse (70:30) flour, cassava starch and amaranth flour in the proportion of 10:60:30. Accompanied by a tomato-based sauce. [a]control: [b]n.a	50 regular consumers	9-point hedonic scale for liking 5-point scale (5: would certainly buy, 3: maybe would buy/maybe not, 1: would certainly not buy)	Average score of 7.2, with 81% of acceptance. For the buying intention, the experimental pasta received an average score of 2.3	Fiorda et al. (2013)
USA Consumer liking	*Spaghetti* 9 samples: unripe plantain (15–30%), chickpea (60–70%) and white corn flour (5–20%) [a]control: 100% durum semolina	30 regular consumers	9-point hedonic scale to assess the flavour, texture, and overall liking	The control spaghetti received the highest score of acceptability, while all the GF spaghetti ranged above the scale median value of 4.5	Flores-Silva et al. (2015)
Uruguay Sensory profile Consumer liking and purchase intention	*Spaghetti* 6 samples: 1: whole cully corn flour; 2: whole capia corn flour (CC); 3: durum wheat semolina; 4: durum wheat semolina; 5: bread wheat flour; and 6: rice flour. [a]control: commercial samples rice-based (gluten-free) or wheat-based.	10 semi-trained assessors for flash profile to generate descriptor terms for CATA (Study 1) 85 individuals (30 celiac and 55 non-celiac) for consumer liking and for purchase intention, relating to the CATA terms created in study 1 (Study 2)	Flash profile to generate descriptor terms for CATA 9-point hedonic scale for consumer acceptability 9-point hedonic scale (1: definitely would not buy, 9: definitely would buy) for purchase intention	38 terms were selected for use at CATA. The CC sample was featured: the celiac consumers used terms denoting positive attributes tasty, smooth, tender, delicious and for special diets – which explains the high scores for acceptability and purchase intention, because they regularly consume rice flour pasta. The opposite happened with non-celiac consumers.	Giménez et al. (2015)

Malaysia Consumer liking	Pasta 5 samples: (i) corn flour, (ii) corn starch, (iii) durian seed flour, (iv) pumpkin flour 25%, and (v) pumpkin flour 50%, compared to [a]control: Commercial GF pasta	30 trained regular panellists	9-point hedonic scale to assess the appearance, odour, colour, firmness, flavour, and overall liking	The addition of 25% pumpkin flour improved GF pasta overall liking	Mirhosseini et al. (2015)
Brazil Consumer liking and Buying intention	*Spaghetti* 1 sample (selected previously- from response surface methodology): 25 g of pasta (0.65 of dry potato pulp; 0.10 of extruded potato pulp and 0.25 of amaranth flour), with tomato sauce [a]control: [b]n.a	80 regular consumers	9-point hedonic scale to assess the appearance, texture, flavour, and odour	Scores above 7 for all evaluated attributes	Bastos et al. (2016)
Not informed Consumer liking	Pasta 9 samples: partial replacement of rice flour by yellow pea flour, chickpea flour, or lentil flour (10, 20, 30%). Served without sauce. [a]control: 100% rice flour	15 semi-trained regular panellists	9-point scale to assess the appearance, colour, flavour, stickiness, and overall 5-point scale (1: poor, 5: good)	All samples showed acceptable scores (values >5) for overall impression.	Bouasla et al. (2017)

(continued)

Table 9.5 (continued)

Country and sensory focus	Gluten-free pasta	Participants	Sensory methodology	Main sensory conclusions	References
Brazil Sensory profile	Pasta 15 samples: 40–60% of sorghum, 15–30% of rice and/or 10–20% of corn and 10–40% of potato starch.t through and experimental design	12 trained regular panellists	Quantitative Descriptive Analysis, applying 9 cm scale to assess the intensity of the attributes appearance, colour, odour, hardness, elasticity, stickiness, grittiness, taste, residual bitterness, and overall quality	The samples containing a higher proportion of sorghum flour and/or corn flour were perceived to be bitter, obtaining lover scores No differences were observed for the intensity of odour, taste, residual bitterness, elasticity, stickiness, grittiness, and overall quality of pasta samples	Ferreira et al. (2016)
Brazil Consumer liking and Intent of purchase	*Tagliarini* 1 selected sample (mixture design): cassava starch (0.55), peach palm flour (0.35), and golden linseed flour (0.10). 25 g samples, with or without tomato sauce (optional)	80 regular consumers	9-point structured hedonic scale to assess the appearance, texture, flavour, and odour liking Intent of purchase	Mean score of 7.7 for all attributes. 47.5% of tasters "would certainly buy" the evaluated gluten-free pasta	Sakurai et al. (2020)
Ecuador Consumer liking	Pasta 3 samples: rice flour (80 to 90%), lupine flour (10 to 30%), whole egg, guar gum	112 regular consumers	9-point hedonic scale, to assess the overall liking, appearance, flavour, and texture preferences	The colour and flavour of the samples were influenced by the addition of lupine flour	Albuja-Vaca et al. (2020)
Turkey Consumer liking	*Penne* 7 samples: Rice semolina, and corn semolina (1:1) + guar gum, quinoa flour (raw/germinated, 10–30% substitution of the flour basis) [a]control: Rice semolina and corn semolina (1:1)	20 regular consumers	7-point hedonic scale to assess the taste, odour, appearance, and overall liking	The use of 20 and 30% of raw or germinated quinoa reduced the appearance score and overall liking	Demir and Bilgiçli (2021)

Brazil Consumer liking	3 samples (selected previously – from response surface methodology): Rice flour (RF) + biofortified sweet potato flour (BSPF) to levels respectively (90:10; 80:20 and 85:15) + hydrolysed soy protein concentrate, sodium carboxymethyl cellulose gum, and monoglycerides.	57 regular consumers	9-point hedonic scale to assess appearance, aroma, texture, and overall liking Colour and texture intensity using a 9-point Just-About-Right scale, (0–4.4 cm: too much light colour and soft, 4.5 cm: JAR, 4.6–9 cm: too much dark colour and firm). Penalty Analysis to assess the raw and cooked pastas: visual and texture colour	According to the penalty analysis, the parameters colour and consistency penalized these averages The sample prepared with 80:20 RF:BSPF, presented the highest overall liking	Scarton et al. (2021)
Thailand Consumer liking	*Spaguetti* 4 samples: rice flour, defatted soy protein (10%), modified starch (3%), and mango peel fibre (MPF, 2.5 to 10%). [a]Control: 100% rice flour	40 regular consumers	5-point hedonic scale to assess the colour, texture, cohesiveness, pasta stability, overall liking	The addition of MPF (7.5–10%) reduced the scores for overall liking and increased the brown colour of the GF pastas	Rungsardthong et al. (2021)

(continued)

Table 9.5 (continued)

Country and sensory focus	Gluten-free pasta	Participants	Sensory methodology	Main sensory conclusions	References
Spain Sensory Texture Profile, quantitative descriptive analysis	Pasta 4 samples: with different levels of seabass concentrate (5–10%), rice flour (40–80%), oat bran (5%), yellow corn flour (45%) and white corn flour (45%). All served without sauce. [a]control: 100% durum wheat pasta (commercial)	10 regular evaluators expert in sensory Assessors	Sensory Texture Profile (0: absence; 5: maximum intensity) to assess the elasticity, hardness, disintegration, graininess, pastiness, and stickiness Quantitative Descriptive Analysis to assess the characteristic aroma of cooked pasta, fish aroma, other odours, hardness, characteristic flavour of cooked pasta, fish flavour, aftertaste, other flavours, intensity in yellow, and the homogeneity of the colour	GF pastas had lower hardness, springiness, gumminess, chewiness, and fracturability, and higher adhesiveness than wheat pasta All GF pastas were characterized by fish aromas and flavours with a certain aftertaste and a lower hardness in comparison with durum pasta.	Aínsa et al. (2021)

[a]Control: formulation developed in the study used for comparison. [b]*n.a.* not available

pasta (Zandonadi et al. 2012) was used. Considering that wheat-based pastas have distinct cooking and sensory characteristics, the comparison with these pastas could not be a good parameter for sensory improvement. It is also necessary some detailing regarding the quantities, temperature of serving, sauce adding and other parameters – also equalizing the experiments with a usual pasta consumption. According to Table 9.5, the usual quantity of samples was 20–25 g of cooked pasta, when described, with addition of tomato sauce in a few studies (Bastos et al. 2016, Sakurai et al. 2020).

The most-mentioned sensory descriptors of GF pastas, described in Fig. 9.5, were appearance, aroma, texture, and overall quality. For studies with descriptive methods, the terms are mainly related to texture, such as hardness, elasticity, or stickiness. The texture is a decisive factor related to pasta consumption and is also related to its cooking quality. Due to the different technological interactions between components – such as hydrocolloids, starches, protein ingredients and fibres – there was a wide variety of possible textures for GF pasta, unlike the gluten-network interaction in wheat-based pastas. Thus, studies about texture profile, as performed by Aínsa et al. (2021), for example, and the evaluation of texture impact in overall liking form an important approach for sensory studies of GF pastas. The JAR scale

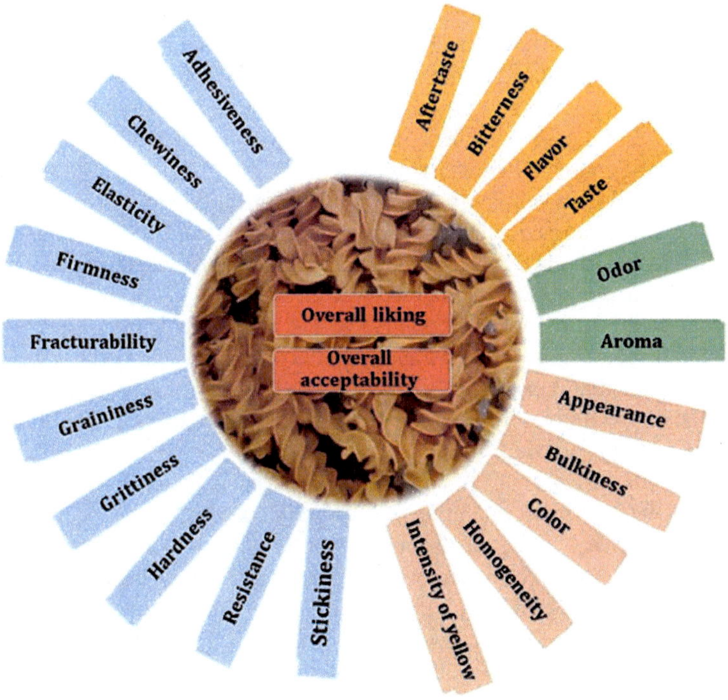

Fig. 9.5 Sensory descriptors used in gluten-free pasta studies (2011–2021). (Source: from authors)

was also used – as seen in Scarton et al. (2021) study, which evaluated *fusilli*-type GF pastas, providing useful information about the ideal consistency and colour according to consumers, demonstrating that the texture impairs the mean scores of other attributes in the evaluation of these pastas.

Few studies have been conducted with trained (Padalino et al. 2011; Mirhosseini et al. 2015; Aínsa et al. 2021) or semi-trained (Giménez et al. 2015; Bouasla et al. 2017) panellists but they did not specify the type of selection and training. Also, studies are still not focused on individuals who regularly consume GF products, which has been discussed in a few articles that point out that GF pasta has a lower degree of liking (Giménez et al. 2015; Aínsa et al. 2021). Thus, research efforts that promote advances in sensory evaluation and identify parameters for GF pastas is a real, current demand that could benefit the productive chain of GF products.

9.8 Conclusions and Topics and Challenges for Further Investigations

Creating GF systems that allow GF bakery and pasta production, as well as developing the quality control of GF foods is a huge task that involves diverse approaches to assess rheological, chemical, physical, nutrient composition, and sensory properties of such products. In some studies, sensory analyses assume a secondary importance, while in others they are the main approach. It is expected that sensory and consumer research will play a pivotal role in GF food research and development in the coming years due to consumer dissatisfaction about currently available products, despite the continued growth of this market.

A challenge for the coming years is to assess GF food consumers to establish whether currently commercial GF bakery and pasta products meet consumer expectations and to identify the key sensory parameters to be targeted during new product development or product reformulation to meet and satisfy consumer expectation. Such studies could provide food scientists and technologists with insights for identifying and responding to consumer needs, both consumers with GRD as well those of the gluten-tolerant population that choose to follow a GF diet. Alongside a better knowledge of the motives that lead these people to adhere to a GF diet, they could also guide them towards healthier food choices.

Recent studies show that GF consumers prefer short list of ingredients, which reinforces the need for reformulation of such products which usually contain a long list of ingredients and additives. Moreover, due to the inherent difficulties, few studies have been done with consumers with CD or other GRD; however, this approach is important to verify whether the developed product meets the requirements of these consumers. Sensory and consumer research with GF consumers will allow the study of different segments of consumers and their preference patterns, driving the developing of consumer-tailored GF foods.

More sensory evaluation is needed with children and adolescents with GRD due to the huge difficulties that they have to accept, adapt, and follow a GF diet (Czaja-Bulsa and Bulsa 2018). This will provide insights regarding their perceptions and needs which could drive the development or improvement of GF foods targeting these consumers.

Important questions still need to be answered: should GF food be compared to GCC? Wheat products are frequently considered as a reference or standard for comparison, although they are clearly different due to the presence of gluten and its unique functionality. Should GF bakery and pasta products be evaluated alone or evaluated as carriers together with spreads and toppings in a more realistic consumption situation?

Still, recent studies have shown that despite its structure and mechanical properties, in-mouth behaviour of a product should be considered in the design of GF foods, as its breakage pattern in the presence of saliva and oral movements are crucial to modulate texture sensations. Further studies about oral processing behaviour and sensations perceived during GF food consumption should help to clarify how eating rate, satiation responses and food intake can be modulated in GF bakery and pasta products.

The future perspective involves extensive sensory and consumer research to narrow the knowledge gap in GF consumer opinions, perceptions, emotions, and behaviour to establish whether currently available GF foods meet consumer expectations at different life stages, and to specially design or reformulate GF bakery and pasta to meet consumer demands for products that combine better flavour, texture, convenience, and health.

Acknowledgments The authors are grateful to the National Council for Scientific and Technological Development (CNPq) for the scholarship by VD Capriles (process 303066/2022-9), FG Santos (process 152121/2022-6), MEA Fernández (process 162127/2021-9), BL Tagliapietra (process 140805/2020-6), M. Scarton (process 140791/2017-5), MTP Clerici (process 312786/2020-4), AC Conti (process 303602/2022-8), the São Paulo Research Foundation (FAPESP) for the scholarship by EV Aguiar (grant 2019/15359-0), and the Coordination for the Improvement of Higher Education Personnel (CAPES) for the scholarship by B. Guedes (process 88887.487836/2020-00).

Conflicts of Interest none.

Funding This work was supported by a grant (2021/06643-7) from São Paulo Research Foundation (FAPESP). "The opinions, hypothesis, conclusions or recommendations contained in this material are the responsibility of the authors and do not necessarily reflect FAPESP's vision".

References

Aguiar EV, Santos FG, Krupa-Kozak U, Capriles VD (2021a) Nutritional facts regarding commercially available gluten-free bread worldwide: recent advances and future challenges. Crit Rev Food Sci Nutr 2021:1–13. Advance online publication. https://doi.org/10.1080/10408398.2021.1952403

Aguiar EV, Santos FG, Centeno ACLS, Capriles VD (2021b) Influence of pseudocereals on gluten-free bread quality: a study integrating dough rheology, bread physical properties and acceptability. Food Res Int 150:110762. https://doi.org/10.1016/j.foodres.2021.110762

Aguiar EV, Santos FG, Faggian L, Araujo MBS, Araújo VA, Conti-Silva AC, Capriles VD (2022) An integrated instrumental and sensory techniques for assessing liking, softness and emotional related of gluten-free bread based on blended rice and bean flour. Food Res Int 154:110999. https://doi.org/10.1016/j.foodres.2022.110999

Aínsa A, Vega A, Honrado A, Marquina P, Roncales P, Gracia JAB, Morales JBC (2021) Gluten-free pasta enriched with fish by-product for special dietary uses: technological quality and sensory properties. Foods 10:3049. https://doi.org/10.3390/foods10123049

Albuja-Vaca D, Yépez C, Vernaza G, Navarrete D (2020) Gluten-free pasta: development of a new formulation based on rice and lupine bean flour (*Lupinus Mutabilis*) using a mixture-process design. Food Sci Technol 40:2–414. https://doi.org/10.1590/fst.02319

Alencar NMM, Araújo VA, Faggian L, Araújo MBS, Capriles VD (2021) What about gluten-free products? An insight on celiac consumers' opinions and expectations. J Sens Stud 36(4):e12664. https://doi.org/10.1111/joss.12664

Ares G, Varela P (2017) Trained vs. consumer panels for analytical testing: fueling a long lasting debate in the field. Food Qual Prefer 61:79–86. https://doi.org/10.1016/j.foodqual.2016.10.006

Axel C, Zannini E, Arendt EK (2017) Mold spoilage of bread and its biopreservation: a review of current strategies for bread shelf life extension. Crit Rev Food Sci Nutr 57(16):3528–3542. https://doi.org/10.1080/10408398.2016.1147417

Bastos GH, Soares Junior MS, Caliari MP, Pereira ALA, Morais CC, Campos MRH (2016) Physical and sensory quality of gluten-free spaghetti processed from amaranth flour and potato pulp. LWT Food Sci Technol 65:128–136. https://doi.org/10.1016/j.lwt.2015.07.067

Bender D, Schönlechner R (2020) Innovative approaches towards improved gluten-free bread properties. J Cereal Sci 91:102904. https://doi.org/10.1016/j.jcs.2019.102904

Bhatt S, Kumari N, Abhishek V et al (2021) Elucidating the role of amaranth flour in formulation of gluten free black rice muffins and its premix: nutritional, physico-chemical and textural characteristics. J Food Meas Charact 15:675–685. https://doi.org/10.1007/s11694-020-00675-y

Borges VC, Fernandes SS, Zavareze ER, Haros CM, Hernandez CP, Dias ARG, Salas-Mellado MM (2021) Production of gluten free bread with flour and chia seeds (Salvia hispânica L). Food Biosci 43:101294. https://doi.org/10.1016/j.fbio.2021.101294

Bouasla A, Wójtowicz A, Zidoune MN (2017) Gluten-free precooked rice pasta enriched with legumes flours: physical properties, texture, sensory attributes and microstructure. LWT Food Sci Technol 75:569–577. https://doi.org/10.1016/j.lwt.2016.10.005

Brazil- Ministry of Health. Law n° 493 of April, 15th (2021) Dispõe sobre os requisitos de composição e rotulagem dos alimentos contendo cereais para classificação e identificação como integral e para destaque da presença de ingredientes integrais. URL https://www.in.gov.br/en/web/dou/-/resolucao-rdc-n-493-de-15-de-abril-de-2021-315225504

Brazil- Ministry of Health. Law n° 54 of November, 12th (2012) Regulamento Técnico sobre Informação Nutricional Complementar, 2012. URL http://bvsms.saude.gov.br/bvs/saudelegis/anvisa/2012/rdc0054_12_11_2012.html

Breshears KL, Crowe K (2013) Sensory and textural evaluation of gluten-free bread substituted with amaranth and montina flour. J Food Res 2(4):1–10. https://doi.org/10.5539/jfr.v2n4p1

Brigagão TCS, Fortes RR, Lourenço CO, Carvalho EEN, Cirillo MÂ, Nachtigall AM, Vilas Boas BM (2021) Optimization of gluten-free muffins made with pineapple peel, banana peel, and pumpkin seed flours. J Food Process Preserv 45:e16037. https://doi.org/10.1111/jfpp.16037

Campo E, Arco L, Urtasun L, Oria R, Mairal AF (2016) Impact of sourdough on sensory properties and consumers' preference of gluten-free breads enriched with teff flour. J Cereal Sci 67:75–82

Cappelli A, Oliva N, Cini E (2020) A systematic review of gluten-free dough and bread: dough rheology, bread characteristics, and improvement strategies. Appl Sci 10:6559. https://doi.org/10.3390/app10186559

Capriles VD, Arêas JAG (2013) Effects of prebiotic inulin-type fructans on structure, quality, sensory acceptance and glycemic response of gluten-free breads. Food Funct 4(1):104–110. https://doi.org/10.1039/c2fo10283h

Capriles VD, Arêas JAG (2014) Novel approaches in gluten-free breadmaking: interface between food science, nutrition and health. Compr Rev Food Sci Food Saf 13(5):871–890. https://doi.org/10.1111/1541-4337.12091

Capriles VD, Santos FG, Arêas JAG (2016) Gluten-free breadmaking: improving nutritional and bioactive compounds. J Cereal Sci 67:83–91. https://doi.org/10.1016/j.jcs.2015.08.005

Capriles VD, Santos FG, Aguiar EV (2021) Innovative gluten-free breadmaking. In: Galanakis C (ed) Trends in wheat and bread making, 1st edn. Academic/Elsevier, Amsterdam, pp 371–404. https://doi.org/10.1016/B978-0-12-821048-2.00013-1

Capriles VD, Santos FG, Fratelli C, Aguiar EV, Muniz DG, Faggian L, Araújo MBS, Arújo VA (2022) Formulação alimentícia sem glúten e seus usos. Brazilian Patent, BR 10 2022 000348 3. Jan 2022

Cayres CA, Ascheri JLR, Couto MAPG, Almeida EL, Melo L (2020) Consumers' acceptance of optimized gluten-free sorghum-based cakes and their drivers of linking and disliking. J Cereal Sci 93:102938. https://doi.org/10.16016/j.jcs.2020.102938

Centeno ACL, Aguiar E, Santos F, Queiroz V, Conti-Silva AC, Krupa-Kozak U, Capriles VD (2021) Defining whole grain sorghum flour and water levels to improve sensory and nutritional quality of gluten-free bread—a factorial design approach. Appl Sci 11:8186. https://doi.org/10.3390/app11178186

Cervini M, Frustace A, Garrido GD, Rocchetti G, Giuberti G (2021) Nutritional, physical and sensory characteristics of gluten-free biscuits incorporated with a novel resistant starch ingredient. Heliyon 7:e06562. https://doi.org/10.1016/j.heliyon.2021

Chauhan A, Saxena DC, Singh S (2015) Total dietary fibre and antioxidant activity of gluten free cookies made from raw and germinated amaranth (*Amaranthus* spp.) flour. LWT Food Sci Technol 63:939–945. https://doi.org/10.1016/j.lwt.2015.03.115

Christ-Ribeiro A, Chiatto LM, Mafaldo CRF, Badiale-Furlong E, Souza-Soares LA (2021) Fermented rice-bran by *Saccharomyces cerevisiae*: nutritious ingredient in the formulation of gluten-free cookies. Food Biosci 40:100859. https://doi.org/10.1016/j.fbio.2020.100859

Codex Alimentarius Commission (1996). Alinorm 97/22 appendix II guidelines for use of nutrition claims. Report twenty-fourth session of the codex committee on food labeling. URL http://www.fao.org/docrep/meeting/005/W1715E/W1715E03.htm#app2

Conte P, Fadda C, Drabińska N, Krupa-Kozak U (2019) Technological and nutritional challenges, and novelty in gluten-free Breadmaking – a review. Polish J Food Nutr Sci 69(1):5–21. https://doi.org/10.31883/pjfns-2019-0005

Czaja-Bulsa G, Bulsa M (2018) Adherence to gluten-free diet in children with celiac disease. Nutrients 10(10):1424. https://doi.org/10.3390/nu10101424

David Wesley S, Bolini HMA, Clerici MTPS (2021) Gluten-free rice & bean biscuit: characterization of a new food product. Heliyon 7(1):e05956. https://doi.org/10.1016/j.heliyon.2021.e05956

Demir B, Bilgiçli N (2021) Utilization of quinoa flour (*Chenopodium quinoa Willd.*) in gluten-free pasta formulation: effects on nutritional and sensory properties. Int J Food Sci Technol 27(3):242–250. https://doi.org/10.1177/1082013220940092

Di Cairano M, Galgano F, Tolve R, Caruso MC, Condelli N (2018) Focus on gluten free biscuits: Ingredients and issues. Trends Food Sci Technol v. 81:203–212. https://doi.org/10.1016/j.tifs.2018.09.006

Dick M, Limberger C, Thys SRC, Rio AO, Flôres SH (2020) Mucilage and cladode flour from cactus (*Opuntia monacantha*) as alternative ingredients in gluten-free crackers. Food Chem 314:126178. https://doi.org/10.1016/j.foodchem.2020.126178

do Nascimento AB, GMR F, dos Anjos A, Teixeira E (2014) Gluten-free is not enough – perception and suggestions of celiac consumers. Int J Food Sci Nutr 65(4):394–398. https://doi.org/10.3109/09637486.2013.879286

do Nascimento AB, GMR F, Teixeira E (2017) We want to be normal! Perceptions of a group of Brazilian consumers with coeliac disease on gluten-free bread buns. Int J Gastron Food Sci 7:27–31. https://doi.org/10.1016/j.ijgfs.2017.01.001

Drub T, Santos FG, Centeno ACLS, Capriles VD (2021) Sorghum, millet and pseudocereals as ingredients for gluten-free whole-grain yeast rolls. Int J Gastron Food Sci 23:100293. https://doi.org/10.1016/j.ijgfs.2020.100293

Duta DE, Culetu A (2015) Evaluation of rheological, physicochemical, thermal, mechanical and sensory properties of oat-based gluten free cookies. J Food Eng 162:1–8. https://doi.org/10.1016/j.jfoodeng.2015.04.002

El Khoury D, Balfour-Ducharme S, Joye IJ (2018) A review on the gluten-free diet: technological and nutritional challenges. Nutrients 10:1410. https://doi.org/10.3390/nu10101410

Fadda C, Sanguinetti AM, Del Caro A, Collar C, Piga A (2014) Bread staling: updating the view. Compr Rev Food Sci Food Saf 13(4):473–492. https://doi.org/10.1111/1541-4337.12064

Ferreira SMR, Mello AP, Anjos MCR, Kruger CCH, Azoubel PM, Alves MAO (2016) Utilization of sorghum, rice, corn flours with potato starch for the preparation of gluten-free pasta. Food Chem 191:147–151. https://doi.org/10.1016/j.foodchem.2015.04.085

Fiorda FA, Soares Junior MS, Silva FA, Souto LRF, Grosmann, M. V. E (2013) Amaranth flour, cassava starch and cassava bagasse in the production of gluten-free pasta: technological and sensory aspects. Int J Food Sci Technol 48(9):1977–1984. https://doi.org/10.1111/ijfs.12179

Flores-Silva PC, Berrios JJ, Pan J, Agama-Acevedo E, Monsalve-Gonzales A, Bello-Pérez LA (2015) Gluten-free spaghetti with unripe plantain, chickpea and maize: physicochemical, texture and sensory properties. CYTA J Food 13(2):159–166. https://doi.org/10.1080/19476337.2014.929178

Fratelli C, Muniz DG, Santos FG, Capriles VD (2018) Modelling the effects of psyllium and water in gluten-free bread: an approach to improve the bread quality and glycemic response. J Funct Foods 42:339–345. https://doi.org/10.1016/j.jff.2018.01.015

Fratelli C, Santos FG, Muniz DG, Habu S, Braga A, Capriles VD (2021) Psyllium improves the quality and shelf life of gluten-free bread. Foods 10(5):954. https://doi.org/10.3390/foods10050954

Fry L, Madden AM, Fallaize R (2018) An investigation into the nutritional composition and cost of gluten-free versus regular food products in the UK. J Hum Nutr Diet 31(1):108–120. https://doi.org/10.1111/jhn.12502

Genevois CE, de Escalada Pla MF (2021) Soybean by-products and modified cassava starch for improving alveolar structure and quality characteristics of gluten-free bread. Eur Food Res Technol 247:1477–1488. https://doi.org/10.1007/s00217-021-03725-x

Genevois CE, Grenóvero MS, de Escalada Pla MF (2021) Use of different proportions of rice milling fractions as strategy for improving quality parameters and nutritional profile of gluten-free bread. J Food Sci Technol 58:3913–3923. https://doi.org/10.1007/s13197-020-04852-1

Giménez MA, Gámbaro A, Miraballes M, Roascio A, Amarillo M, Sammán N, Lobo M (2015) Sensory evaluation and acceptability of gluten-free Andean corn spaghetti. J Sci Food Agric 95:186–192. https://doi.org/10.1002/jsfa.6704

Giuberti G, Rocchetti G, Sigolo S, Fortunati P, Lucini L, Gallo A (2018) Exploitation of alfalfa seed (*Medicago sativa* L.) flour into gluten-free rice cookies: nutritional, antioxidant and quality characteristics. Food Chem 239:679–687. https://doi.org/10.1016/j.foodchem.2017.07.004

Gomez C, Colina J (2019) Formulation of gluten-free cupcake with hydrocolloids for people with celiac disease. Bioact Compd Health Dis 2(6):134–148. https://doi.org/10.31989/bchd.v2i6.630

Haas RV, Homem RV, Farias DV, Schmidt HO, Rockett FC, Venzke JG, Jomori MM, Kist TL, Rios AO, VRD O (2022) Potential of teff (Eragrostis tef) flour as an ingredient in gluten-free cakes: chemical, technological and sensory quality. Int J Food Sci Technol 57:2051–2059. https://doi.org/10.1111/ijfs.15431

Hamdani AM, Wani IA, Bhat NA (2020) Gluten free cookies from rice-chickpea composite flour using exudate gums from acacia, apricot and karaya. Food Biosci 35:100541. https://doi.org/10.1016/j.fbio.2020.100541

Hanci O, Jeanes YM (2019) Are gluten-free food staples accessible to all patients with coeliac disease? Frontline Gastroenterol 10:222–228. https://doi.org/10.1136/flgastro-2018-101088

Jeong D, Hong JS, Liu Q, Choi H-D, Chung H-J (2021) The effects of different levels of heat-treated legume flour on nutritional, physical, textural and sensory properties of gluten muffins. Cereal Chem 98:392–404. https://doi.org/10.1002/cche.10379

Kaur M, Sandhu KS, Arora A, Sharma A (2015) Gluten free biscuits prepared from buckwheat flour by incorporation of various gums: physicochemical and sensory properties. LWT Food Sci Technol 62:628–632. https://doi.org/10.1016/j.lwt.2014.02.039

Kock HL, Magano NN (2020) Sensory tools for the development of gluten-free bakery foods. J Cereal Sci 94:102990. https://doi.org/10.1016/j.jcs.2020.102990

Konuk Takma D, Ülkeryıldız Balçık E, Sahin-Nadeem H (2021) Physicochemical and sensory properties of gluten-free cupcakes added with fig seeds pomace flour. J Food Process Preserv 45:e15619. https://doi.org/10.1111/jfpp.15619

Lawless HT, Heymann H (2010) Introduction. In: Lawless HT, Heymann H (eds) Sensory evaluation of food: principles and practices, 2nd edn. Springer, New York, pp 1–18

Levent H, Sayaslan A, Yesil S (2021) Physicochemical and sensory quality of gluten-free cakes supplemented with grape seed, pomegranate seed, poppy seed, flaxseed, and turmeric. J Food Process Preserv 45:e1514. https://doi.org/10.1111/jfpp.15148

Locke JEC, Gonzalez LC, Loubes MA, Tolaba MP (2019) Optimization of rice bread formulation by mixture design and relationship of bread quality to flour and dough atributes. LWT – Food Sci Technol 113:108299. https://doi.org/10.1016/j.lwt.2019.108299

Mancebo CM, Rodriguez P, Gómez M (2016) Assessing rice flour-starch-protein mixtures to produce gluten free sugar-snap cookies. LWT Food Sci Technol 67:127–132. https://doi.org/10.1016/j.lwt.2015.11.045

Manley Duncan (2011) Manley's Technology of Biscuits, Crackers and Cookies. Fourth Edition. Elsevier Ltd. https://www.sciencedirect.com/book/9781845697709/manleys-technology-of-biscuits-crackers-and-cookies#book-info

Masure HG, Fierens E, Delcour JA (2016) Current and forward looking experimental approaches in gluten-free bread making research. J Cereal Sci 67:92–111. https://doi.org/10.1016/j.jcs.2015.09.009

Matos ME, Rosell CM (2015) Understanding gluten-free dough for reaching breads with physical quality and nutritional balance. J Sci Food Agric 95(4):653–661. https://doi.org/10.1002/jsfa.6732

Melini V, Melini F (2018) Strategies to extend bread and GF bread shelf-life: from sourdough to antimicrobial active packaging and nanotechnology. Fermentation 4(1). https://doi.org/10.3390/fermentation4010009

Milde LB, Ramallo LA, Puppo MC (2012) Gluten-free bread based on tapioca starch: texture and sensory studies. Food Bioprocess Technol 5:888–896. https://doi.org/10.1007/s11947-010-0381-x

Mir SA, Bosco SJD, Shah MA, Santhalakshmy S, Mir MM (2017) Effect of apple pomace on quality characteristics of brown rice based cracker. J Saudi Soc Agric 16:25–32. https://doi.org/10.1016/j.jssas.2015.01.001

Mirhosseini H, Rashid NFA, Amid BT, Cheong KW, Kazemi M, Zulkurnain M (2015) Effect of partial replacement of corn flour with durian seed flour and pumpkin flour on cooking yield, texture properties, and sensory attributes of gluten free pasta. LWT Food Sci Tech 63(1):184–190. https://doi.org/10.1016/j.lwt.2015.03.078

Morais EC, Cruz AG, Faria JAF, Bolini HMA (2014) Prebiotic gluten-free bread: sensory profiling and drivers of liking. LWT Food Sci Technol 55(1):248–254. https://doi.org/10.1016/j.lwt.2013.07.014

Nath P, Kale SJ, Kaur C, Chauhan OP (2018) Phytonutrient composition, antioxidant activity and acceptability of muffins incorporated with red capsicum pomave powder. J Food Sci Tech 55(6):2208–2219. https://doi.org/10.1007/s13197-018-3138-6

Nespeca LS, da Silva Paulino HF, Barlati Vieira da Silva T, Bona E, Leimann FV, LLM M, FAR C, Droval AA, RHB F (2021) How does the replacement of rice flour with flours of higher nutritional quality impact the texture and sensory profile and acceptance of gluten-free chocolates cakes? Int J Food Sci Technol 56:2019–2029. https://doi.org/10.1111/ijfs.14833

Neves ECA, Moysés BA, Neves DA, Campelo PH, Clerici MTPS (2021) Sustainable and regional gastronomy: cassava leaves as a potential ingredient for gluten-free biscuits. Res Soc Dev 10:e12010313071. https://doi.org/10.33448/rsd-v10i3.13071

O'Shea N, Arendt E, Gallagher E (2014) State of the art in gluten-free research. J Food Sci 79:R1067–R1076. https://doi.org/10.1111/1750-3841.12479

Padalino L, Mastromatteo M, Sepielli G, Nobile M (2011) Formulation optimization of gluten-free functional spaghetti based on maize flour and oat bran enriched in b-glucans. Materials 12:2119–2135. https://doi.org/10.3390/ma4122119

Paesani C, Bravo-Núñez A, Gómez M (2020) Effect of extrusion of whole-grain maize flour on the characteristics of gluten-free cookies. LWT Food Sci Technol 132:109931. https://doi.org/10.1016/j.lwt.2020.109931

Pio Ávila B, Cardozo LO, Alves GD, Gularte MA, Monks J, Elias MC (2019) Consumers' sensory perception of food attributes: identifying the ideal formulation of gluten- and lactose-free brownie using sensory methodologies. J Food Sci 84(12):3707–3716. https://doi.org/10.1111/1750-3841.14845

Potter R, Stojceska V, Plunkett A (2014) An investigation of the consumer perception on the quality of the gluten and wheat free breads available on the UK market. Food Measure 8:362–372. https://doi.org/10.1007/s11694-014-9199-y

Radočaj O, Dimić E, Tsao R (2014) Effects of hemp (*Cannabis sativa* L.) seed oil PressCake and decaffeinated green tea leaves (*Camellia sinensis*) on functional characteristics of gluten-free crackers. J Food Sci 79:C318–C325. https://doi.org/10.1111/1750-3841.12370

Radünz M, Camargo TM, Nunes CFP, Pereira EDS, Ribeiro JA, Hackbart HCDS (2021) Gluten-free green banana flour muffins: chemical, physical, antioxidant, digestibility, and sensory analysis. J Food Sci Technol 58(4):1295–1301. https://doi.org/10.1007/s13197-020-04638-5

Roman L, Belorio M, Gomez M (2019) Gluten-free breads: the gap between research and commercial reality. Compr Rev Food Sci Food Saf 18:690–702. https://doi.org/10.1111/1541-4337.12437

Rosell CM, Marco C, García-Alvárez J, Salazar J (2011) Rheological properties of rice-soybean protein composite flours assessed by mixolab and ultrassound. J Food Process Eng 34:1838–1859

Rungsardthong V, Namprakob P, Korkerd S, Lamsal B (2021) Physical and cooking properties of extruded rice spaghetti supplemented with mango peel fibre. Curr J Appl Sci Technol 11:230–239. https://doi.org/10.14456/jcst.2021.24

Sakurai CN, Rodrigues AMC, Pires MB, SILVA HM (2020) Quality of pasta made of cassava, peach palm and golden linseed flours. Food Sci Technol 40:1–234. https://doi.org/10.1590/fst.09119

Santos FG, Capriles VD (2021) Relationships between dough thermomechanical parameters and physical and sensory properties of gluten-free bread texture during storage. LWT Food Sci Technol 139:110577. https://doi.org/10.1016/j.lwt.2020.110577

Santos FG, Fratelli C, Muniz DG, Capriles VD (2018) Mixture design applied to the development of chickpea-based gluten-free bread with attractive technological, sensory, and nutritional quality. J Food Sci 83:188–197. https://doi.org/10.1111/1750-3841.14009

Santos FG, Aguiar EV, Rosell CM, Capriles VD (2021a) Potential of chickpea and psyllium in gluten-free breadmaking: assessing bread's quality, sensory acceptability, and glycemic and satiety indexes. Food Hydrocoll 113:106487. https://doi.org/10.1016/j.foodhyd.2020.106487

Santos FG, Aguiar EV, Braga ARC, Alencar NMM, Rosell CM, Capriles VD (2021b) An integrated instrumental and sensory approach to describe the effects of chickpea flour, psyllium, and their combination at reducing gluten-free bread staling. Food Pack Shelf Life 28:100659. https://doi.org/10.1016/j.fpsl.2021.100659

Scarton M, Ribeiro T, Godoy HT, Behrens JH, Campelo PH, Clerici MTPS (2021) Gluten free pasta with natural ingredient of color and carotene source. Res Soc Dev 10:e21310413959. https://doi.org/10.33448/rsd-v10i4.13959

Schmelter L, Rohm H, Struck S (2021) Gluten-free bakery products: cookies made from different Vicia faba bean varieties. Future Foods 4:100038. https://doi.org/10.1016/j.fufo.2021.100038

Sedej I, Sakaca M, Mandić A, Misan A, Pestorić M, Simurina O, Canadanovic-Brunet J (2011) Quality assessment of gluten-free crackers based on buckwheat flour. LWT – Food Sci Technol 44:694–699. https://doi.org/10.1016/j.lwt.2010.11.010

Silva DW, Bolini HMA, Clerici MTPS (2021) Gluten-free rice & bean biscuit: characterization of a new food product. Heliyon 7:05956. https://doi.org/10.1016/j.heliyon.2021.e05956

Sulieman AA, Zhu K, Peng W, Hassan HA, Obadi M, Siddeeg A, Zhou H (2019) Rheological and quality characteristics of composite gluten-free dough and biscuits supplemented with fermented and unfermented *Agaricus bisporus* polysaccharide flour. Food Chem 271:193–203. https://doi.org/10.1016/j.foodchem.2018.07.189

Taghdir M, Mazloomi SM, Honar N, Sapandi M, Ashourpour M, Salehi M (2016) Effect of soy flour on nutritional, physicochemical, and sensory characteristics of gluten-free bread. Food Sci Nutr 5(3):1–7

Torbica A, Hadnadev M, Dapčević HT (2012) Rice and buckwheat flour characterisation and its relation to cookie quality. Food Res Int 48:277–283. https://doi.org/10.1016/j.foodres.2012.05.001

Tsatsaragkou K, Protonotariou S, Mandala I (2016) Structural role of fibre addition to increase knowledge of non-gluten bread. J Cereal Sci 67:58–67. https://doi.org/10.1016/j.jcs.2015.10.003

Valitutti F, Iorfida D, Anania C, Trovato CM, Montuori M, Cucchiara S, Catassi C (2017) Cereal consumption among subjects with celiac disease: a snapshot for nutritional considerations. Nutrients 9:396. https://doi.org/10.3390/nu9040396

Varela P, Ares G (2012) Sensory profiling, the blurred line between sensory and consumer science. A review of novel methods for product characterization. Food Res Int 48:893–908

Whole grains council (2021) Whole grain stamp. https://wholegrainscouncil.org/whole-grain-stamp

Xu J, Zhang Y, Wang W, Li Y (2020) Advanced properties of gluten-free cookies, cakes, and crackers: a review. Trends Food Sci Technol 103:200–213. https://doi.org/10.1016/j.tifs.2020.07.017

Zandonadi RP, Botelho RBA, Gandolfi L, Ginani SJ, Montenegro FM, Pratesi R (2012) Green Banana pasta: an alternative for gluten-free diets. J Acad Nutr Diet 112:1068–1072. https://doi.org/10.1016/j.jand.2012.04.002

Ziobro R, Witczak T, Juszczak L, Korus J (2013) Supplementation of gluten-free bread with non-gluten proteins—effect on dough rheological properties and bread characteristic. Food Hydrocoll 32(2):213–220

Chapter 10
Regulation and Labelling. Methods of Analysis for the Determination of Gluten in Foods

Carolina Cagnasso, Silvina Marquez, and Laura Beatriz López

Abbreviations

AFC	Argentine Food Code
ANMAT	Food and Medical Technology
AOECS	Association Of European Coeliac Societies
CFDA	China Food and Drug Administration
CGL	Crossed Grain Logo
DES	Eutectic solvents
DNA	Deoxyribonucleic acid
ELISA	Enzyme-linked Immunoassay
EU	European Union
FAO	Food and Agriculture Organisation of the United Nations
FDA	Food and Drug Administration
LC-MS	Mass spectrometry
MAFF	Ministry of Agriculture, Forestry, and Fisheries
MALDI	Matrix-assisted-laser-desorption ionization
SEREMI	Regional Ministerial Secretariat
PCR	Polymerase chain reaction
POD	Peroxidase
Q	Quadruple
RSDr	Relative standard deviation
TACC	Trigo (wheat), Avena (oat), Cebada (barley) and Centeno (rye)
TOF	Time of flight
WGPAT	Working Group on Prolamin Analysis and Toxicity
WHO	World Health Organisation
WTO	World Trade Organisation

C. Cagnasso · S. Marquez · L. B. López (✉)
Universidad de Buenos Aires, Facultad de Farmacia y Bioquímica, Buenos Aires, Argentina
e-mail: ccagnasso@docente.ffyb.uba.ar; smarquez@docente.ffyb.uba.ar; laulop@ffyb.uba.ar

M. F. de Escalada Pla, C. E. Genevois (eds.), *Designing Gluten Free Bakery and Pasta Products*, https://doi.org/10.1007/978-3-031-28344-4_10

10.1 Introduction

The global trade of food is a diverse and complex operation. The expansion and diversification of the food trade resulted in an increasing number of countries that are becoming both significant importers and exporters of food. It is obvious that food requirements should be harmonise globally and there is a growing need for international guidelines and rules. In the particular case of gluten-free foods there is no unified international legislation and different countries have adopted their own regulations. In general, many countries follow CODEX ALIMENTARIUS standards, however many exceptions can be found, for example Chile, Australia or Japan among others. The aim of this chapter is to give an overview of the international legislation and the different methods available for gluten detection and the scope of each of them. Therefore, the chapter information is presented beginning with the *Codex Alimentarius* definitions and practices as reference and continuing with the legislations of other countries by alphabetic order.

10.2 Codex Alimentarius

It consists of a joint program established in 1963 by FAO (Food and Agriculture Organisation of the United Nations) and WHO (World Health Organisation).

The Codex Alimentarius Commission is an intergovernmental Organisation that currently consists of 189 Codex Members, 188 Member Nations and 1 Member Organisation of the European Union (EU).

It is responsible of the development of food standards its objectives are: to protect the health of consumers (safety); defend the right of consumers to purchase genuine food, ensure fair trade practices that do not represent technical barriers to commerce, and develop scientifically justified standards.

The Codex Alimentarius has influenced on National Regulations since it serves as a reference for updating national legislation (for example: Argentine Food Code). It is also used as a reference to establish regional standards (for example MERCOSUR, EU, USMCA). Internationally, it is used as a reference for the World Trade Organisation (WTO) to resolve international disputes.

In relation to gluten-free foods, in 1979 Codex Alimentarius published the Codex Standard on Foods for Special Diets Intended for Gluten-Intolerant People, Codex Stan 118-1979. This Standard has been amended in 1983 and 2015 and revised in 2008 (Codex Alimentarius 2015). The products covered by this standard are described as follows:

10.2.1 Gluten-Free Foods

Gluten-free foods are dietary foods

(a) consisting of or made only from one or more ingredients which do not contain wheat (i.e. all Triticum species, such as durum wheat, spelt, and khorasan wheat, which is also marketed under different trademarks such as KAMUT), rye, barley, oats or their crossbred varieties, and the gluten level does not exceed 20 mg/kg in total, based on the food as sold or distributed to the consumer, and/or
(b) consisting of one or more ingredients from wheat (i.e. all Triticum species, such as durum wheat, spelt, and khorasan wheat, which is also marketed under different trademarks such as KAMUT), rye, barley, oats or their crossbred varieties, which have been specially processed to remove gluten, and the gluten level does not exceed 20 mg/kg in total, based on the food as sold or distributed to the consumer.

10.2.2 Foods Specially Processed to Reduce Gluten Content to a Level Above 20 Up to 100 mg/kg

These foods consist of one or more ingredients from wheat (i.e., all Triticum species, such as durum wheat, spelt, and khorasan wheat, which is also marketed under different trademarks such as KAMUT), rye, barley, oats or their crossbred varieties, which have been specially processed to reduce the gluten content to a level above 20 up to 100 mg/kg in total, based on the food as sold or distributed to the consumer.

Decisions on the marketing of products described in this section may be determined at the national level.

Oats can be tolerated by most but not all people who are intolerant to gluten. Therefore, the allowance of oats that are not contaminated with wheat, rye or barley in foods covered by this standard may be determined at the national level.

In relation to the labelling, the norm establishes:

The term "gluten-free" shall be printed in the immediate proximity of the name of the product in the case of products described in section Gluten-free foods.

The labelling of products described in section Foods specially processed to reduce gluten content to a level above 20 up to 100 mg/kg should be determined at the national level. However, these products must not be called gluten-free. The labelling terms for such products should indicate the true nature of the food and shall be printed in the immediate proximity of the name of the product.

A food which, by its nature, is suitable for use as part of a gluten-free diet, shall not be designated "special dietary", "special dietetic" or any other equivalent term. However, such a food may bear a statement on the label that "this food is by its nature gluten-free" provided that it complies with the essential composition provisions for gluten-free (not exceed 20 mg/kg) and considering that such a statement does not mislead the consumer. More detailed rules in order to ensure that the consumer is not misled may be determined at national level.

The limit values in gluten free foods results from considering two factors: the minimum toxic dose that causes harmful effects on the intestinal mucosa (50 mg/day) and an estimation of the possible daily consumption of gluten through foods that contain traces of it. It should be considered that most foods that do not contain any of the unsuitable grains may contain traces of gluten due to contamination during their manufacture, which, depending on the amount ingested, may represent a non-negligible source of gluten. The cut-off point of 20 mg/kg leaves a wide safety margin so as not to exceed the maximum intake of 50 mg/day of gluten, even without even reaching the threshold of 10 mg/day considered to be of maximum safety (Ministerio de Salud de la Nación Argentina 2010).

In relation to methods of analysis and sampling, the norm establishes:

10.2.3 General Outline of the Methods

- The quantitative determination of gluten in foods and ingredients shall be based on an immunologic method or other method providing at least equal sensitivity and specificity.
- The antibody used should react with the cereal protein fractions that are toxic for persons intolerant to gluten and should not cross-react with other cereal proteins or other constituents of the foods or ingredients.
- Methods used for determination should be validated and calibrated against a certified reference material, if available.
- The detection limit has to be appropriate according to the state of the art and the technical standard. It should be 10 mg gluten/kg or below.
- The qualitative analysis that indicates the presence of gluten shall be based on relevant methods (e.g. ELISA-based methods, DNA methods).

10.2.4 Method for Determination of Gluten

The methodology established by CODEX is the Enzyme-linked Immunoassay (ELISA) R5 Mendez Method (Codex Standard 234-1999 2019).

10.3 Regulation of Gluten-Free Foods in Different Countries

10.3.1 Argentina (Argentine Republic)

In Argentine, the legislation that contemplates gluten-free foods is found in Chapter XVII of the Argentine Food Code (AFC) in articles 1383 and 1383 bis (Argentine Food Code 2021).

The AFC defines "gluten-free food" as prepared only with ingredients that due to their natural origin and the application of good manufacturing practices, which prevents cross contamination, do not contain prolamins from wheat, from all Triticum species, such as spelt (*Triticum spelta* L.), kamut (*Triticum polonicum* L.), of durum wheat, rye, barley, oats or their crossed varieties. The gluten content may not exceed the maximum of 10 mg/kg.

Analytical methodology based on Codex STAN 118-79 (adopted in 1979, amended in 1983; revised in 2008) ELISA R5 Méndez enzyme-linked immunosorbent assay should be used to verify gluten-free status. It also includes all those that the National Health Authority evaluates and accepts in the future.

These products will be labelled with the name of the product followed by the indication "gluten-free" ("libre de gluten") and must also include the legend "Without TACC" ("sin TACC") near the name of the product with characters of good enhancement, size and visibility. "TACC" is Trigo (wheat), Avena (oat), Cebada (barley) and Centeno (rye).

The elaboration of the products must comply with the requirements of the AFC for gluten-free foods for the purposes of inclusion in the label the legend "Without TACC".

For the approval of gluten-free foods, manufacturers and/or importers must submit to the Health Authority of their jurisdiction:

- analysis that supports the status of "gluten-free" granted by an official body or entity with official recognition.
- a good manufacturing practices program, in order to ensure non-contamination with derivatives of wheat, oats, barley and rye in the processes, from the reception of raw materials to the commercialization of the final product.

The gluten-free products that are marketed in Argentine must have printed on their containers or wrappers, in a clearly visible way, a symbol, which consists of a circle with a cross bar on three wheat spikes and the legend "Without TACC" in the bar admitting two variants, one in black and white and the other in colour (red, yellow, white and black). They may bear, in addition to the mandatory symbol, two other optional symbols: the international crossed grain stamp and the Argentine Coeliac Association symbol (AFC 2021).

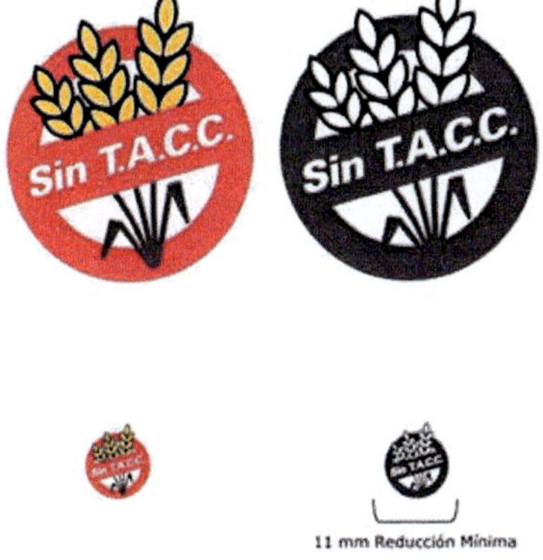

In Argentine all foods registered as gluten-free have the mandatory symbol on their labels. In addition, some of them present one or both optional symbols.

The National Administration of Medicines, Food and Medical Technology (ANMAT), an entity that belongs to the Ministry of Health, carries out the control of gluten-free foods at national level. There is a Gluten-Free Food Laboratory-Based Surveillance Program within the framework of the comprehensive inspection plan for establishments, food products, and materials in contact with food. The objective of this program is to compile information about the presence and concentration of gliadins, labelling of gluten-free foods, and to identify trends and possible areas of intervention. It is applied in foods that are marketed in Argentine, which are included in the Integrated List of Gluten-Free Foods, and gluten-free foods that are marketed only in a municipality or province (Comprehensive Inspection Plan 2021).

10.3.2 *Australia and New Zealand*

The regulation of food quality and integrity in Australia and New Zealand is governed primarily by the Australia New Zealand Food Standards Code (Food Standards Code [FSANZ] 2021). The Food Code is given the force of law in each of the Australian and New Zealand states and territories through local Food Acts.

Compliance with the Food Code is mandatory for all food products imported, manufactured, supplied and sold in Australia and New Zealand. Responsibility for enforcing the Food Code lies in local food authorities in the states and territories (Allred and Reid 2021).

The food code stipulates what terms are permitted in relation to gluten on food packages or menus in Australia:

- "Gluten-free" – contains no detectable gluten
- "Low gluten" – contains no more than 200 mg/kg of gluten
- "Contains/is high in gluten" – contains more than 200 mg/Kg of gluten

Other terms such as "no added gluten", "gluten friendly", "gluten removed", "coeliac friendly" or "99% gluten-free" are not permitted under the Code.

If claiming "gluten-free" or "low gluten", then the amount of gluten needs to be included in the Nutritional Ingredients Panel (Environmental Health Unit 2021).

A "gluten-free" claim cannot be accompanied by a cross contact statement such as (NSW Food Authority 2011):

- "May contain traces of gluten"
- "May be present gluten"
- "Made in a facility that also processes gluten"
- "Made with equipment processing gluten"

Coeliac New Zealand's Crossed Grain Logo (CGL) Trademark confirms that products that display the CGL symbol also state that it is "gluten-free" and meet the FSANZ criteria of "no detectable gluten". The Crossed Grain symbol is the certified trademark owned by Coeliac New Zealand for the certification of products produced and licensed in New Zealand and sold in New Zealand or Australia (Coeliac New Zealand 2021).

There is also another symbol that can be found and is endorced by a coeliac association of Asutralia.

The authorized methods to analyse gluten content are R5 Sandwich ELISA and G12 ELISA. For hydrolysed samples (e.g. beers, fermented sauces etc.) a Competitive -R5 -ELISA test kit needs to be used (Coeliac Australia 2021). Foods labelled as "gluten-free" must not contain any detectable gluten; and no oats or their products; or cereals containing gluten that have used malt or their products. Non detectable meaning less than equals 3 mg/kg which is the detectable level of the methods (Australian Food and Grocery Council 2021).

10.3.3 Brazil (Federative Republic of Brazil)

Brazilian legislation is limited. In RDC-RESOLUTION N°. 40 of 8 February 2002, gluten is defined as a set of proteins present in wheat, oats, barley, malt and rye (Resolution RDC N° 40, 2002). Law N°10674 of 2003 establishes that all industrial food must contain on its label the phrase "contains gluten" (*"contém Glúten"*) or "does not contain gluten" (*"não contém Glúten"*) as appropriate. This phrase must be present on the food label as well as on posters and publicity materials in characters that stand out, clear and easy to read. The cut-off point and the analytical methodology to be used were not established in the law (Law N°10674, 2003).

10.3.4 Canada

The legislation governing the labelling of gluten-free foods in Canada can be found in the Food and Drug Regulation (FDR, 2021). The reference to "gluten-free" labelling is found in section B.24.018. Although it does not define what a "gluten-free food" is, it can be inferred that it is the food that does not contain any gluten protein or modified gluten protein, including any gluten protein fraction. Section B.01.010.1(1) defines gluten as any protein from the grain of barley, oats, rye, triticale, wheat or the grain of a hybrid strain that is created from at least one of these cereals. In addition, any modified gluten protein, including any gluten protein fraction that is derived from the grain of any of the above-mentioned cereals or their hybrids. Section B.24.018 states that it is prohibited to label, package, sell or advertise a food in a manner that may create the impression that it is a gluten-free food when it does not comply with the above. Although no specific threshold value is mentioned in the regulation, Health Canada recognises the Codex Alimentarius Standard (Codex Stan 118-1979), which states that the gluten content of foods labelled "gluten-free" should not exceed 20 mg/kg (Health Canada, 2012).

Health Canada accepts gluten-free oats, i.e. oats that have been specially produced to ensure that they contain no more than 20 mg/kg of gluten from wheat, rye, barley or their hybrid strains. To facilitate the identification of uncontaminated oats, Health Canada has created a marketing authorisation that allows gluten-free oats and foods made with gluten-free oats as ingredients to be labelled as "gluten-free".

Health Canada recognises the effectiveness of ELISA-based methods for detecting the presence of gluten, specifically the Mendez antibody (R5 antibodies) that allow the detection and quantification of gluten in processed foods. However, Health Canada will continue to assess analytical methods that are specific to the detection and quantification of gluten in processed foods and will provide further guidance on the applicability of these methods.

10.3.5 Chile (Republic of Chile)

In Chile, the legislation related to gluten-free foods is found in the SANITARY REGULATION OF FOODS DTO. N° 977/96 (D.OF. 13.05.97) TITLE XXVIII.- OF FOODS FOR SPECIAL DIETS Paragraph VI.- Of foods for gluten-free diets, articles 516, 517 y 518 (Sanitary Regulation of Foods, 2021).

Gluten-free food is one that is prepared only with ingredients that due to their natural origin and the application of good manufacturing practises - which prevent cross contamination - do not contain prolamins from wheat, from all *Triticum* species such as spelt (*Triticum spelta L.*), kamut (*Triticum polonicum L.*), durum wheat, rye, barley, nor their cross varieties, as well as oats.

The manufacturers of these foods must comply with the requirements established in this Regulation to include in the label the legend "gluten-free". They must have a program of good manufacturing practices, in order to ensure non-contamination with derivatives of wheat, rye, barley and oats in the processes, from the reception of raw materials to the commercialization of the final product.

It also includes that gluten-free flours intended for baking, as well as gluten-free bread, must contain the vitamins and minerals established for wheat flour. The established values are: thiamine 6.3 mg/kg, riboflavin 1.3 mg/kg, niacin 13.0 mg/kg and iron 30.0 mg/kg. Iron must be added in the form of ferrous sulphate. If it is not possible, ferrous fumarate can be used as long as equivalence with ferrous sulphate is maintained. It should also contain 1.8 mg/kg of folic acid, but it is accepted that it is present in a range of 1.0 to 2.6 mg/kg.

All gluten-free foods must be nutritionally labelled in accordance with the provisions of the general labelling and the corresponding article of this Regulation.

The term "gluten-free"and the logo or symbol of the crossed grain symbol, may only be used when the result of the laboratory analysis of the food product does not exceed 5 milligrams of gluten, of established cereals, per kilogram of the product ready for its delivery to the final consumer. The Institute of Public Health of Chile will establish the analytical technique to be used.

The expression "gluten-free"("libre de gluten") will be labelled near the name of the product, with characters of good enhancement, size and visibility.

The proposed analysis methodology is the Official AOAC Method 2012.01 which allows the determination of gliadin as a measure of gluten in foods containing wheat, rye and barley. It consists of a sandwich-type enzyme immunoassay with R5 monoclonal antibody for the quantitative gluten analysis (prolamins) in foods, AOAC Official Methods of Analysis (2012). Cp. 32 (Gluten Analysis in Food, 2018).

In gluten-free products it can be seen the crossed grain symbol or the Official trademark logo of the gluten-free certification program of the Chilean Coeliac Society (Corporación de Apoyo al Celíaco, COACEL).

Companies that produce and sell gluten-free foods have been audited since 2019. The Regional Ministerial Secretariat (SEREMI) corresponding to each region carries out this task.

10.3.6 China (People's Republic of China)

China Food and Drug Administration (CFDA), food products are regulated by different CFDA departments from drugs and biological products. The statutory basis for food regulation is the PRC (People's Republic of China) Food Safety Law (2015). Due to a recent structural change, CFDA is now part of the State Administration for Market Regulation.

There is no specific regulation for gluten-free foods in China. The standard applied to the labelling of prepackaged foods to be offered directly or indirectly as such to consumers is GB 7718-2011 "General Rules for the Labelling of Prepackaged Foods" (GAIN, 2011) which recommends the labelling of foods containing sensitising substances such as gluten. This regulation does not explicitly mention gluten-free products but for export products the CODEX STAN 118-1979 may be applicable.

10.3.7 European Union

Commission Implementing Regulation (EU) N° 828/2014 of 30 July 2014 regulates the information provided to consumers on the absence or reduced presence of gluten in foods (Commission Implementing Regulation-EU, 2014).

Gluten is defined as a protein fraction from wheat (means any *Triticum* species.), rye, barley, oats or their crossbred varieties and derivatives thereof, to which some persons are intolerant, and which is insoluble in water and 0.5 M sodium chloride solution. Within this legislation, there are two categories of food, "gluten-free" and "very low gluten". The statement "gluten-free" may only be made where the food as sold to the final consumer contains no more than 20 mg/kg of gluten. The statement "very low gluten" may only be made where the food, consisting of or containing one or more ingredients made from wheat, rye, barley, oats or their crossbred varieties which have been specially processed to reduce the gluten content, contains no more than 100 mg/kg of gluten in the food as sold to the final consumer.

It should be noted that some people with intolerance to gluten can include oats in their diet without an adverse effect on their health. However, a major concern is the contamination of oats with wheat, rye or barley that can occur during grain harvesting, transport, storage and processing. Therefore, there are additional requirements for food containing oats. Oats contained in a food presented as "gluten-free" or "very low gluten" must have been specially produced, prepared and/or processed in a way to avoid contamination by wheat, rye, barley, or their crossbred varieties and the gluten content of such oats cannot exceed 20 mg/kg.

When the food complies with the requirements specified for each category it may be labelled with the claim "gluten-free" or "very low gluten" as appropriate.

In addition, the food information may be accompanied by the statements "suitable for people intolerant to gluten" or "suitable for coeliacs". Furthermore, in the case where foods are specially produced, prepared and/or processed to reduce the gluten content of one or more gluten-containing ingredients or to replace gluten-containing ingredients by other naturally gluten-free ingredients, the above mentioned food information may be accompanied by the claims "formulated specifically for people intolerant to gluten" or "formulated specifically for coeliacs".

It is important to note that food information on the absence or reduced presence of gluten in infant formulae and follow-on formulae is prohibited.

The regulation does not specify an official methodology for quantifying gluten.

There is also no official logo for labelling gluten-free foods regulated by The Commission of the European Communities. Although, depending on the country where the food is marketed, different logos certified by non-profit organisations can be observed. The most important is the one licensed by the Association Of European Coeliac Societies (AOECS). This Association is an independent, non-profit organisation representing people affected by coeliac disease or dermatitis herpetiformis across Europe and beyond (AOECS 2021). AOECS is an umbrella organisation of European national coeliac societies, aiming to represent 40 enrolled member societies on an international stage. AOECS has developed the European Licensing System, which can be licensed by AOECS members in their national territories. This licence allows the use of the Crossed Grain Stamp on the basis of compliance with common standards. This symbol is owned by the UK Coeliac Association, which has made it available to AOECS and its member associations.

The symbol may be depicted in any colour and shall always be accompanied by the registration or licence code to show that it is being used with permission from the licensor. This code consists of 8 alphanumeric digits and must be visible together with the logo according to the established format: XX-YYY-ZZZ. In products containing oat the code includes AVENA/OATS-XX-YYY-ZZZ (European Licensing System, 2017).

XX = Country code
YYY = Code of the producer and/or company owning the brand.
ZZZ = Product code.

10.3.8 India (Republic of India)

The Food Safety and Standards Authority of India sets the legislation related to food products. Gluten-free foods consist of or are made of one or more ingredients containing rice, millets, ragi, pulses or legumes. A food which, by its nature, is suitable for use as part of a gluten-free diet shall not be named as "special dietary", "special dietetic" or any other equivalent term, however, such food may bear a statement on the label that "this food is by its nature gluten-free". For the purpose of labelling a product as gluten-free, when such a product is analysed, the gluten levels shall be below 20 mg/kg as per the method declared by the Organisation for Economic Co-operation and Development or the Association of Official Agricultural Chemists. The term "gluten-free"shall be printed in the immediate proximity of the name of the product in the case of products. In the case that gluten-free products are manufactured in a plant where non gluten-free products are also made, this must be declared in the label like: "Processed in a plant where gluten containing products are manufactured" (FSSAI, 2018).

10.3.9 Israel (State of Israel)

The food control service of the Ministry of Health is the regulatory agency responsible for the development of food standards and regulations dealing with foods sold in Israel, including novel foods. A food may be labelled with the words "gluten-free" if it meets the following conditions: the rate of gluten in it is not greater than or equal to 20 mg/kg; it was manufactured under appropriate manufacturing conditions as defined in the Public Health Order to the satisfaction of the Director; the necessary steps were taken to ascertain that the level of gluten in the ingredient and the food shall not exceed 20 mg/kg. No person shall produce a food that contains or has added to it gluten at a ratio above 20 mg/kg, nor import nor market it, unless the list of ingredients of the food includes the name of the plant that is the source of the gluten and the words "contains gluten" (Public Health Order, 2011).

10.3.10 Japan

Japan has excellent labelling requirements for food allergens, and restaurant chains make lists of which items on the menu may possess a problem. The Japanese Ministry of Agriculture, Forestry, and Fisheries (MAFF) has created regulations for listing certain allergens in packaged food. "Wheat-free" is one of the claims regulated but unfortunately this doesn't specifically include gluten. It is important to notice that wheat is mandatory to list but not rye, malt, barley, or oats (MAFF, 2011). This is problematic given the prominence of barley in Japanese foods, including as an ingredient in miso and vinegar, an addition to rice dishes, and *mugicha* (barley tea), which is popular in the summer.

While rice is the traditional staple food of Japanese cuisine (and doesn't contain gluten), in modern times there are many Japanese foods that are prepared with wheat and other ingredients containing gluten.

There is no regulation for gluten-free labelling in Japan. Manufacturers can use such claim, but even in cases where a gluten-free labelling is used (based on the 20 mg/kg standard used overseas), it is thought to be necessary to put a note such as "This labelling does not mean the product does not include wheat allergen". When "gluten-free"is claimed in a labelling for food including wheat allergen, it is likely that consumers will assume that the wheat allergen is not included, so following the rules of the Act against Unjustifiable Premiums and Misleading Representations, it is likely to become an issue.

In response to the growing demand for gluten-free products, Japan began operating the world's first certification system for "non-gluten" rice flour in June 2018. Under this certification system, certification bodies grant the "non-gluten rice flour certification" mark to rice flour that uses rice produced in Japan, contains 1 mg/kg or less gluten (a much stricter criterion than that for gluten-free products) and is produced in a factory with stable production and shipping systems (Osamu 2020).

The methods approved for testing are: Nippon Ham FASTKIT ELISA Ver. III Wheat, Prima Ham Allergen I ELISA II Wheat and Morinaga Institute of Biological Science, Inc. FASPEK ELISA II Wheat (gliadin) (GAIN, 2017).

10.3.11 Korea (Republic of Korea)

The Ministry of Food and Drug Safety sets the Foods Labelling Standards. The "gluten-free" claim is allowed for products that do not use wheat, rye, barley, oat or crossbreed of such grains and whose total gluten content in the finished product is not more than 20 mg/kg. It is also allowed for products with ingredients that are made by removing gluten from the aforementioned grains, such that the total gluten content in the finished product is not more than 20 mg/kg (Ministry of Food and Drug Safety, 2016).

10.3.12 Mexico (United Mexican States)

In Mexico, the legislation that regulates gluten-free foods is The Official Mexican Standard NOM-086-SSA1-1994 for foods and non-alcoholic beverages with modifications in their composition (Official Mexican Standard, 1994).

It defines gluten-free food as products from which gluten has been removed. Gluten is also defined as those proteins found in wheat, triticale, rye, barley or oats. Gluten-free foods include foods in which the ingredients that naturally contain gluten have been replaced by others that do not contain gluten, and foods that contain any of the aforementioned cereals as ingredients but have been treated to remove gluten.

This Standard also states that gluten-free products that replace staple foods such as flour or bread must provide approximately the same amount of vitamins and minerals as equivalent foods with gluten. The minimum addition to be made in wheat flour and nixtamalized maize flour is 5 mg/kg of thiamine, 3 mg/kg of riboflavin, and 35 mg/kg of niacin, folic acid 2 mg/kg, 40 mg/kg of iron and 40 mg/kg of zinc. Both ferrous sulphate and ferrous fumarate can be used as a source of iron (Official Mexican Standard, 2008).

It is stipulated that the labelling of these foods must be done with the claim "gluten-free"("SIN GLUTEN") near the product name. In addition, they must clarify the nature and origin of the starch or starches used (Official Mexican Standard, 1994).

For these products, the total nitrogen content of the cereal grains used that contain gluten must not exceed a value of 0.05 g/100 g expressed in dry matter (Official Mexican Standard, 1994).

10.3.13 Paraguay (Republic of Paraguay)

The Paraguayan legislation regulating the labelling of gluten-free products, including food, is Law No. 6072 of 2018 (Law N° 6072, 2018). It defines gluten as the protein present in wheat, oats, barley and rye, identified by the acronym T.A.C.C. for its initials in Spanish. It establishes that those products aimed at the coeliac population that are marketed in the country must comply with the requirements established in this law and its respective regulations and must have the legend "gluten-free"("sin gluten"), "no gluten contains" ("no contiene gluten") or "T.A.C.C-free" ("sin T.A.C.C.") printed clearly and visibly on their packaging, wrappers, labels or signs. In addition, the national symbol identifying gluten-free products, must be displayed in a visible place on domestically produced products.

Alternative versions are also available and will only be used when it is not possible to reproduce the colours of the main version. (Application Manual for the Gluten-Free Product Identification Logo, 2018).

The law establishes that the Ministry of Public Health and Social Welfare is in charge of setting the cut-off value, taking into account the values published periodically by Codex Alimentarius; establishing the mechanisms of analysis and certification and the monitoring systems. In addition, it is responsible for approving certificates for imported gluten-free products and for compiling a register of gluten-free products to facilitate access to information for the public (Law N° 6072, 2018). This information is not available because until December 2021, the law has not yet been regulated.

10.3.14 Russia (Russian Federation)

In 2012 Russia became a member of the World Trade Organization and this led a number of changes in compliance with international norms and standards. Many of Russian foods and trade regulations had been changed or are still in the process of being reformed, largely due to a policy of integration pursued by the Customs Union of Russia, Belarus and Kazakhstan. But, as a member of Eurasian Economic Community, Russia is also engaged not only in harmonisation throughout the Customs Union but also Kyrgyzstan and Tajikistan, and Armenia, Moldova and Ukraine as observer countries. Russia also continues to coordinate policy reforms closely with the European Union, its primary trade partner, ultimately bringing Russian food and sanitary norms closer to international standards (e.g. Codex) (Shamtsyan, 2014).

The food regulation agency responsible for the food safety in Russia is the Rosselkhoznadzor (Federal Service for Veterinary and Phytosanitary Surveillance) and the Rospotrebnadzor (Federal Service for Supervision of Consumer Rights Protection and Human Welfare). The Russian Federation has several federal laws regarding foodstuffs, including those of foreign origin. Apart from these mandatory requirements, safety and identification are described in sanitary and regulatory documents such as Sanitary Rules and Regulations (SanPiN), national standards (GOST) and other technical regulations. In total, there are more than 700 State laws and standards and governmental orders regulating food production in Russia. In the particular case of labelling requirements primary legislation for "General

Requirements for Consumer Information Regarding Foodstuffs" (GOST P51074-2003) incorporates Codex Alimentarius International Food-Packaging Standards. It covers all special requirements for nutrition labelling and seeks to incorporate international standards to prevent trade barriers from arising. It is intended to provide objective and trustworthy methods for assessing the quality and safety of Russian products (Shamtsyan, 2014).

In 2010 the Customs Union Commission (hereinafter referred to as the Commission), that includes an Agreement on Uniform Principles and Rules of Technical Regulation in the Republic of Belarus, the Republic of Kazakhstan and the Russian Federation decided to: 1. Adopt the Technical Regulations of the Customs Union "Food Products Labelling" (TR CU 022/2011). That regulation discloses that for food products containing grain ingredients it is allowed to place the words "Do not contain gluten" after the food product content in the event grain ingredients containing gluten were not used or gluten was removed (Custom Union Commission, 2011).

In Russia, the word for gluten is "клейковина" and for gluten-free is "без глютена". In order for these products to be labelled as gluten-free, it is necessary to analyse the level of gluten in accordance with TR CU 027/2012 "On the safety of certain types of specialised food products, including dietary therapeutic and preventive dietary nutrition." According to this regulation, gluten-free food products must be made from one or more ingredients that do not contain wheat, rye, barley, oats or their crossbred variants and/or must consist or be made in a special way (to reduce gluten level) from one or more components obtained from wheat, rye, barley, oats or their crossbred variants, while the level of gluten in the ready-to-eat product is not more than 20 mg/kg (Ushakova et al., 2021).

Regarding the labelling, the international symbol for gluten-free food safety, that was created in 1965 by the British Coeliac Association ("Crossed Grain Symbol") can be used only after obtaining a licence from the St. Petersburg Society of Coeliac Diseases and it is the only copyright holder of the Crossed Grain Stamp in the Russian Federation (San Petersburg coeliac society, 2021).

10.3.15 United States of America

The legislation governing gluten-free foods is found in the Code of Federal Regulations, Title 21, section §101.91 (21CFR101.91) (Code of Federal Regulations, 2021).

In this section gluten is defined as the proteins that naturally occur in a "gluten-containing grain", i.e. any species belonging to the genus *Triticum* (wheat), *Secale* (Rye) and *Hordeum* (Barley) and their crossbred hybrids and that may cause adverse health effects in persons with coeliac disease.

It may bear the labelling claim "gluten-free" the food that inherently does not contain gluten or does not contain any one of the following:

- An ingredient that is a gluten-containing grain.
- An ingredient that is derived from a gluten-containing grain and that has not been processed to remove gluten.
- An ingredient that is derived from a gluten-containing grain and that has been processed to remove gluten, if the use of that ingredient results in the presence of 20 mg/kg or more gluten in the food.

Other claims permitted are "no gluten", "free of gluten", or "without gluten".

A food bearing the term "wheat" in the list of ingredients or the statement "contains wheat" in its labelling, and also bearing the statement "gluten-free"or any of its synonyms will be deemed misbranded unless the word "wheat" in the list of ingredients or the statement "contains wheat" is immediately followed by an asterisk referring to another asterisk in close proximity to the ingredient statement with the following sentence: "Wheat has been processed to enable this food to meet the Food and Drug Administration (FDA) requirements for gluten-free foods".

The regulation does not require manufacturers to place the voluntary gluten-free claim in any specific location on the food label. There is also no official symbol accredited by the FDA (Food and Drug Administration, 2021).

FDA uses routine post-market monitoring activities to enforce the gluten-free food labelling regulation. These activities include sampling; periodic inspections of food manufacturing facilities; food label reviews; follow-up on consumer and industry complaints reported; and, when needed, gluten analyses of food samples.

Any foods that carry the label "gluten-free," "no gluten," "free of gluten," or "without gluten" must contain less than 20 mg/kg of gluten.

The regulation allows each manufacturer to select the most appropriate test methods for controlling this limit, considering the type of foods they produce. Manufacturers are not obligated to use one specific method to check gluten content in their foods. FDA recommends the use of scientific valid methods for validating the gluten test results in order to be reliable and consistent. FDA has currently identified two scientific valid methods. Both are sandwich enzyme-linked immunosorbent assays (ELISA)-based methods (R5 antibody-based ELISA of R-Biopharm® and Wheat Protein ELISA Kit (Gliadin) of Morinaga Institute of Biological Science, Inc). There are not currently available scientifically valid methods to detect gluten in fermented and hydrolysed foods (Food and Drug Administration, 2021). In this case, the manufacturer of such foods bearing the "gluten free" claim must make and keep records regarding the fermented or hydrolysed food demonstrating adequate assurance that:

- The food is gluten-free before fermentation or hydrolysis.
- The manufacturer has adequately evaluated their processing for any potential gluten cross-contact; and
- Where a potential for gluten cross-contact has been identified, the manufacturer has implemented measures to prevent the introduction of gluten into the food during the manufacturing process.

The same recommendations apply to foods containing one or more fermented or hydrolysed ingredients (Code of Federal Regulations, 2021).

10.3.16 Uruguay (Oriental Republic of Uruguay)

The legislation related to gluten-free foods is found in the National Bromatological Regulation, Chapter 29 (National Food Regulation, 1994). Gluten-free foods are among the foods modified in their protein composition. They are those that contain as ingredients wheat, rye, barley or oats or cross varieties of those species from which all the gluten has been removed or those in which all ingredients normally present and that contain gluten have been replaced by gluten-free ingredients. They are foods made to meet the needs of people who do not tolerate gluten. It defines gluten as the prolamin fraction found in wheat, barley, rye and oats or cross varieties of these species and their derived products, which some people do not tolerate.

It establishes that gluten-free foods, which are used to replace important staple foods, such as flour or bread, must supply the same amount of vitamins and minerals as the original foods used to replace them. In Uruguay, wheat flour is fortified/enriched with dehydrated ferrous sulphate or ferrous fumarate 30 mg/kg (as elemental Fe) and with folic acid 2.4 mg/kg (Decree N° 130/006, 2006).

The labelling of "gluten-free" foods may indicate that they "do not contain gluten" and use the international coeliac symbol. When a food contains only natural gluten-free cereals in its composition, it may be labelled as "naturally gluten-free". When a food labelled "gluten-free"contains starch, the source of the starch must be declared on the label.

In commercial gluten-free products, the crossed grain symbol can be seen.

From the Municipality of Montevideo, the Food Regulation Service is working on the control of companies that manufacture and sell gluten-free foods, to guarantee their safety and provide security to the coeliac population.

10.3.17 Summary of Gluten Containing Grains Contemplated on the Legislation and Gluten Limits of Each Country

Country	Gluten containing grains	Limits
Argentine	Wheat, from all Triticum species, such as spelt (*Triticum spelta* L.), kamut (*Triticum polonicum* L.), of durum wheat, rye, barley, oats or their crossed varieties	No more than 10 mg/kg of gluten
Australia and New Zealand	Wheat, rye, barley, oats and spelt	"Gluten-free" – contains no detectable gluten "low gluten" – contains no more than 200 mg/kg of gluten "Contains/is high in gluten" – contains more than 200 mg/kg of gluten
Brazil	Wheat, oats, barley, malt and rye	No limits stablish in the legislation

Country	Gluten containing grains	Limits
Canada	Barley, oats, rye, triticale, wheat or the grain of a hybrid strain that is created from at least one of these cereals	Not more than 20 mg/kg of gluten recommended by Health Canada (no limits stablish in the legislation)
Chile	Wheat, from all *Triticum* species such as spelt (*Triticum spelta L.*), kamut (*Triticum polonicum L.*), durum wheat, rye, barley, nor their cross varieties, as well as oats	Not more than 5 mg/kg of gluten
China	There is no specific regulation for gluten-free foods in China, for export products the CODEX may be applicable.	
European Union	Wheat (means any *Triticum* species.), rye, barley, oats or their crossbred varieties and derivatives thereof	Gluten-free: Not more than 20 mg/kg of gluten Very low gluten: Not more than 100 mg/kg of gluten.
India	A gluten-free foods is defined as a one containing one or more of these: Rice, millets, ragi, pulses, and legumes. The only reference that is made is to gluten containing grains is about wheat	Gluten free: not more than 20 mg/kg Low gluten: Gluten levels between 20 and 100 ppm
Israel	Wheat, rye, barley, oat or crossbreed of such grains	Not more than 20 mg/kg of gluten
Japan	There is no regulation for gluten-free labelling in Japan There is a specific regulation for "wheat-free" There is a specific regulation for "non-gluten" rice flour	For gluten-free certify rice: no more than 1 mg/kg or gluten
Korea	Wheat, rye, barley, oat or crossbreed of such grains	Not more than 20 mg/kg of gluten
Mexico	Wheat, triticale, rye, barley or oats	Not more than 0.05 g total nitrogen/100 g expressed in dry matter
Paraguay	Wheat, oats, barley and rye	No limits stablish in the legislation
Russia	Wheat, oats, barley and rye	Not more than 20 mg/kg of gluten
United States of America	*Triticum* (wheat), *Secale* (rye) and *Hordeum* (barley)	Not more than 20 mg/kg of gluten
Uruguay	Wheat, rye, barley or oats or cross varieties	No limits stablish in the legislation

10.4 Methods of Analysis for the Determination of Gluten in Food

Methods based on the detection of proteins or DNA are available for the determination of gluten in food (Osorio et al., 2019).

The most used methods that allow the detection of gluten proteins are immunological methods such as enzyme-linked immunosorbent assay (ELISA) and lateral flow immunochromatography; and physicochemical methods such as mass spectrometry coupled with chromatography (Diaz-Amigo and Popping, 2010).

Well-defined reference material and a reliable method are needed to allow a correct recovery of the target analyte. The method must be validated so that it meets the usual criteria of sensitivity, specificity, accuracy and precision. It is important to consider possible cross-reactivity, the possible effects of the matrix and the treatment to which the food under study was subjected (Popping et al., 2010).

10.4.1 ELISA Methods

Elisa Immunoassays are the most frequently used methods (D'Aiutolo et al., 2018; Osorio et al., 2019). Sandwich and competitive ELISA kits are commercially available. In the sandwich ELISA, two antibodies are used, the primary antibody and the secondary antibody linked to an enzyme. In this test, the direct binding of the allergen to the two antibodies is established, leaving the analyte "trapped" between them.

In competitive ELISA, the sample is incubated with the primary antibody (preincubated) and then this preparation is added on top of an antigen-coated surface. The free primary antibody not bound to the allergen in the sample, is able to bind the antigen-coated surface. Finally, the amount of free primary antibody, now bound to the antigen in the well, is detected by a second enzyme-labelled antibody. The more primary antibody detected, the less allergen the sample contains.

The most widely used ELISA assay format is the sandwich. This type of capture assay is called a "sandwich" assay because the analyte to be measured is bound between two primary antibodies, each detecting a different epitope of the antigen, the capture antibody and the detection antibody. The sandwich ELISA format is highly used because of its sensitivity and specificity. In allergen detection, this type of ELISAs are used because the target proteins have at least two epitopes which can be detected by the antibodies. The competitive format is chosen for the determination of small fragments or small analytes, which may have only one epitope (Popping et al., 2010).

ELISA is a versatile technique since different types of antibodies with different specificities can be combined, different types of assays can be developed: competitive or sandwich, several buffers and extraction solutions are used. Regarding the latter, some solutions contain denaturing and reducing agents that make possible to solubilize protein aggregates. These are initially incompatible with the assay because they can affect antibodies and antibody antigen binding. However, if they are used very dilute, they do not affect assay performance (Ito et al., 2016; Cellerino et al., 2020). ELISA is a quantitative technique that allows the quantification of concentrations suggested as safe. The limits of quantification of these kits are below the clinical thresholds.

As a biological test it is sensitive to changes in the structure of the allergen. If polyclonal antibodies are used, it is possible to detect allergens with a certain degree of modification. On the other hand, if monoclonal antibodies are used the detection of the analyte can be difficult if the protein structure has been modified. There may be unwanted false positives due to cross-reaction of the antibodies with non-target proteins or due to nonspecific binding with other components of the food. This test is useful for unprocessed ingredients and for some specific matrices with processed ingredients.

There is automated equipment that generates high throughput for routine analysis with a large number of samples. They can be quantitative, but results vary among commercial kits. This is due to the lack of standardisation that includes specificity of the antibodies used, calibration material, sample extraction solution and units in which the results are expressed.

Gluten detection can be difficult in some samples using ELISA methods, for example: highly hydrolysed or fermented samples, oils or derivatives (lecithin, tocopherols, phytosterols), highly processed products subjected to high temperatures and high pressure and in dressings (very acidic, low pH). For example, it is not possible to achieve a good extraction of allergenic proteins in oils, it is a complex matrix to analyse.

There are some specific kits for hydrolysed or fermented products, for these samples it must be used these kits and not kits for general foods. In highly processed products, it must be verified with a positive control that the allergen can be detected. In products with very low pH the proteins precipitate, they can form aggregates, therefore the correct extraction must be ensured.

Regarding the limits of quantification of the different commercial ELISA kits, all of them present low and safe limits, around 2.5–5 mg/kg of gluten, depending on the commercial kit.

10.4.2 Lateral Flow Immunochromatography

The sample flows by capillary action along a nitrocellulose membrane, to reach a line in which the specific antibody has been adsorbed. There, the reaction occurs giving rise to an antibody antigen coloured complex. Non-specific antibodies are found in the control line. It is characterized by being a qualitative or semi-quantitative method that does not require the use of equipment. The reading is visual and is often used to control surfaces and work or production environments. In addition, it can be saved as a document. They are fast, portable and easy to use. They are often associated with the handling of swabs and they are mainly used for verification of cleaning methods. Samples with high analyte concentrations can show a Hook effect, this implies that highly positive samples can show a negative result (D'Aiutolo et al., 2018; Popping et al., 2010).

The sensitivity of some commercially available gliadin dipsticks is sufficient enough for gluten analysis. As example, one commercial kit has the following limits: Surfaces approx. 1.6–3 μg gluten/100 cm^2, cleansing water (without cleansing reagent) approx. 10 ng/mL gluten, cleansing water (with cleansing reagent) approx.

50–100 ng/mL gluten. Another commercial kit has these limits: 5, 10, 20 mg/kg gluten (raw and finished products), 35 ppb gluten (rinse water), and 4 μg/25 cm^2 (swab testing).

10.4.3 *Liquid Chromatography Coupled with Mass Spectrometry*

Chromatography followed by mass spectrometry allows the direct detection of the analyte without the need to resort to an intermediate (antibodies in the ELISA). An enzymatic digestion of the proteins under study is carried out resulting in several peptides. The peptides of interest are selected and used as a "fingerprint" of the allergen avoiding cross reactivity and false positives in allergen detection. The selection of peptides is based on their abundance and their stability in processed foods. Liquid chromatography is performed to separate peptide fragments of different sizes. The next stage consists of the ionization of the peptides (electron ionization, ionic bombardment, MALDI: Matrix-assisted-laser-desorption ionization or electrospray ionization). The subsequent measurement of the mass/charge ratio is carried out by means of the mass spectrometer: Quadruple (Q), Ion trap (Ion-trap), Time of flight (TOF), Fourier transformation. Typically performed in tandem, which increases sensitivity, resolution, and accuracy: QQQ, Q/TOF; TOF/TOF. This method allows to confirm the unequivocal presence of the allergen in the sample while it is not affected by modifications in the structure of the proteins. It presents a wide range of extraction possibilities with respect to ELISA, including those that could affect antibody antigen binding.

It has a sensitivity similar to ELISA (mg/kg) and allows analyte quantifications to be carried out. The main disadvantage is the high cost of the equipment. In addition, the method set-up and the analysis require highly qualified personnel. It is a robust confirmatory method in court and it is considered a Gold Standard method according to internationally recognized consortia, such as EuroPrevall - MoniQa - iFAAM (D'Aiutolo et al., 2018).

Mass spectrometry is good for confirmation purposes rather than for screening analysis. Moreover, it is likely to be best suited to regulatory agencies or academic labs rather than food manufacturers (Diaz-Amigo and Popping, 2010; Osorio et al., 2019; Popping et al., 2010).

10.4.4 *Technologies Based on DNA- PCR and Real Time PCR*

It is possible to amplify DNA from foods containing gluten by means of PCR. Specific oligonucleotides are needed to serve as primers. Since in food there may be components that inhibit PCR (for example polyphenols), a prior extraction of these compounds must be done before performing PCR. It is rare to obtain false positive results due to the inadequate choice of primers or the similarity of the sequence to be amplified with other species. DNA can be amplified by end-point PCR, which is qualitative (i.e. detects the presence of a specific DNA sequence), or by real time PCR, which is quantitative, provided that a suitable reference material is used. The application of this technique for the detection of gluten is controversial since it does not detect the gluten proteins themselves and the concentration of DNA may not correlate with the presence of these proteins or with their concentration.

They are easier to develop than other biological assays, since all the necessary components are commercially available and do not require animal inputs or maintenance of cell lines. However, they require laboratory infrastructure such as dedicated rooms and this is not practical for industry or standard food analysis laboratories. DNA and proteins have different stability properties in different food processing procedures (Diaz-Amigo C, Popping B. 2010).

PCR is an alternative tool to ELISA methods for screening purposes and especially for confirmation of ELISA results. The PCR method is complementary to ELISA (D'Aiutolo et al., 2018; Osorio et al., 2019; Popping et al., 2010).

In summary:

- Immunoassays (ELISA test and Lateral flow immunochromatography): These are simple tests that are easily applied in the industry because the necessary technical qualification is low, and they do not require expensive equipment. Their great advantage is that they are direct and specific. They are based on the detection of the allergenic protein by specific antibodies. They are the most recommended for industry and analysis laboratories if there is a standardised kit.
- Molecular techniques (PCR): These are more complex tests, which imply greater qualification and more expensive equipment. They are specific but indirect tests. They detect the presence of DNA, not proteins. They are suitable in cases where commercial immunochemical tests are not available or when the sample undergoes severe heat treatments.
- Techniques of chromatography associated with mass spectrometry (LC-MS): It is a methodology that implies an instrument with a very high cost, specialised and experienced operators. They are specific and direct. They are based on the specific detection of peptides of the allergenic protein by means of mass spectrometry analysis. They are well suited as confirmatory methods and for the standardisation of reference methods.

10.4.5 Extraction of Gluten from Food Matrices

Since gluten is made up of prolamin and glutelin fractions, a possible solvent for extraction is an alcoholic solution of ethanol or propanol. It is efficient for the extraction of prolamins but not for extracting glutelins that have disulphide bridges. To improve the efficiency of gluten extraction, the addition of denaturing agents and reducing agents should be used. This is particularly important in foods that have undergone a heat treatment that can cause aggregation and formation of disulphide bridges. The R5 ELISA method utilises the so-called "cocktail" extraction solution consisting of 2-mercaptoethanol and guanidine hydrochloride reagents in phosphate buffered saline, which enables the extraction of gluten from heated or cooked food (Xhaferaj et al., 2020).

Ito K et al. (2016), used an extraction solution that contains sodium dodecyl sulphate as denaturing agent and sodium sulphite as reducing agent. This original extraction solution enables target protein to be solubilized even though it was previously insolubilized by food processing. The ELISA based on the SDS/0.1 M sulphite extraction solution has been authorized as the revised official method for food allergen analysis in Japan (Ito et al., 2016).

An alternative to gluten extraction in processed and unprocessed foods is to use new generation ionic liquids called deep eutectic solvents (DES). Due to their low toxicity, biodegradability and cost effectiveness, they are often used as alternatives to organic solvents, following the principles of green chemistry. Some examples of these solvents are different choline chloride-based DESs (Svigolj et al., 2017), and diluted fructose-citric acid (Lores et al., 2017).

10.4.6 AOAC Official Method 2012.01

Different legislations establish the AOAC official method 2012.01 as a gluten control methodology, including Codex Alimentarius, Argentina, Chile, Russia and New Zealand among others. This method was proposed and published in 2012 in Gliadin as a Measure of Gluten in Foods Containing Wheat, Rye, and Barley—Enzyme Immunoassay Method Based on a Specific Monoclonal Antibody to the Potentially coeliac Toxic Amino Acid Prolamin Sequences: Collaborative Study (Immer and Haas-Lauterbach, 2012). The Working Group on Prolamin Analysis and Toxicity (WGPAT) organised a collaborative study to confirm whether the two R5 antibody-based ELISA test kits are able to detect gliadin in the lower mg/kg level. Twenty laboratories investigated 12 blind-coded samples, spiked and naturally contaminated, to show the possibility of determining traces of gliadin in heat-treated or non-heat-treated foods by ELISA. It was recommended that the method be accepted by AOAC as Official First Action. In 2016 it was revised to update title as part of Final Action vote (change "foods containing wheat, rye, and barley" to "rice- and corn-based foods"). In March 2017 a modification of the wash solution to substitute thimerosal in the washing buffer with mercury-free preserving agent bronidox L, D(b) was included.

The method is based on an enzyme immunoassay format using a monoclonal antibody that can determine gliadin derived from wheat and related prolamins derived from rye and barley. It is important to highlight that the monoclonal antibody used in this method corresponds to R5 developed by Enrique Méndez's working group (Valdés et al. 2003).

The antibody binds to the potentially coeliac toxic amino acid sequence QQPFP (glutamine-glutamine-proline-phenylalanine-proline) and to related sequences, which exist on all the gliadin subunits (Osman et al., 2001). The antibody detects prolamins in non-heated and heated food by using an additional specific extraction method (cocktail solution). No cross-reactivity exists in oats, maize, rice, millet, teff, buckwheat, quinoa, and amaranth.

Prolamins from food are extracted by using a cocktail solution containing β-mercaptoethanol (250 mM) and guanidine hydrochloride (2 M) described by García et al. 2005, following an extraction with 80% ethanol. This extraction cocktail is more efficient to extract cross-linked prolamins present in heat-treated foods. Also, the cocktail is compatible with the R5 antibody ELISA method, since 2-mercaptoethanol at the concentration used does not affect the functionality of the immobilised R5 monoclonal antibodies (Popping et al., 2010). After centrifugation, the supernatant is used in a second- step sandwich method. The analyte is incubated in monoclonal antibody-coated wells forming an antibody–antigen complex. In a second step, an antibody peroxidase (POD) conjugate reacts with the complex to form an antibody–analyte–antibody complex. A chromogen/substrate reaction with the immobilised POD labelled conjugate determines the bound analyte. Non immobilised components are removed by washing between steps. The response of sample extracts is compared with response observed with calibration standards.

10.4.7 AOAC Official Method 2014.03

This method was proposed and published in 2015 in Gluten in Rice Flour and Baked Rice Products by G12 Sandwich ELISA: First Action 2014.03 (Halbmayr-Jech et al., 2015).

The Protein and Enzymes Technical Committee of American Association of Cereal Chemists initiated a collaborative study to confirm whether the G12 antibody-based sandwich ELISA test kit was able to detect gluten in the lower mg/kg level. Twenty laboratories investigated 24 heat-treated and non-heat-treated blind-coded samples with incurred gluten levels up to 100 mg/kg. The method has been validated for testing foods to conform to the defined Codex thresholds for gluten in gluten-free products at less than 20 mg gluten/kg. The collaborative study showed that low levels of gluten could be detected by G12 Sandwich ELISA with reproducibility RSDR of 32% and repeatability RSDr of 16%. Incurred samples showed a recovery between 62 and 135%.

The AOAC Official Method 2014.03 Gluten in Rice Flour and Rice-Based Food Products G12 Sandwich ELISA, First Action 2014, Final Action 2018 was posted on March 9, 2015 and February 9, 2018.

The method is based on an enzyme immunoassay format using a monoclonal G12 antibody that can determine gluten derived from wheat, rye, barley, and cross-bred varieties. The G12 antibody binds to the coeliac toxic amino acid sequence QPQLPY and related sequences in rye and barley. The antibody detects prolamins in unheated and heated food by using a specific proprietary extraction solution. No cross-reactivity has been determined to maize, rice, teff, millet, buckwheat, quinoa, amaranth and soy. Gluten is extracted from samples using proprietary extraction solutions containing reducing agents followed by ethanol extraction. After centrifugation the supernatant is used in a sandwich enzyme-linked immunoassay. When incubated on monoclonal antibody-coated microwells, the analyte is forming an antibody-antigen complex. After a washing step, an enzyme-conjugated monoclonal antibody is applied to the well and incubated. After a second washing step, an enzyme substrate is added, and blue colour develops. The intensity of the colour is directly proportional to the concentration of gluten in the sample or standard. A stop solution is then added which changes the colour from blue to yellow. The microwells are measured optically using a microwell reader with a primary absorbance filter of 450 nm (OD450). The optical densities of the samples are compared to the standards and an interpolated result is determined.

The G12 antibody is a monoclonal antibody that targets a toxic fragment of gluten that triggers the auto-immune reaction in coeliac patients. This antibody was raised against an α2-gliadin fragment that is 33 amino acids long and a principal contributor to gluten immunotoxicity. This 33-mer is highly resistant to breakdown by digestive enzymes and is, therefore, a suitable molecule for the use as an analytical marker.

This method in addition to being approved by AOAC was approved by AACC (AACC International Approved Method 38–52.01).

10.5 Conclusions

It can be concluded that several advances were developed related to detecting and quantifying gluten content in natural and processed foods in the last 20 years. It could allow to standardize methodology internationally for the corresponding food control. Nevertheless, no unified international legislation for gluten-free products could be adopted by the different countries till the moment, affecting global food trading and people with coeliac disease that travel to foreign countries.

Acknowledgments UBACYT 20020190100121BA

References

Allred L, Reid J (2021) Gluten-free products: what you need to know about international requirements in Food Safety Magazine. Available in: https://www.food-safety.com/articles/7043-gluten-free-products-what-you-need-to-know-about-international-requirements. Accessed 28 Dec 2021

AOAC Official Methods of Analysis (2012) AOAC Official Method 2012.01Gliadin as a measure of Gluten in rice- and corn-based foods enzyme immunoassay method based on a specific monoclonal antibody to the potentially celiac toxic amino acid prolamine sequences. First Action 2012 Final Action 2016. 2017 AOAC International

AOECS (2021) Association of european coeliac societies. Available in: https://www.aoecs.org. Accessed 28 Dec 2021

Application Manual for the Gluten-Free Product Identification Logo (2018) National Institute of Food and Nutrition. Available in: https://drive.google.com/file/d/1caTfSbS2NmxAhK8FdJg0-vhMgDBJCbXj/view?usp=sharing. Accessed 28 Dec 2021

Argentine Food Code (2021) Chapter XVII. Available in: https://www.argentina.gob.ar/sites/default/files/anmat_caa_capitulo_xvii_actualiz_2021-01.pdf. Accessed 28 Dec 2021

Australian Food and Grocery Council, Allergen Bureau (2021) Food industry guide to allergen management and labelling. For Australia and New Zealand. Available in: https://allergenbureau.net/wp-content/uploads/2021/04/FIGAML_April_2021_F1.pdf. Accessed 28 Dec 2021

Cellerino K, Binaghi MJ, Ambrosi V y López LB (2020) Detection of traces of soy and milk in gluten-free products: development of two competitive enzyme immunoassays. Acta Bioquím Clín Latinoam 54 (4): 395–406

Code of Federal Regulations (2021) Title 21, Volume 2, Section § 101.91. Available in https://www.ecfr.gov/current/title-21/chapter-I/subchapter-B/part-101. Accessed 28 Dec 2021

Codex Alimentarius (2015) Standard for foods for special dietary use for persons intolerant to gluten CXS 118-1979. Adopted in 1979. Amended in 1983 and 2015. Revised in 2008. Codex Alimentarius, Roma, Italia. Available in: http://www.fao.org/fao-who-codexalimentarius/shproxy/en/?lnk=1&url=https%253A%252F%252Fworkspace.fao.org%252Fsites%252Fcodex%252FStandards%252FCXS%2B118-1979%252FCXS_118e_2015.pdf. Accessed 28 Dec 2021

Codex Standard 234-1999 (2019) Recommended methods of analysis and sampling. Codex Alimentarius Commission. Available in: https://www.fao.org/fao-who-codexalimentarius/sh-proxy/en/?lnk=1&url=https%253A%252F%252Fworkspace.fao.org%252Fsites%252Fcodex%252FStandards%252FCXS%2B234-1999%252FCXS_234e.pdf. Accessed 28 Dec 2021

Coeliac Australia (2021) Making a gluten free claim 2021. Available in: https://www.coeliac.org.au/s/for-business/making-a-gf-claim. Accessed 28 Dec 2021

Coeliac New Zealand (2021) Licence the crossed grain logo through CNZ. Available in: https://coeliac.org.nz/. Accessed 28 Dec 2021

Commission Implementing Regulation-EU (2014) N° 828/2014 On the requirements for the provision of information to consumers on the absence or reduced presence of gluten in food. Available in: https://eur-lex.europa.eu/legal-content/EN/TXT/PDF/?uri=CELEX:32014R0828&from=en. Accessed 28 Dec 2021

Comprehensive Inspection Plan (2021) Available in:https://www.argentina.gob.ar/anmat/regulados/alimentos/plan-integral-fiscalizacion/programas-alimentos. Accessed 28 Dec 2021

Customs Union Commission (2011) Decision N.811. Moscow. Available in: https://ec.europa.eu/food/system/files/2016-10/ia_eu-ru_sps-req_decision-881_en.pdf. Accessed 28 Dec 2021

D'Aiutolo C, Da Silva L, González C, López L, López MC, Polenta G (2018) Manual for the implementation of the "Guide for the management of allergens in the food industry". In Buenos Aires (ed) Allergens in food platform

Ministerio de Salud De la Nación Argentina Dirección de Calidad de los Servicios de Salud (2010) Punto de corte de alimentos libres de gluten Informe Técnico Científico de Evaluación de Tecnología Sanitaria (ITC). Available in: https://bancos.salud.gob.ar/sites/default/files/2018-10/0000000633cnt-11-irest-pto-gluten.pdf

Decree N° 130/006 (2006) Cereals. Production of wheat flours enriched with vitamins and minerals. Available in: https://www.impo.com.uy/bases/decretos/130-2006. Accessed 28 Dec 2021

Diaz-Amigo C, Popping B (2010) Analytical testing as a tool for the enforcement of future regulatory thresholds for food allergens. J AOAC Int 93(2):434–441. https://doi.org/10.1093/jaoac/93.2.434

Environmental Health Unit (2021) Labelling guidelines for food businesses. Wyndham CityAvailable in: https://www.wyndham.vic.gov.au/sites/default/files/2021-08/Food%20Labelling%20Guidelines.pdf. Accessed 28 Dec 2021

European Licensing System (2017) Federation of Associations of Coeliacs of Spain. Available in: https://celiacos.org/wp-content/uploads/2019/02/Reglamento-General-ELS-Rev.-02.17.pdf. Accessed 28 Dec 2021

FDR (2021) Food and drug regulation C.R.C., c. 870. Available in: https://laws-lois.justice.gc.ca/eng/regulations/C.R.C.,_c._870/index.html. Accessed 28 Dec 2021

Food and Drug Administration (2021) Questions and answers on the gluten-free food labeling final rule. Available in: https://www.fda.gov/food/food-labeling-nutrition/questions-and-answers-gluten-free-food-labeling-final-rule. Accessed 28 Dec 2021

Food Standards Code (2021) Available in: https://www.foodstandards.gov.au/code/Pages/default.aspx. Accessed 28 Dec 2021

FSSAI (2018) Food safety and standards authority of India. Gluten Free Foods, Guidance Note N°. 09/2018. Available in: https://fssai.gov.in/upload/uploadfiles/files/Guidance_Note_Ver2_Gluten_Free_31_10_2019_Revised_10_02_2020.pdf. Accessed 28 Dec 2021

GAIN (2011) General rules for nutrition labeling of prepackaged foods. Available in: https://www.fsis.usda.gov/sites/default/files/media_file/2021-02/gb-7718-2011-part-i.pdf. Accessed 28 Dec 2021

GAIN (2017) GAIN report number JA7094 rice flour standards and labelling guidelines established. Available in: https://apps.fas.usda.gov/newgainapi/api/report/downloadreportbyfilename?filename=Rice%20Flour%20Standards%20and%20Labelling%20Guidelines%20Established_Tokyo_Japan_6-28-2017.pdf. Accessed 28 Dec 2021

García E, Llorente M, Hernando A, Kieffer R, Wieser H, Méndez E (2005) Development of a general procedure for complete extraction of gliadins for heat processed and unheated foods. Eur J Gastroenterol Hepatol 17:529–539

Gluten Analysis in Food (2018) Institute of public health. Available in: https://www.ispch.cl/sites/default/files/prestacion/2010/03/8310299.pdf. Accessed 28 Dec 2021

Halbmayr-Jech E, Rogers A, Don C, Prinster M (2015) Gluten in rice flour and baked rice products by G12 Sandwich ELISA: First Action 2014.03. J AOAC Int 98(1):103–111. https://doi.org/10.5740/jaoacint.14-197

Health Canada (2012) Health canada's position on gluten-free claims. Available in: https://www.canada.ca/en/health-canada/services/food-nutrition/food-safety/food-allergies-intolerances/celiac-disease/health-canada-position-gluten-free-claims.html. Accessed 28 Dec 2021

Immer U, Haas-Lauterbach S (2012) Gliadin as a measure of gluten in foods containing wheat, rye, and barley—enzyme immunoassay method based on a specific monoclonal antibody to the potentially celiac toxic amino acid prolamin sequences: collaborative study. J AOAC Int 95(4):1118–1124. https://doi.org/10.5740/jaoacint.CS2012_01

Ito K, Yamamoto T, Oyama Y, Masahiro O (2016) Food allergen analysis for processed food using a novel extraction method to eliminate harmful reagents for both ELISA and lateral-flow tests. Anal Bioanal Chem 408(22):5973–5984

Law N° 6072 (2018) Establishing control measures for gluten-free products. Available in: https://www.bacn.gov.py/archivos/8495/Ley%2060722018..pdf. Accessed 28 Dec 2021

Law No 10674 (2003) It obliges food products on the market to provide information on the presence of gluten, as a preventive measure and to control coeliac disease. Available in: http://www.planalto.gov.br/ccivil_03/leis/2003/l10.674.htm. Accessed 28 Dec 2021

Lores H, Romero V, Costas I, Bendicho C, Lavilla I (2017) Natural deep eutectic solvents in combination with ultrasonic energy as a green approach for solubilisation of proteins: application to gluten determination by immunoassay. Talanta 162:453–459. https://doi.org/10.1016/j.talanta.2016.10.078

MAFF (2011) Japanese ministry of agriculture, forestry, and fisheries. Available in: https://www.maff.go.jp/e/policies/standard/jas/law.html. Accessed 28 Dec 2021

Ministry of Food and Drug Safety (2016) Public announcement N°. 2016-45, foods labelling standards (Korea). Available in: https://www.zm.gov.lv/public/ck/files/PVD/Eksports/Korea%20Foods_Labelling_Standards(N°_2016-45).pdf. Accessed 28 Dec 2021

National Food Regulation (1994) National food regulation. In: Chapter 29. Uruguay. Available in: https://www.impo.com.uy/bases/decretos-reglamento/315-1994/29. Accessed 28 Dec 2021

NSW Food Authority (2011) Presence of gluten in foods labelled 'gluten-free'. Available in: https://www.foodauthority.nsw.gov.au/sites/default/files/_Documents/scienceandtechnical/gluten_survey_report_2011.pdf. Accessed 28 Dec 2021

Official Mexican Standard (1994) NOM-086-SSA1-1994. Goods and services. Food and non-alcoholic beverages with modifications in their composition. Nutritional specifications. Available in: http://dof.gob.mx/nota_detalle.php?codigo=4890075&fecha=26/06/1996. Accessed 28 Dec 2021

Official Mexican Standard (2008) NOM-247-SSA1-2008. Products and services. Cereals and cereal products. Cereals, cereal flours, meal, semolina or semolina. Foodstuffs based on: cereals, edible seeds, flours, semolina or semolina or their mixtures. Bread products. Health and nutritional provisions and specifications. Test methods. Available in: http://dof.gob.mx/nota_detalle.php?codigo=5100356&fecha=27/07/2009. Accessed 28 Dec 2021

Osamu S (2020) World's First "Non-Gluten" Rice Flour World's First "Non-Gluten" Rice Flour. Highlighting Japan. Available in: https://www.maff.go.jp/e/policies/agri/attach/pdf/riceflour-5.pdf. Accessed 28 Dec 2021

Osman A, Uhlig H, Valdes I, Amin M, Mendez E, Mothes T (2001) A monoclonal antibody that recognizes a potential coeliac-toxic repetitive pentapeptide epitope in gliadins. Eur J Gastroenterol Hepatol 13:1189–1193

Osorio C, Mejías J, Rustgi S (2019) Gluten detection methods and their critical role in assuring safe diets for celiac patients. Nutrients 11(12):2920

Popping B, Diaz-Amigo C, Hoenicke K (eds) (2010) Molecular biological and immunological techniques and applications for food chemists, 1st edn. Wiley, Hoboken

PRC (People's Republic of China) Food Safety Law (2015) Available in: http://faolex.fao.org/docs/pdf/chn154228.pdf. Accessed 28 Dec 2021

Public Health Order (2011) Public health order (Food) (Gluten Labelling), 5756-1996, Amendment 2011, Israel

Resolution RDC N° 40 (2002) National health surveillance agency. Available in: https://bvsms.saude.gov.br/bvs/saudelegis/anvisa/2002/rdc0040_08_02_2002.html. Accessed 28 Dec 2021

San Petersburg Coeliac Society (2021) Available in: https://celiac.spb.ru/. Accessed 28 Dec 2021

Sanitary Regulation of Foods (2021) DTO. N° 977/96 (D.OF. 13.05.97) Title XXVIII.- of foods for special diets Párrafo VI.-. Available in: https://dipol.minsal.cl/wp-content/uploads/2021/03/RSA-DECRETO_977_96_act-02-02-2021.pdf. Accessed 28 Dec 2021

Shamtsyan M (2014) Food legislation and its harmonization in Russia. J Sci Food Agric 94:1966–1969

Svigelj R, Bortolomeazzi R, Dossi N, Giacomino A, Bontempelli G, Toniolo R (2017) An effective gluten extraction method exploiting pure choline chloride-based deep eutectic solvents (ChCl-DESs). Food Anal Methods 10:4079–4085

Ushakova Y, Rysmukhambetova G, Ziruk I, Belova M, Sadygova M (2021) IOP. Development criteria for gluten-free foods. Conf Ser Earth Environ Sci 723:032067

Valdés I, García E, Llorente M, Méndez E (2003) Innovative approach to low-level gluten determination in food using a novel sandwich enzyme linked immunosorbent assay protocol. Eur J Gastroenterol Hepatol 15(5):465–474. https://doi.org/10.1097/01.meg.0000059119.41030.df

Xhaferaj M, Alves T, Ferreira M, Scherf K (2020) Recent progress in analytical method development to ensure the safety of gluten-free foods for celiac disease patients. J Cereal Sci 96(103114):1–11. https://doi.org/10.1016/j.jcs.2020.103114

Index

M. F. de Escalada Pla, C. E. Genevois (eds.), *Designing Gluten Free Bakery and Pasta Products*, https://doi.org/10.1007/978-3-031-28344-4